MATERNAL CARDIAC CARE

A GUIDE TO MANAGING PREGNANT WOMEN WITH HEART DISEASE

MATERNAL CARDIAC CARE

A GUIDE TO MANAGING PREGNANT WOMEN WITH HEART DISEASE

John H. Wilson, MD, FACC, FHRS
Section Head of Cardiology, retired
Cincinnati, Ohio;
Director Electrophysiology, retired
Good Samaritan Hospital
Cincinnati, Ohio
Director Device Clinic
Electrophysiology
TriHealth
Cincinnati, Ohio

William T. Schnettler, MD, FACOG
Chairman
Department of Obstetrics and Gynecology
Good Samaritan Hospital
Cincinnati, Ohio;
Director
Center for Maternal Cardiac Care
TriHealth
Cincinnati, Ohio

Adam M. Lubert, MD
Pediatric Cardiologist
Cincinnati Children's Hospital Medical Center
Cincinnati, Ohio

Andrea Girnius, MD
Assistant Professor of Clinical Anesthesiology
Anesthesiology
University of Cincinnati
Cincinnati, Ohio

ELSEVIER

Elsevier
1600 John F. Kennedy Blvd.
Ste 1800
Philadelphia, PA 19103-2899

MATERNAL CARDIAC CARE: A GUIDE TO MANAGING
PREGNANT WOMEN WITH HEART DISEASE

ISBN: 978-0-323-82464-4

Notice

Practitioners and researchers must always rely on their own experience and knowledge in evaluating and using any information, methods, compounds or experiments described herein. Because of rapid advances in the medical sciences, in particular, independent verification of diagnoses and drug dosages should be made. To the fullest extent of the law, no responsibility is assumed by Elsevier, authors, editors or contributors for any injury and/or damage to persons or property as a matter of products liability, negligence or otherwise, or from any use or operation of any methods, products, instructions, or ideas contained in the material herein.

Senior Content Strategist: Nancy Anastasi Duffy
Senior Content Development Manager: Somodatta Roy Choudhury
Publishing Services Manager: Deepthi Unni
Senior Project Manager: Manchu Mohan
Book Designer: Ryan Cook

Printed in India

Last digit is the print number: 9   8   7   6   5   4   3   2   1

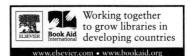

To our mothers, our spouses, all the women who came through our program, and Margo, the nurse practitioner who coordinates our Maternal Cardiac Care program.

In recent years, the all-cause mortality rate of pregnancy for women in the United States has been increasing. The reasons for this are complex but are attributable in part to increases in obesity and substance abuse. Unfortunately, mortality rates for women with cardiac disease are also rising, in part because more women with serious cardiac disease are electing to have children. The complexity of caring for these women and their babies has created a need for specialized maternal cardiac care facilities and health care teams with expertise in both cardiac care and high-risk obstetrics.

Establishing a maternal cardiac care program is challenging. It requires the commitment of a number of key specialists, including (at a minimum) obstetricians dedicated to high-risk care, cardiologists with expertise in adult congenital disease, obstetric anesthesiologists, and cardiac surgeons. We find it advantageous to also include pulmonologists, electrophysiologists, and an expert in substance abuse. These are just the physician specialists.

Our team obviously involves nurses, and we have obstetrics nurses and a cardiology and cardiothoracic surgery nurse coordinator present at our team meetings. In addition, we have a social worker and a clinic and scheduling coordinator present at biweekly and monthly meetings (depending on the number of cases) to discuss new patients and generate care plans. At these same meetings, we also review updates on all current patients. We try to have as many members of the team present as possible. In addition to the core members, a number of other subspecialists are called on as needed, including nephrologists, endocrinologists, infectious disease specialists, neurologists, and psychiatrists.

Obviously, a maternal cardiac care program requires a huge commitment of resources, which cannot be financially compensated in its entirety. However, the need is clearly there because the number of patients with serious cardiac disease who become pregnant continues to rise.

ACKNOWLEDGEMENTS

We wish to acknowledge: Dr. Gruschen Veldtman for reviewing the manuscript while he was at Cincinnati Children's Hospital Medical Center, and Celia F. Berg, creative partner Two Herons Consulting, for editing the manuscript.

CONTRIBUTORS

Jay Conhaim, MD
Pediatrician
General Pediatrics
University of Cincinnati Medical Center
Cincinnati, Ohio

Andrea Girnius, MD
Assistant Professor of Clinical Anesthesiology
Anesthesiology
University of Cincinnati
Cincinnati, Ohio

Kristin Horton, MD
Assistant Professor
Department of Anesthesiology
University of Cincinnati Medical Center
Cincinnati, Ohio

Helen Jones, PhD
Associate Professor
Physiology and Functional Genomics
University of Florida
Gainesville, Florida

Timothy K. Knilans, MD
Director
Clinical Cardiac Electrophysiology and Pacing
Cincinnati Children's Hospital
Cincinnati, Ohio;
Professor
UC Department of Pediatrics
University of Kentucky
Lexington, Kentucky

Adam M. Lubert, MD
Pediatric Cardiologist
Cincinnati Children's Hospital Medical Center
Cincinnati, Ohio

Erin M. Miller, MS
Genetic Counselor
The Heart Institute
Cincinnati Children's Hospital Medical Center
Cincinnati, Ohio

Helen Pappas, MD, FASA
Assistant Professor
Anesthesiology
Northwestern University
Chicago, Illinois

William T. Schnettler, MD, FACOG
Chairman
Department of Obstetrics and Gynecology
Good Samaritan Hospital
Cincinnati, Ohio;
Director
Center for Maternal Cardiac Care
TriHealth
Cincinnati, Ohio

J. Michael Smith, MD
Chief
Cardiac Surgery
College of Medicine
Cincinnati, Ohio

Jane C. Whalen, DNP, APRN.CNS, CCNS-CSC, CCRN
Advanced Practice Nurse II
Cardiothoracic Surgery
TriHealth
Cincinnati, Ohio

John H. Wilson, MD, FACC, FHRS
Section Head of Cardiology, retired
Cincinnati, Ohio;
Director Electrophysiology, retired
Good Samaritan Hospital
Cincinnati, Ohio;
Director Device Clinic
Electrophysiology
TriHealth
Cincinnati, Ohio

CONTENTS

Physiologic Adaptations to Pregnancy

John H. Wilson, MD, FACC, FHRS

For women with cardiac disease, the physiologic changes associated with pregnancy can impact the health of the mother and baby and affect the course of gestation and delivery. Many of these normal changes are driven by hormonal alterations initiated by the placenta (such as rising levels of estrogen and progesterone, which increase continuously during pregnancy), and they help optimize fetal growth, protect the mother from delivery complications, and contribute to a successful pregnancy. This chapter reviews some of the physiologic changes that occur during pregnancy, emphasizing issues that may affect patients with underlying heart disease. The changes discussed include those to the cardiovascular system, respiratory system, hematologic and immune systems, renal system, gastrointestinal (GI) system, and placenta.

CARDIOVASCULAR SYSTEM

Physiologic changes to the cardiovascular system during pregnancy include blood volume expansion, edema, increased cardiac output, hemodynamic changes during labor, hemodynamic changes during the postpartum period, and vascular changes in the uterus.

Blood Volume Expansion

Optimal cardiac function requires a balance between preload, afterload, heart rate, and contractility. During pregnancy, there is a dramatic increase in blood volume, which equates to an increase in cardiac preload. Starting at 6 to 8 weeks of gestation, maternal blood volume increases by up to 50% above nonpregnant values. This increase may be enhanced by multiple gestation, or it may be blunted in pregnancies complicated by fetal growth restriction, hypertension, or preeclampsia. The increase in plasma volume is greater than the increase in red cell mass (~18%), leading to a lowered hematocrit, sometimes described as "the physiologic anemia" of pregnancy. Evidence suggests that the decreased blood viscosity facilitates placental perfusion and lowers the workload of the heart, and the absence of this "physiologic anemia" may lead to higher rates of stillbirth and fetal growth restriction. The increased plasma volume is partly caused by changes in the maternal hypothalamus–pituitary–adrenal axis, which lowers the threshold for renin, aldosterone, and antidiuretic hormone release, leading to retention of both sodium and water. Additionally, the increased vascular capacitance caused by the smooth muscle–relaxing effect of progesterone and other vasodilators allows for the increased systemic release of these hormones without concomitant negative feedback. Water retention is greater than sodium retention, explaining the mild reduction in sodium concentration that occurs in pregnant women (135–138 mEq/L compared with 135–145 mEq/L in nonpregnant women). These changes peak near the beginning of the third trimester.

Edema of Pregnancy

During normal pregnancy, total body water increases by 6 to 8 L. An estimated 4 to 6 L of this increase is extracellular, with 2 to 3 L being interstitial. Additionally, colloid osmotic pressure decreases, and capillary hydrostatic pressure increases. The hormonal changes of pregnancy also lead to increased water in the ground substance of connective tissue. Thus, it is not surprising that up to 80% of women with normal pregnancies manifest peripheral edema, particularly in the third trimester. Obese women, older women, and multiparous women all tend to develop more pronounced edema. In about half of women, the edema is limited to the lower extremities. In the other half, it is more generalized, involving the hands and the face. The edema can be sporadic or persistent, with both types occurring with approximately equal frequency.

The edema of pregnancy is not necessarily a negative occurrence. Women with edema tend to have babies of slightly greater birthweight, although the babies are not edematous. They have a lower incidence of low-birthweight babies and a slightly reduced rate of perinatal mortality compared with women who do not develop edema.

The increased plasma volume results in the development of normal physical examination findings unique to pregnancy, and an understanding of these will help to identify true perturbations in the cardiovascular system. Although the development of mild or moderate peripheral edema is common among women in the late second and third trimesters, the severe or earlier development of edema may indicate a failure of the cardiovascular system to tolerate the increase in plasma volume. Women with diminished systolic cardiac function or severely regurgitant valvular disease may manifest early and severe peripheral edema. Similarly, the increased blood flow through the heart may cause a functional heart murmur often described as a "systolic flow murmur." It is often characterized as a systolic crescendo–decrescendo murmur of a grade 1 or 2, loudest with auscultation over the left-second intercostal space. An additional sound also may be heard bilaterally along the mid-clavicular line and represents the "mammary soufflé" associated with increased blood volume perfusing the breasts. Diastolic murmurs, harsh or loud murmurs, clicks, and rubs are abnormal and warrant a cardiac work-up.

Certain laboratory, imaging, and electrocardiogram findings are associated with the increased plasma volume seen in pregnancy. Hemoglobin concentration declines an average of 1.5 to 2.0 g/dL, such that the Centers for Disease Control and Prevention has defined true anemia during pregnancy as a hemoglobin less than 11.0 g/dL during the first and third trimesters and less than 10.5 g/dL during the second trimester. Chest x-ray findings may include enlargement of the cardiac silhouette and great vessels, and echocardiography may identify increased chamber dimensions and mild valve regurgitation. Coinciding with the increased cardiac chamber sizes, the nature of the electrical circuitry within the heart changes subtly. The electrocardiogram changes include mild sinus tachycardia, left-axis deviation, mild ST segment changes, and the development of small Q waves and T-wave inversions (especially in leads III and AVF). Findings outside of these expected physiologic changes suggest the presence of underlying disease or intolerance to the increase in plasma volume.

Increased Cardiac Output

In part because of the increased preload and the operation of Starling's law, which states that contractility of the heart will increase as it is stretched by increased volume, cardiac output increases by 30% to 50% in a normal pregnancy. The increase in stroke volume is coupled with an increase in heart rate during pregnancy, which also contributes to increased cardiac output. The heart rate increases progressively throughout pregnancy and reaches a maximum of 20% to 25% over prepregnancy values in the third trimester. The increased heart rate is largely caused by an increase in sympathetic tone and a decrease in parasympathetic tone. The combination of the increases in stroke volume and heart rate results in a progressively increasing cardiac output that begins in the first trimester and peaks by 28 to 32 weeks' gestation. The increases in heart rate and cardiac output are greater, 5.2 L/min versus 5.6 L/min, during subsequent pregnancies than during the first. The maternal cardiac output can change with body position. Various body positions and postures may cause the gravid uterus to obstruct the vena cava, resulting in diminished venous return and significant reductions in cardiac output (Fig. 1.1).

Although cardiac remodeling occurs during pregnancy, such that left ventricular wall thickness increases by about 28% and left ventricular mass increases by 52%, the contractility of the cardiomyocytes themselves does not increase. Rather, systemic and pulmonary resistance diminishes, contributing to the important rise in cardiac output. Diminished resistance is partly caused by increases in the serum concentration of progesterone, nitric oxide

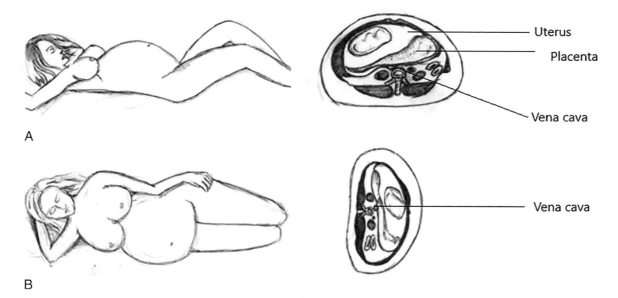

Fig. 1.1 A, Compression of the vena cava in a supine position. **B,** Compression is relieved by a left lateral position.

(NO), and prostaglandins. NO and prostaglandins, such as prostacyclin (PGI_2), are vasodilators with direct relaxing effects on the endothelium. Somewhat counterintuitively, the maternal circulation also demonstrates increases in blood levels of both renin and angiotensin. However, there appears to be a decreased responsiveness to the pressor effects of these hormones, such that, despite their elevated serum concentrations in pregnancy, systemic vascular resistance diminishes.

Changes in left atrial function have been evaluated using two-dimensional speckle tracking. These studies demonstrate that whereas left atrial reservoir and booster pump functions increase in pregnancy, left atrial conduit function decreases.

Vascular resistance reaches its lowest point at 20 to 24 weeks' gestation. The decrease in vascular resistance leads to physiologic hypotension. After the nadir is reached, vascular resistance increases, approaching prepregnancy values by term. Thus, blood pressure falls throughout the first and early second trimesters but increases in concert with the changes in vascular resistance toward term—often returning to prepregnancy values or even slightly higher.

Increases in cardiac output, coupled with a redistribution of blood flow to the organs most vital for optimal maternal and fetal health (Fig. 1.2), provide additional oxygen uptake, heat dissipation, and excretion of metabolic waste. Uterine blood flow increases 10-fold throughout gestation, and the percentage of total cardiac output received increases from 2% before pregnancy to 10% at term. Pulmonary blood flow increases by approximately 30% by term, but no change in pulmonary artery pressure is seen. Blood flow to the brain increases by about 10%. Skin perfusion doubles in the second and third trimesters to provide improved heat exchange. By the second trimester, renal blood flow has increased by roughly 30% with a concomitant rise in the glomerular filtration rate (GFR) for the purposes of clearing metabolic wastes. As pregnancy progresses, it increases further to as much as 50% to 60%. An increase in distribution of cardiac output to the breasts occurs during pregnancy in anticipation of lactation and the need to provide nourishment to the newborn.

The increased cardiac demand and redistribution of cardiac output result in several common symptoms that can be considered normal for pregnancy. As early as the first trimester, patients may experience mild shortness of breath and occasional palpitations lasting a few seconds. They may find it more difficult to tolerate exercise, and their breathing may become more labored when climbing several flights of stairs. Other common symptoms are skin flushing and the sensation of feeling

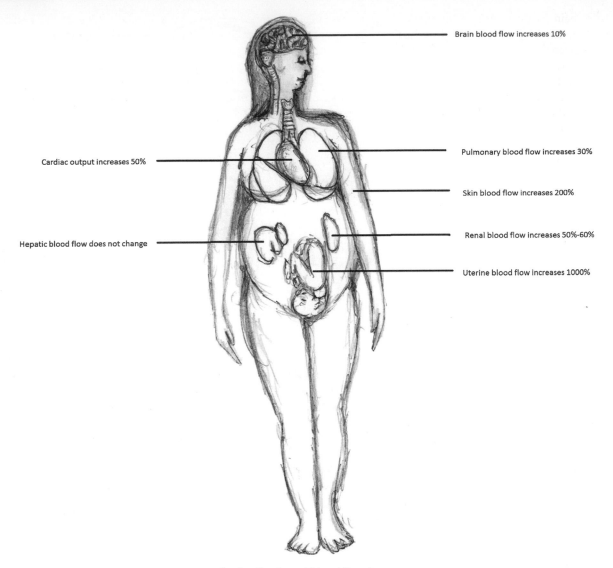

Brain blood flow increases 10%

Cardiac output increases 50%

Pulmonary blood flow increases 30%

Skin blood flow increases 200%

Hepatic blood flow does not change

Renal blood flow increases 50%-60%

Uterine blood flow increases 1000%

Fig. 1.2 Redistribution of blood flow in pregnancy.

warm. However, chest pain is not common and should never be considered normal for pregnancy. Palpitations that last minutes rather than seconds also should be considered pathologic. In addition, the inability of a nonobese woman to climb one flight of stairs without marked shortness of breath warrants concern.

Hemodynamic Changes During Labor

During labor and delivery, the contraction of uterine muscle expels blood from the veins and venules within the uterus, resulting in a cyclic increase in blood volume

of 300 to 500 mL with each contraction, the "autotransfusion effect." Uterine contractions also may change the shape of the uterus, decreasing the pressure placed on the inferior vena cava and improving venous return. As a result, stroke volume is augmented, and cardiac output increases approximately 30% during labor. In addition, the increased cardiac output may be attributed to an increase in heart rate associated with the catecholamine surge from pain and anxiety. Regional analgesia has been shown to blunt the expected rise in cardiac output, perhaps partly caused by the reduced catecholamine surge from pain partly caused by the reduced venous return that occurs because of the vasodilation of the lower body. Depending on the woman's level of anxiety and pain as well as her position, blood pressure may increase by up to 15% with uterine contractions.

Delivery is associated with a significant loss of maternal blood volume. Routine vaginal and cesarean delivery may result in losses of up to 10% and 30%, respectively, of maternal blood volume. Nevertheless, cardiac output continues to increase in the first hour or two after delivery because of the reduced vena caval compression and the autotransfusion effect from the involuted uterus. Over the subsequent 2 to 6 weeks, cardiac output returns to prelabor values. Heart rate and blood pressure increases are quite variable, depending on multiple factors, including pain levels and type of anesthesia.

Labor and delivery represent periods of heightened risk for women unable to accommodate the increased venous return and cardiac output, including women with mitral stenosis or left ventricular systolic dysfunction.

During the peripartum period, all women have an increased risk of aortic dissection or rupture. In the 6 months before delivery and for 3 months postpartum, the risk is increased by a factor of 4. This is of particular concern for women with aortopathies (e.g., Marfan syndrome, Loeys-Dietz syndrome, and the vascular type of Ehlers-Danlos syndrome), who are already at risk for aortic dissection. It is intuitive that the hemodynamic changes of pregnancy, including increased heart rate and stroke volume, would increase stress on the aorta, but many other factors likely contribute as well. The compression of the gravid uterus on the aorta increases outflow resistance. Pregnancy also causes many hormonal changes that affect the walls of the blood vessels, and these may result in a weakening of the blood vessel wall that predisposes it to aortic rupture and dissection. In women with aortopathies, any signs or symptoms suggesting cardiac compromise—shortness of breath, chest pain or pressure, upper back pain, oxygen desaturation, narrowing pulse pressure, or tachycardia and hypotension—warrant a thorough cardiovascular evaluation.

Hemodynamic Changes During the Postpartum Period

The hemodynamic changes slowly return to prepregnancy values over several weeks. In the first 3 days postpartum, the increased blood volume and cardiac output decrease by 10%. The physiologic anemia of pregnancy resolves over a period of several weeks. Within 2 weeks, the systemic vascular resistance increases by 30%, returning to prepregnancy values, and a brief period of mild bradycardia may occur. Stroke volume and cardiac output completely return to prepregnancy levels over a period of 24 weeks. Left atrial and left ventricular dimensions return to normal after 24 weeks, as does left ventricular mass.

Vascular Changes in the Uterus

Maternal vascular adaptation to pregnancy is critically important to expand the capacity for blood flow through the placenta to meet the needs of the developing fetus. Failure of the maternal vasculature to properly adapt can result in hypertensive disorders of pregnancy, such as preeclampsia.

A variety of growth factors and cytokines are involved in the vascular adaptation to pregnancy. Maternal recognition of pregnancy and vascular adaptation to it begins at embryo implantation. Extravillous trophoblast migration initiates remodeling of the spiral arteries in the decidua of the uterus during the first trimester, forming low-flow, high-volume vessels and sinuses that allow placental villi to bathe in maternal blood. In the second trimester, myometrial spiral arteries are remodeled from high-resistance coiled vessels to dilated low-resistance vessels. Transformation of the myometrial spiral arteries both increases the volume and slows the rate of blood flow to the intervillous space of the developing placenta. This allows exchange of gases and facilitated transport of nutrients to the fetal circulation.

As previously discussed, pregnancy causes an increase in maternal blood volume, increased cardiac output, and a drop in systemic vascular resistance. Because of the decrease in vascular resistance, the blood pressure typically does not increase. Vascular resistance drops throughout the body, but there is a disproportionately larger drop in vascular resistance in the uterine circulation. The result is a greater proportion of the cardiac output going to the uteroplacental unit to meet the needs of the developing placenta and fetus. Compared with the nonpregnant state, uterine blood flow during pregnancy increases an estimated 30- to 50-fold. The drop in vascular resistance is partly caused by remodeling of the spiral arterioles and partly caused by uterine vascular remodeling and sustained vasodilation.

Angiogenesis in the uterus occurs during the menstrual cycle and during pregnancy. It occurs as the result of growth factors and cytokines, but other factors, such as the hormones of pregnancy (human chorionic gonadotropin, estradiol, and progesterone), also likely stimulate angiogenesis. Angiogenesis during pregnancy results in an increase in overall vessel cross-sectional area and therefore a drop in vascular resistance in the uterus. Other physiologic adaptations of the uterine vasculature also occur during pregnancy. These include outward hypertrophy and vessel lengthening. Outward hypertrophy is an increase in vessel diameter, typically through vascular smooth muscle cell hypertrophy. The maternal uterine arteries are also thought to elongate. The net result of outward hypertrophy is decreased resistance to blood flow. Vessel lengthening increases resistance, but the net result of these changes is a drop in vascular resistance that shunts blood to the uterus and placenta, ensuring adequate gas, nutrient, and waste exchange during pregnancy.

Throughout pregnancy, but especially from midgestation through parturition, adequate uteroplacental blood flow is highly dependent on vasodilation. Pregnancy-induced increases in endothelial cell vasodilator production are necessary to maintain a healthy pregnancy. These vasodilator substances are produced by the placenta and locally throughout the circulation. If the production of vasodilating substance is inadequate, hypertension will result. During pregnancy, the ability of the endothelium of the uterine arteries to produce vasodilators in response to various stimuli is increased. Changes in the response to post-receptor signaling is such that the endothelial cells have greater and more sustained signaling responses to vasodilator-stimulating signals, such as hormones, and to shear or mechanical stress. A common activating mechanism for many vasodilators is elevation of cellular ionized calcium (Ca^{2+}). One important way Ca^{2+} responses can be amplified and sustained is by promoting intercellular signaling through gap junctions. When more coordinated and synchronous signaling events are achieved, there is not only an increase in vasodilator output per cell but also a recruitment of neighboring cells to respond to external stimuli. More specifically, periodic, transient Ca^{2+} burst events have been shown in endothelial cells in response to vasodilatory stimuli. These events are highly dependent on gap junction coupling through the connexin 43 (Cx43) isoform. The following paragraphs discuss how common vasodilators are regulated in pregnancy to maintain adequate uterine blood flow to the placenta.

Nitric oxide production in the endothelium is catalyzed by the enzyme endothelial nitric oxide synthase (eNOS). A soluble gas, NO diffuses from the endothelium to the vascular smooth muscle, promoting cyclic guanosine monophosphate (cGMP) production, which relaxes the smooth muscle. Phosphorylation of eNOS at specific sites (S1179 and S617) increases the sensitivity of eNOS to Ca^{2+}-dependent activation. Both these phosphorylation events have been shown to occur in uterine artery endothelial cells during pregnancy in response to vasodilatory stimuli. In pregnancy, eNOS levels are increased in the uterine artery endothelium, but in the absence of Ca^{2+} signaling, this does not enhance NO production.

Prostacyclin is a potent vasodilator derived from endothelial arachidonic acid metabolism. In general, the impact of PGI_2 on vascular tone can best be explained by the ratio of thromboxane (TX) A2 to PGI_2. TXA2 acts as a vasoconstrictor on the vascular smooth muscle, and PGI_2 functions as a vasodilator. There is strong evidence that PGI_2 plays an important role in pregnancy-adapted vasodilator responses.

Endothelium-derived hyperpolarizing factor (EDHF) also has been implicated as important in endothelial cell-mediated vasodilator production in pregnancy. It has become clear, however, that EDHF is not a single factor but a spectrum of responses that are neither NO nor PGI_2 mediated but that nonetheless result in smooth muscle relaxation. As with NO and PGI_2, Ca^{2+} signaling plays an important part in mediating at least some forms of EDHF production.

Estrogen has many important effects on maternal vascular adaptations to pregnancy. It assists in angiogenesis at the implantation site, which is essential for maintaining early pregnancy. As gestation continues and the critical regulator of vascular resistance switches from angiogenesis to vasodilation, estrogen promotes vasodilator production. However, estrogen alone is not effective at activation of Ca^{2+} signaling. The effects of estrogen on NO and PGI_2 production may be more through genomic regulation of estrogen receptors, ERα and ERβ, by directly promoting eNOS and cyclooxygenase 1 (COX-1) expression. Exposure of endothelial cells to estrogen increases eNOS and COX-1 expression and therefore raises vasodilatory capacity. Estrogen also may promote vascular endothelial growth factor (VEGF) production by endothelial cells and thus indirectly support vascular remodeling.

Progesterone levels rise through pregnancy, elevating rapidly as the gestation nears term and then falling dramatically at parturition. Early in pregnancy, progesterone likely plays a role in decidualization at the implantation site because a progesterone receptor is expressed in the endothelium of the decidua. Higher progesterone levels in early pregnancy correlate with lower blood pressures later in pregnancy, though it may not be causative. Progesterone is also able to promote vasodilator production through stimulation of eNOS (and thus NO production) as well as increased expression of activity of COX-1, which regulates PGI_2 production.

The role of androgens in pregnancy adaptation is poorly understood, although they may play a role as a negative regulator of blood flow in preeclampsia.

Both NO and PGI_2 have been shown to induce the production and secretion of both cGMP and cyclic adenosine monophosphate (cAMP) in vascular smooth muscle. Cyclic nucleotides (cAMP and cGMP) are best known as inhibitors of vascular tone in vascular smooth muscle, but they also can play an important role in promoting adaptation of endothelium. Part of maintaining uterine blood flow through sustained vasodilation requires upregulation of functional Cx43 in the plasma membrane. Cyclic nucleotides are known to drive Cx43 expression inside the cell as well as connexisome movement into gap junction plaques in the plasma membrane. Observations suggest that vascular function may become self-reinforcing through a cyclic nucleotide feed-forward loop that amplifies and sustains vasodilator production. Cyclic nucleotides spilling from the uterus also may explain pregnancy-adaptive effects in the systemic circulation, where substantial increases in cyclic nucleotides are detectable and cause increased and sustained Ca^{2+} signaling.

Normal pregnancy is now recognized to be a mild inflammatory state. Immune cells and their byproducts are known to interact with invading trophoblasts and endothelial cells. In early pregnancy, immune cells play an important role in the implantation and establishment of the placenta. The decidua is known to contain a large number of immune cells, including helper T cells, natural killer cells, dendritic cells, and macrophages. These cells are known to produce many growth factors and cytokines including VEGF, tumor necrosis factor α, and interleukin (IL)-1β, IL-6, and IL-8, all of which may be important in establishing placentation and the neovascularization that accompanies it. These immune cell–derived growth factors and cytokines are important for vascular remodeling to provide adequate blood supply to the placenta. VEGF is also known as a somewhat weak agonist for vasodilator production (through its ability to weakly mobilize Ca^{2+}), and this may be beneficial for late-pregnancy support of uterine blood flow.

RESPIRATORY SYSTEM

Physiologic changes to the respiratory system during pregnancy include both functional and anatomic adaptations. These changes strive to achieve optimal maternal oxygenation and ventilation, but they may produce symptoms that practitioners should be knowledgeable about when caring for pregnant women with underlying heart disease.

Functional Adaptations

The maternal respiratory rate usually remains constant, but tidal volume increases by 30% to 50%, leading to a similar increase in minute ventilation. One hypothesis proposes that increased progesterone levels may raise the sensitivity to carbon dioxide in the respiratory center of the medulla, thus driving this increase in ventilation and improving maternal exhalation of the fetus's metabolic byproducts. Even with a normal respiratory rate, up to 70% of pregnant women complain of some degree of labored breathing or shortness of breath. These symptoms tend to begin early in the second trimester and plateau at the beginning of the third trimester, often worsening when the woman is sitting. Unfortunately, they are also present in situations of cardiac compromise and represent common indications for cardiac evaluation in pregnancy. Differentiating normal physiologic adaptations from a pathologic process can be challenging, but certain findings upon questioning and examination can prove helpful. Cough, fever, pain, hemoptysis, and sputum production should raise concern about an underlying pathology. In addition, in situations of normal physiologic adaptation, the lung exam should be clear of rales, consolidation, wheezing, and diminished breath sounds. Chest x-ray findings should be normal, with the exception of increased aeration, slight enlargement of the cardiac silhouette, and an increase in the subcostal angle.

The normal respiratory adaptation of increased minute ventilation reduces the partial pressure of carbon dioxide ($PaCO_2$) to 27 to 32 mmHg and increases the partial pressure of oxygen (PaO_2) to 100 to 110 mm Hg. As a result, the maternal pH is slightly alkalotic, with a mean value between 7.40 and 7.45. Functional residual capacity decreases by up to 20%, owing largely to decreases in expiratory reserve volume and residual volume caused by the upwardly displaced diaphragm. Consequently, the pregnant woman is left with less reserve during periods of hypoxia. Inspiratory capacity is slightly increased, but the total lung capacity is slightly decreased from 4.2 L to 4.0 L. Airway resistance remains unchanged in pregnancy, as does the forced expiratory volume in 1 second (FEV_1).

Alveolar diffusing capacity rises about 10% in the first trimester but returns to baseline during the second and third trimesters. All of these functional adaptations serve to create a gradient whereby the maternal compartment is rich in oxygen and low in CO_2, with an oxyhemoglobin disassociation curve shifted to optimize diffusion across the placenta and the fetal compartment.

Anatomic Adaptations

During pregnancy, the thoracic cage has been reported to increase in circumference by 5 to 7 cm, and the chest diameter can increase by 2 cm. Flaring of the ribs, such that the subcostal angle (the angle between the right- and left-sided cartilage associated with the 7th to 10th ribs) increases from an average of 68 degrees to an average of 103 degrees (at term), also occurs. The enlarging uterus pushes up the diaphragm by 4 to 5 cm, possibly leading to bibasilar alveolar collapse and atelectasis. The vasodilatory effect of increased serum progesterone is thought to also cause increased vascularity and hyperemia of the upper respiratory mucosa, often leading to epistaxis and nasal congestion, and it may potentially affect the absorption of inhaled medications.

Pleura

Asymptomatic pleural effusions may occur in up to 23% of women in the immediate postpartum period.

HEMATOLOGIC AND IMMUNE SYSTEMS

Hematologic and immune adaptations of pregnancy serve to balance two seemingly contradictory goals: optimal nourishment of the growing and somewhat "foreign" fetoplacental unit and protection of the mother from the physiologic stresses of hemorrhage and exposure to "nonself" cells. As previously discussed, these adaptations strive to optimize maternal oxygen-carrying capacity and uteroplacental perfusion, but they also allow immunologic tolerance to the growing conceptus and establish a homeostatic state capable of tolerating potentially catastrophic blood loss. Hemostasis requires complex interactions between platelets, coagulation factors, and the vascular endothelium. Although most women maintain normal platelet counts throughout pregnancy, mean platelet counts may drop, particularly during the third trimester. Roughly 5% of pregnant women develop a mild gestational thrombocytopenia that rarely nadirs below 100,000/mcL. In contrast, in women with immune thrombocytopenia, thrombotic thrombocytopenic purpura, preeclampsia, antiphospholipid antibody syndrome, and drug-induced thrombocytopenia, platelet counts are typically lower than 100,000/mcL. Immediately postpartum, platelet counts begin to increase, returning to baseline 3 to 4 weeks postpartum. Platelet function is usually unchanged in normal pregnancy. Pregnancy is a known hypercoagulable state with a 12-fold increased risk for venous thromboembolism caused both by vascular stasis and an increase in clotting factors VII, VIII, X and XII; fibrinogen; and von Willebrand factor. Whereas factor XI decreases by 30% and protein S activity decreases, both plasminogen activator and plasminogen activator inhibitor levels increase, resulting in reduced fibrinolysis during pregnancy. However, fibrin split products, such as D-dimer, increase markedly in pregnancy with levels in late pregnancy up to 10-fold higher than in the nonpregnant state. Therefore, D-dimer levels are not reliable in predicting thromboembolism in pregnant patients. Factor V, prothrombin, antithrombin III, and protein C activities usually do not change. Resistance to activated protein C increases in the second and third trimesters. Routine coagulation panels remain normal. By 8 to 12 weeks postpartum, changes in clotting factor levels return to prepregnancy levels.

In addition to the increased production of red blood cells, pregnant women demonstrate increased white blood cell (WBC) counts caused by increased erythropoietin and bone marrow granulopoiesis. The increase in WBC counts begins in the second month of pregnancy and plateaus in the second or third trimester, at which time WBC counts range from 9000/mcL to 15,000/mcL. The increased WBC counts of normal pregnancy can sometimes make the diagnosis of infection challenging. In labor and immediately after delivery, WBC counts often rise, and counts as high as 25,000/mcL may be seen in women without evidence of infection. The increase in WBCs is mainly caused by an increase in neutrophils. Lymphocyte and basophil counts remain unchanged. Eosinophil counts generally increase slightly. Monocytes, which are involved in preventing fetal allograft rejection, are increased. The total WBC count returns to normal by the sixth day postpartum.

RENAL SYSTEM

An understanding of the physiologic adaptations in the renal system is also important when caring for pregnant women with underlying cardiac disease. The kidneys increase in length and volume, and the ureters dilate from the relaxing effect of progesterone and compression of the gravid uterus. This is most often more dramatic in the right ureter owing to the physiologic dextrorotation (rightward rotation) of the gravid uterus. A physiologic "hydronephrosis of pregnancy" can be seen in up to 80% of pregnant women. As early as 14 weeks of pregnancy, both renal blood flow and GFR increase by 50%, probably because of the vasodilation of arterioles. The increase in GFR leads to decreased serum creatinine concentration. Creatinine levels above 0.8 mg/dL during pregnancy may indicate renal dysfunction. By 4 weeks postpartum, the increased GFR returns to baseline. Aldosterone levels are also increased during pregnancy. Serum aldosterone levels increase and contribute to the retention of sodium. During a normal pregnancy, sodium gain is estimated at 900 to 1000 mEq. However, because the retention of water is even greater, sodium concentration and osmolality drop. Sodium concentration drops 4 tot 5 mEq/L, and osmolality falls to about 270 mOsm/kg. Total body stores of potassium also increase during pregnancy by about 320 mEq.

In pregnancy, there is an increase in the urinary excretion of proteins, most notably after 20 weeks' gestation. The rise in proteinuria peaks at about 20 weeks' gestation. The diagnosis of proteinuria during pregnancy is made when the protein levels exceed 300 mg/24 hours, which is twice the upper limit of normal in nonpregnant women.

GASTROINTESTINAL SYSTEM

Physiologic changes in the GI system that occur during pregnancy may affect the absorption and metabolism of certain medications. Gastric emptying is delayed during pregnancy, and small intestinal transit time is increased. The gastric pH increases, which may reduce the absorption of acidic drugs.

Changes in the liver generally cause increases in cytochrome p450 levels, a family of oxidative liver enzymes responsible for the metabolism of many drugs. Accordingly, the clearance of agents metabolized by these enzymes may be enhanced. The clearance of digoxin, which is renally excreted, is significantly increased because of increased renal blood flow. Digoxin is primarily bound to albumin. Other physiologic changes that may alter drug metabolism during pregnancy are the reduction in plasma proteins (especially albumin) and an increase in maternal adipose tissue. Increased blood volume results in a larger volume of distribution for all agents. Nausea and vomiting, common during pregnancy, also may affect pharmacologic therapies.

PLACENTA

The placenta is a temporary organ that connects the developing fetus to the uterine wall via the umbilical cord. It is a fetomaternal organ with two components: the fetal placenta (chorion frondosum), which develops from the same blastocyst that forms the fetus, and the maternal placenta (decidua basalis), which develops from the maternal uterine tissue. Via its connection to the mother's blood stream, the placenta is involved in nutrient uptake, thermoregulation, waste elimination, and gas exchange. It has immune and endocrine functions as well. The placenta is an important producer of the hormones that support pregnancy. It metabolizes a number of substances and can release metabolic products into maternal or fetal circulations. The placenta's role in maintaining a healthy pregnancy and its potential role in pregnancy complications are discussed in Chapter 35.

BIBLIOGRAPHY

Adams JQ, Alexander AM. Alterations in cardiovascular physiology during labour. *Obstet Gynecol.* 1958;12(5):542–549.

Awe R, Nicotra M, Newsome T, Viles R. Arterial oxygenation and alveolar-arterial gradients in term pregnancy. *Obstet Gynecol.* 1979;53(2):182–186.

Bader R, Bader M, Rose D, Braunwald E. Hemodynamics at rest and during exercise in normal pregnancy as studied by cardiac catheterization. *J Clin Invest.* 1955;34: 1524–1536.

Bieniarz J, Yoshida T, Romero-Salinas G, Curuchet E, Caldeyro-Barcia R, Crottogini J. Aortocaval compression by the uterus in late human pregnancy. IV. Circulatory homeostasis by preferential perfusion of the placenta. *Am J Obstet Gynecol.* 1969;103:19–31.

Borghi C, Esposti D, Immordino V, et al. Relationship of systemic hemodynamics, left ventricular structure and function, and plasma natriuretic peptide concentrations during pregnancy complicated by preeclampsia. *Am J Obstet Gynecol.* 2000;183:140–147.

Chandra S, Tripathi A, Mishra S, Amzarul M, Vaish A. Physiological changes in hematological parameters during pregnancy. *Indian J Hematol Blood Transfus.* 2012;28(3): 144–146.

Cheung K, Lafayette R. Renal physiology of pregnancy. *Adv Chronic Kidney Dis.* 2013;20(3):209–214.

Clark S, Cotton D, Lee W, et al. Central hemodynamic assessment of normal term pregnancy. *Am J Obstet Gynecol.* 1989;161:1439–1442.

Contreras G, Gutiérrez M, Beroiza T, et al. Ventilatory drive and respiratory muscle function in pregnancy. *Am Rev Respir Dis.* 1991;144(4):837–841.

Davey D, Macnab M. Plasma adrenaline, noradrenaline, and dopamine in pregnancy hypertension. *Br J Obstet Gynaecol.* 1981;88:611–618.

Davidson J. Kidney function in pregnant women. *Am J Kidney Dis.* 1987;9:248–252.

Duvekot J, Cheriex E, Pieters F, Menheere P, Peeters L. Early pregnancy changes in hemodynamics and volume hemostasis are consecutive adjustments triggered by a primary fall in systemic vascular tone. *Am J Obstet Gynecol.* 1993;169:1382–1392.

Elkus R, Popovicj J. Respiratory physiology in pregnancy. *Clin Chest Med.* 1992;13(4):555–565.

Feinsilver S, Hertz G. Respiration during sleep in pregnancy. *Clin Chest Med.* 1992;13(4):637–644.

Gazioglu K, Kaltreider N, Rosen M, Yu P. Pulmonary function during pregnancy in normal women and in patients with cardiopulmonary disease. *Thorax.* 1970;25: 445–450.

Gee J, Packer B, Millen J, Robin E. Pulmonary mechanics during pregnancy. *J Clin Invest.* 1967;46:945–952.

Geva T, Mauer M, Striker I, Kirshon B, Pivarnik J. Effects of physiologic load of pregnancy on left ventricular contractility and remodeling. *Am Heart J.* 1997;133:53–59.

Grindheim G, Toska K, Estensen M, Rosseland L. Changes in pulmonary function during pregnancy: a longtitudinal cohort study. *Br J Obstet Gynaecol.* 2012;119(1):94–101.

Hendricks C, Quilligan E. Cardiac output during labor. *Am J Obstet Gynecol.* 1956;71:953–972.

Hunter S, Robson S. Adaptation of the maternal heart in pregnancy. *Br Med J.* 1992;68:540–543.

Hytten F. Blood volume changes in normal pregnancy. *Clin Haematol.* 1985;14(3):601–612.

Katz R, Karliner J, Resnik R. Effects of a natural volume overload state (pregnancy) on left ventricular performance in normal human subjects. *Circulation.* 1978;58:434–441.

Kjeldsen J. Hemodynamic investigations during labour and delivery. *Acta Obstet Gynecol Scand Suppl.* 1979;89:1–252.

Lees M, Taylor S, Scott D, Kerr M. A study of cardiac output at rest during pregnancy. *J Obstet Gynaecol Br Commonw.* 1967;74(3):319–328.

Liberatore S, Pistelli R, Patalano F, et al. Respiratory function during pregnancy. *Respiration.* 1984;46(2):145–150.

Lund C, Donovan J. Blood volume during pregnancy. Significance of plasma and red cell volumes. *Am J Obstet Gynecol.* 1967;98:394–403.

Mabie W, DiSessa T, Crocker L, Sibal B, Arheart K. A longitudinal study of cardiac output in normal human pregnancy. *Am J Obstet Gynecol.* 1994;170:849–856.

Metcalfe J, Romney S, Ramsey L, Reid D, Burwell C. Estimation of uterine blood flow in normal human pregnancy at term. *J Clin Invest.* 1955;34(11):1632–1638.

Milne J, Mill R, Coutts J, Macnaughton M, Moran F, Pack A. The effect of human pregnancy on the pulmonary transfer factor for carbon monoxide as measured by the single breath method. *Clin Sci Mol Med.* 1977;53(2):271–276.

Mone S, Sanders S, Colan S. Control mechanism for physiological hypertrophy of pregnancy. *Circulation.* 1996;94: 667–672.

Morschauser TJ, Ramadoss J, Koch JM, et al. Local effects of pregnancy on connexin proteins that mediate Ca2+-associated uterine endothelial NO synthesis. *Hypertension.* 2014;63(3):589–594.

Natrajan P, McGarrigle H, Lawrence D, Lachelin G. Plasma adrenaline and noradrenaline levels in normal pregnancy and pregnancy-induced hypertension. *Br J Obstet Gynaecol.* 1982;89:1041–1045.

Peck T, Arias F. Hematologic changes associated with pregnancy. *Clin Obstet Gynecol.* 1979;22(4):785–798.

Pirani B, Campbell D, MacGillivray I. Plasma volume in normal first pregnancy. *J Obstet Gynaecol Br Commonw.* 1973;80:884–887.

Pritchard J. Changes in blood volume during pregnancy and delivery. *Anesthesiology.* 1965;26:393–399.

Pritchard J, Rowland R. Blood volume changes in pregnancy and the puerperium III. Whole body and large vessel hematocrits in pregnant and nonpregnant women. *Am J Obstet Gynecol.* 1964;88:391–395.

Robson S, Dunlop W, Boys R, Hunter S. Cardiac output during labour. *Br Med J (Clin Res ED).* 1987;295: 1169–1172.

Robson S, Hunter S, Boys R, Dunlop W. Serial study of the factors influencing changes in cardiac output during human pregnancy. *Am J Physiol*. 1989;256:H1060–H1065.

Rovinsky J, Jaffin H. Cardiovascular hemodynamics in pregnancy. I. Blood and plasma volumes in multiple pregnancy. *Am J Obstet Gynecol*. 1965;93:1–15.

Sanghavi M, Rutherford JD. Cardiovascular physiology of pregnancy. *Circulation*. 2014;130(12):1003–1008.

Senadheera S, Bertrand PP, Grayson TH, Leader L, Murphy TV, Sandow SL. Pregnancy-induced remodeling and enhanced endothelium-derived hyperpolarization-type vasodilator activity in rat uterine radial artery: transient receptor potential vanilloid type 4 channels, caveolae and myoendothelial gap junctions. *J Anat*. 2013;223(6): 677–686.

Stephansson O, Dickman P, Johansson A, Cnattingius S. Maternal hemoglobin concentration during pregnancy and risk of stillbirth. *JAMA*. 2000;284(20):2611–2617.

Taylor D, Lind T. Red cell mass during and after normal pregnancy. *Br J Obstet Gynaecol*. 1964;86:364–370.

Templeton A, Kelman G. Maternal blood gases (PaO_2--PaO_2), physiological shunt and VD/VT in pregnancy. *Br J Anaesth*. 1976;48(10):1001–1004.

Thomsen J, Fogh-Anderson N, Jaszczak P. Atrial natriuretic peptide, blood volume, aldosterone, and sodium excretion during twin pregnancy. *Acta Obstet Gynecol Scand*. 1994;73:14–20.

Ueland K, Metcalfe J. Circulatory changes in pregnancy. *Clin Obstet Gynecol*. 1975;18(3):41–50.

Ueland K, Novy M, Peterson E, Metcalfe J. Maternal cardiovascular dynamics IV. The influence of gestational age on the maternal cardiovascular response to posture and exercise. *Am J Obstet Gynecol*. 1969;104:856–864.

Ueland K. Maternal cardiovascular dynamics VII. Intrapartum blood volume changes. *Am J Obstet Gynecol*. 1976;126:671–677.

Weinbergerr S, Weiss S, Cohen W, Weiss J, Johnson T. Pregnancy and the lung. *Am Rev Respir Dis*. 1980;121(3): 559–581.

Yoshimura T, Yoshimura M, Yasue H, et al. Plasma concentration of atrial natriuretic peptide and brain natriuretic peptide during normal human pregnancy and the post-partum period. *J Endocrinol*. 1994;140:393–397.

2

The Cardiac Physical Examination in Pregnancy

John H. Wilson, MD, FACC, FHRS

The many physiologic changes that occur in pregnancy are reflected in the cardiac physical examination. In this chapter, we note changes the practitioner should expect and the timing of those changes, with respect to respiratory rate and pattern, chest wall, lung sounds, pulse, blood pressure, jugular venous pressure, apical impulse, heart sounds, murmurs, and extremities.

RESPIRATORY RATE AND PATTERN

Although minute ventilation increases in pregnancy, the change is mainly caused by an increase in tidal volume; respiratory rate does not change. The increase in tidal volume is caused by an increase in both inspiratory and ventilatory drive and is achieved chiefly by greater displacement of the rib cage.

CHEST WALL

During pregnancy, the enlarging uterus increases the end-expiratory abdominal pressure, displacing the diaphragm upward by as much as 4 cm. Diaphragmatic excursion is not impaired and actually increases by up to 2 cm. The chest height becomes shorter, but the other thoracic dimensions increase, which serves to maintain constant lung capacity. During pregnancy, the thoracic cage has been reported to increase in circumference by 5 to 7 cm, and the chest diameter can increase by 2 cm. Flaring of the ribs, such that the subcostal angle increases from an average of 68 degrees to an average of 103 degrees (at term), also occurs.

LUNG SOUNDS

The lung sounds in pregnancy remain unchanged. The presences of rales, rhonchi, or wheezes should alert the clinician to pathology.

PULSE

The resting heart rate tends to increase; resting heart rates in the 90s are common. The heart rate increases progressively throughout pregnancy, reaching a maximum of 20% to 25% over prepregnancy values in the third trimester. The increased heart rate is largely caused by an increase in sympathetic tone and a decrease in parasympathetic tone. Because of the increased cardiac output of pregnancy, bounding pulses are frequently observed. Bounding pulses develop between 12 and 15 weeks of gestation and persist until roughly 1 month postpartum. An irregular pulse caused by ectopic beats is also common because both premature atrial and premature ventricular contractions increase in frequency during pregnancy.

BLOOD PRESSURE

In pregnancy, blood pressure tends to be lower than in the nonpregnant state. Blood pressure decreases early in the first trimester because of a drop in peripheral vascular resistance, and it continues to drop slowly until 22 to 24 weeks gestation. After 22 to 24 weeks, blood pressure gradually increases to prepregnancy levels.

JUGULAR VENOUS PRESSURE

Beginning at 20 weeks' gestation, the jugular venous pressure rises slightly.

APICAL IMPULSE

A prominent nondisplaced apical impulse is common throughout pregnancy.

HEART SOUNDS

The first component of the first heart sound is caused by mitral valve closure, and the second component is caused by tricuspid closure. The hyperdynamic state of pregnancy accentuates the first heart sound; both components become louder, with the most obvious increase occurring between 12 to 20 weeks of gestation. The first heart sound remains loud until about 32 weeks, when its intensity decreases in some patients. It returns to prepregnancy intensity 2 to 4 weeks postpartum. Exaggerated splitting of the first heart sound, on the order of 30 to 45 msec, is also noted and follows the same time course as the increase in intensity. In pregnancy, both valves close earlier, but the shortening of mitral closure time is greater, leading to the exaggerated split.

The second heart sound changes little; its intensity is not significantly increased. The relationship of the two components of the second heart sound (first component, aortic closure; second component, pulmonic closure) does not change until after 30 weeks. From 30 weeks until delivery, there is blunted respiratory splitting caused by the gravid uterus restricting venous blood return to the right heart. A third heart sound has been reported in up to 80% of pregnant women. Auscultation of a fourth heart sound is reported in about 16% of normal pregnant women.

MURMURS

Pregnancy increases cardiac output; the high-velocity flow through the heart can create turbulence, which produces a heart murmur. Systolic ejection murmurs are reported in more than 90% of pregnant women. The intensity of the murmur is 2/6 (faint but audible on first placing the stethoscope on the chest) in 80% of women and 1/6 (only audible after listening carefully for some time) in the remainder. Eighty-five percent of these murmurs are heard best along the left sternal border from the second to fifth ribs, but they can generally be heard widely over the precordium. This physiologic murmur of pregnancy intensifies with inspiration in some patients, suggesting that it is "right sided" and originates from the pulmonary artery. In other patients, it is intensified by expiration, suggesting that it is "left sided" and may originate from the aorta. These systolic murmurs disappear very quickly after delivery, and in two-thirds of patients they are gone by 8 days postpartum.

Diastolic murmurs have been detected in 20% of patients. Described as soft and medium to high pitched, they are best heard along the left sternal border. It is thought that diastolic murmurs are also caused by increased flow and not incompetence of the semilunar valves.

The time interval of the appearance and disappearance of the physiologic murmurs of pregnancy does not correlate closely with changes in cardiac output, suggesting etiologic factors other than increased blood flow. Two possibilities are the variations in blood viscosity and the physical state of the walls of the great vessels, which change during pregnancy.

Other sounds produced during normal pregnancy include the cervical venous hum, heard along the right upper sternal border and produced by increased venous return, and the mammary souffle, which may be continuous or heard only during systole. These sounds can be obliterated, often by compression of the central vein above the sound. The mammary souffle is produced by increased mammary blood flow and is usually heard in the right- or left-second intercostal space, about 1 cm from the sternum. The mammary souffle can be modified or obliterated by varying the pressure on the chest piece of the stethoscope, which helps distinguish it from murmurs of cardiac origin. A mammary souffle can be heard in about 14% of pregnant women; the majority (70%) are continuous, and the rest are heard only during systole.

EXTREMITIES

Peripheral edema is common, and some evidence of it may be found in up to 80% of normal women at some time during pregnancy.

BIBLIOGRAPHY

Cutforth R, MacDonald C. Heart sounds and murmurs in pregnancy. *Am Heart J.* 1966;71:741–747.

Gourgoulianis K, Karantanas A, Diminikou G, Molyvdas P. Benign postpartum pleural effusion. *Eur Respir J.* 1995;8:1748–1750.

Hegewald M, Crapo R. Respiratory physiology in pregnancy. *Clin Chest Med.* 2011;32:1–13.

LoMauro A, Aliverti A. Respiratory physiology of pregnancy. *Breathe.* 2015;11(4):297–301.

MacGillivray I, Rose G, Row B. Blood pressure survey in pregnancy. *Clin Sci.* 1969;37:395–399.

Sanghavi M, Rutherford J. Cardiovascular physiology of pregnancy. *Circulation.* 2014;130(12):1003–1008.

3

Obstetric Care for Nonobstetricians

William T. Schnettler, MD, FACOG, John H. Wilson, MD, FACC, FHRS

Obstetricians use standard terminology to assess a woman's pregnancy history: gravidity is the total number of pregnancies, and parity is the total number of pregnancies carried to a viable gestational age (24 weeks). Parity is further divided into number of term, preterm, spontaneously aborted, electively aborted, and ectopic pregnancies. Obstetricians also document the number of living children. When reviewing pregnancy history, it is important to note the outcome of each pregnancy, the mode of delivery, birthweight(s), and whether there were any pregnancy complications. The term *nulliparous* is used to describe a woman who has never given birth. The term *primiparous* means having given birth to only one child. The term *multiparous* means having given birth to more than one child.

Signs and symptoms of pregnancy include the following:

Quickening: the sensation of fetal movement

Chadwick's sign: the bluish hue of the cervix on examination

Linea nigra: a dark coloration of the skin at the midline from the umbilicus down to the mons pubis

Palmer erythema

Telangiectasias

Nausea and vomiting

Pregnancy is usually confirmed by a urine test for beta human chorionic gonadotropin (bHCG). A positive result is a level greater than 50 mIU/mL. bHCG levels rise by 50% every 48 hours up to a peak level of 100,000 to 2,000,000 mIU/mL by 10 weeks.

Gestation is calculated from the last menstrual period (LMP). The estimated time of delivery is 40 weeks. A term delivery is considered to occur between 37 and 42 weeks. A preterm delivery is one that occurs before 37 weeks. A fetus is considered viable after 24 weeks. Menstrual-based dating should be accepted only when it is confirmed by ultrasound biometric measurements.

Gestational time points are calculated from the time of conception. Conception is the fusion of the ova and sperm and takes place in the ampullary portion of the fallopian tube. Implantation of the blastocyst into the lining of the uterus occurs at 5 to 7 days. The term *embryo* is used to describe the conceptus from conception until 10 weeks. Between 10 weeks and delivery, the term *fetus* is used. After delivery until 1 year of age, the term *infant* is used.

Events in pregnancy are traditionally categorized by dividing pregnancy into three trimesters (Table 3.1).

Other terms that are frequently used to describe the gestational age are provided in Table 3.2.

Gestational age can be evaluated in several ways. In routine practice, the mainstays are levels of bHCG and ultrasonography. Because bHCG rises by at least 50% every 48 hours (to a peak of 100,000–2,000,000 mIU/mL by 10 weeks), its level can be tracked to ensure the viability of the early pregnancy and to track gestational age. In what is called the discriminatory zone, when the bHCG is about 2500 mIU/mL (roughly 5 weeks after the LMP), transvaginal ultrasonography (TVUS) imaging should identify an intrauterine gestational sac. Fetal cardiac activity is first detected by TVUS at about 6 weeks and later auscultated by a handheld Doppler at about 12 weeks. Ultrasound biometry is used to assess the fetal growth as it relates to established nomograms by gestational age.

Pregnant women should increase caloric intake to 2500 calories/day for singleton gestations and to 2700 to 3000 calories/day for twin gestations. Supplemental iron, at a dosage of 30 mg/day of elemental iron, is recommended in the second trimester. Folate supplementation, given in a dosage of 400 mcg/day, has been shown to reduce the risk of neural tube defects. For women with a history of seizure disorder and women who have had a previous child with a neural tube defect, a dosage of 4 g/day is recommended.

TABLE 3.1 The Three Trimesters of Pregnancy

Trimester	Gestational Age
First	Conception until 13 weeks, 6 days gestational age
Second	14 weeks to 27 weeks, 6 days gestational age
Third	28 weeks to delivery

TABLE 3.2 Terms to Describe Gestational Age at Delivery

Term	Gestational Age
Abortion	<20 weeks, 0 days
Previable preterm birth	20 weeks, 0 days to 23 weeks, 0 days
Preterm birth	23 weeks, 0 days to 36 weeks, 6 days
Early term birth	37 weeks, 0 days to 38 weeks, 0 days
Full-term birth	39 weeks, 0 days to 40 weeks, 6 days
Late-term birth	41 weeks, 0 days to 41 weeks, 6 days
Postterm birth	42 weeks, 0 days and beyond

TABLE 3.3 Recommendations for Weight Gain During Pregnancy

Prepregnancy Weight	Recommended Weight Gain (lb)
Underweight women (BMI <18.5)	28–40
Normal weight women (BMI 18.5–24.9)	25–35
Overweight women (BMI 25.0–29.9)	15–25
Obese women (BMI >30.0)	11–20

BMI, Body mass index.

Recommendations for weight gain during pregnancy are provided in Table 3.3.

Obstetric care may be divided into three phases: prenatal, perinatal, and postnatal. Prenatal care involves maternal education and distinguishing pregnancies that are likely to be uncomplicated from those in which maternal or fetal factors predict a higher likelihood of complications or the need for special care. A history and physical examination can identify potential maternal and fetal risk factors. Standard laboratory assessments performed during the first trimester include complete blood count (CBC), blood type and screen, rapid plasma regain (RPR), rubella immunity, hepatitis B surface antigen, human immunodeficiency virus (HIV), urinalysis and culture, gonorrhea, chlamydia, purified protein derivative, and Pap smear. Appointment frequency is monthly until 28 weeks, then every 2 weeks until 36 weeks, and weekly thereafter. At each visit, it is routine to check fetal heart tones, measure fundal height, perform urine dipstick assessment (protein, glucose, ketones), and obtain weight and blood pressure. At 28 weeks, standard laboratory assessment includes repeat measurement of CBC, blood type and screen, and RPR as well as an initial gestational diabetes screen (50-g Glucola drink followed by serum glucose measurement 1 hour after consumption; cut-off is 130 mg/dL). At 35 to 37 weeks' gestation, it is standard to perform a group B streptococcus vaginal swab.

Modern obstetric care involves routine use of fetal ultrasound. Standard ultrasound assessments include:

First trimester: confirmation of viable intrauterine pregnancy and assistance in gestational age assessment using measurement of the crown–rump length of the fetus. One can also measure the nuchal translucency at this time.

Second trimester: standard anatomic survey performed at roughly 20 weeks' gestation to assess for fetal anomalies and growth

Follow-up ultrasound assessments may be performed thereafter depending on maternal or fetal risk factors or concerns that may arise.

Many pregnant women experience annoying symptoms that do not necessarily imply pregnancy complications. These include leg edema, varicosities and hemorrhoids (caused by impaired venous drainage), and frequent urination (caused by pressure on the bladder by the uterus). Common gastrointestinal symptoms include constipation and esophageal reflux. Back pain and inguinal pain that are worse when walking (round ligament pain) are frequent complaints. Some women experience unusual food cravings (pica). Dehydration may occur. Many women complain of Braxton Hicks contractions.

Maternal risk factors include age (younger than 18 or older than 40 years old) and a body mass index less than 17 or over 35. Previous medical diseases of particular concern are hypertension, diabetes and other endocrine diseases, cardiac disease, pulmonary disease, renal impairment, neurologic conditions, connective tissue disorders, anemia or clotting disorders, cancer, HIV, group B streptococcus carriage, and psychiatric illness.

A history of complications in previous pregnancies may predict a complicated delivery. These include prior cesarean section, preeclampsia or eclampsia, gestational diabetes, obstetric cholestasis, postnatal depression, previous miscarriage, previous preterm delivery, stillborn or neonatal death, or a baby with fetal growth retardation or a congenital abnormality.

Fetal screening includes identifying singleton or multiple pregnancies, confirming gestation, confirming viability, and ascertaining certain risks such as Down syndrome.

Subsequent visits are used to evaluate maternal and fetal well-being. Typically, they include checking maternal blood pressure, providing a urine dipstick for proteinuria and glycosuria analysis, determining fetal viability, and estimating fundal height. Later in pregnancy, it is important to determine fetal position and degree of pelvic engagement of the fetus. A typical follow-up schedule includes visits at 16, 18 to 20, 28, 34, and 38 weeks. If delivery has not occurred by 40 weeks of gestation, the obstetrician will usually initiate a plan for inducing labor.

Any time medications are used in pregnancy, consideration must be given to potential harmful effects on the fetus. The therapies listed in Table 3.4 are generally considered safe.

Normal vaginal delivery, commonly referred to as labor, is typically divided into three stages. The first stage, which persists until the cervix is fully dilated at 10 cm, is typically divided into two phases. The latent phase is the period prior to cervical dilation of 3 cm; its duration varies. The active phase occurs after the cervix has dilated to 3 cm, at which point it begins to dilate at a more consistent rate of about 1.2 cm/hr. The active phase persists until delivery of the baby during the second stage of labor. The second stage includes a passive component (descent of the fetal head) and an active component (pushing); the latter allows delivery of the baby. The third stage of labor is delivery of the placenta, which can take up to 30 minutes. Signs of placental separation include an increase in umbilical cord length, a gush of blood, and uterine fundal rebound. The hour after delivery is often referred to as the fourth stage of labor.

TABLE 3.4	Safe Pregnancy Medications
Condition	**Safe Treatment Options**
Pain	Tylenol, hydration, heating pad (only in second and third trimesters)
Headache	Tylenol, prochlorperazine, promethazine, low-dose beta-blocker, Fioricet (episodic)
Nausea or vomiting	Vitamin B_6, ginger, prochlorperazine, promethazine, metoclopramide, ondansetron (outside of first trimester), corticosteroids (outside of first trimester)
Muscle cramping or pain	Cyclobenzaprine (outside of first trimester)
Depression or anxiety	Nonmedical therapies such as behavioral modification, exercise, and therapy are preferred. If medication is required, selective norepinephrine reuptake inhibitors are preferred (e.g., venlafaxine or desvenlafaxine)

During labor, contractions—which are felt best at the fundus—should last about 45 to 60 seconds and occur with a frequency of three in 10 minutes.

If the first stage of labor is prolonged, usually defined as slower than 1.2 cm/hr of cervical dilation in a nulliparous woman, or less than 1.5 cm/hr in a multiparous woman, amniotomy or administration of Pitocin is recommended. It is also appropriate to use an intrauterine pressure catheter to monitor contraction strength. Failure to progress is defined as no progress in cervical dilation despite 4 hours of adequate labor (<200 Montevideo units [MVUs]). Montevideo units are a method of measuring uterine performance during labor. Each unit is equal to 1 mm Hg, and they are measured over a 10-minute period. Montevideo units are calculated by summing the individual contraction intensities in a 10-minute period. The peak pressure during each contraction is measured, and the baseline value is subtracted. The value for each contraction in a 10-minute period is then summed. Generally, a value above 200 MVUs is considered necessary for adequate labor during the active phase.

In women who have not received an epidural anesthetic, the second stage of labor is considered prolonged if it last more than 2 hours in a nulliparous woman or 1 hour in a multiparous woman. Epidural anesthesia lengthens the normal duration of the second stage of labor. For nulliparous women who have received an epidural, a second-stage duration of more than 3 hours is considered prolonged; for multiparous women who have received an epidural, a second-stage duration of more than 2 hours is considered prolonged.

Table 3.5 lists terms are used to describe the descent of the baby through the vaginal canal.

Assisted vaginal delivery involves using instruments, such as forceps, to deliver the baby; it is used if labor is prolonged or if the mother has a contraindication to pushing. Like all medical intervention, the use of forceps to assist delivery has both benefits and risks. The major benefit of using forceps is that the operator will have a secure grip on the baby with less risk of fetal injury overall. The risks include maternal pelvic floor injury and the potential for injury of the fetal face and skull. Forceps-assisted deliveries are divided into outlet forceps, low forceps, and midforceps deliveries. Outlet forceps should be used only when the scalp is visible, the skull is on the pelvic floor, and the position is either occiput anterior or posterior. The mother's bladder should be drained, and she must have received adequate anesthesia. Rotation of the fetus should be limited to a maximum of 45 degrees. A low forceps delivery is when

the scalp has reached station 2 but the skull is not on the pelvic floor. Midforceps deliveries are when the scalp is at station 2 or higher but the head has engaged; they should be performed only by highly skilled clinicians. An alternative to the use of forceps is a vacuum-assisted delivery, which carries less risk for maternal trauma but higher risks of both failure to achieve delivery and fetal trauma, such as cephalohematoma and lacerations. The requirements for vacuum-assisted delivery are the same as for outlet forceps.

Fetal monitoring with heart rate monitoring and ultrasound throughout labor and delivery is standard. A nonstress test (NST) assesses "reactivity" of the fetal heart rate (FHR) by witnessing two accelerations of 15 beats/min for 15 seconds in a 20-minute FHR strip. If nonreactive, the baby may be sleeping; give the mother juice and repeat for another 20 minutes or perform a biophysical profile (BPP). Sedatives, narcotics, and central nervous system or cardiovascular abnormalities are causes of a nonreactive NST. The following are guidelines for interpreting the FHR strip:

Reassuring findings: variability or beat-to-beat variation of 5 to 25 beats/min above and below the baseline; baseline falls between 110 and 160 beats/min

Early decelerations: subtle deceleration of the FHR that begins and ends with the contraction, a sign of head compression; no treatment is required

Variable decelerations are more jagged and look like a V on the printout, a sign of cord compression; they can occur at any time point in relation to the contraction; may treat with an amnioinfusion

Late decelerations begin at peak of contraction and end after contraction is finished – a sign of uteroplacental insufficiency; must begin in utero resuscitation and assess for whether vaginal delivery is likely

A BPP uses data on heart rate and ultrasound to assess fetal well-being; 8 points is a good score. Four points or less indicates that the fetus in trouble. The point scoring system is listed in Table 3.6.

Other methods of assessing fetal well-being include

Modified BPP = NST and amniotic fluid index

Contraction stress test: nipple stimulation or oxytocin; shows three uterine contractions in 10 minutes to be adequate; a negative result means no late decelerations

Fetal scalp electrode: placed when a more accurate recording of heart rate is needed; do not use in mothers with herpes simplex virus (HSV), HIV, or hepatitis C

TABLE 3.5 Terms Used to Describe Descent of a Baby	
Term	**Definition**
Position	OA (occiput anterior), OP (occiput posterior), LOT (left occiput transverse), ROT (right occiput transverse)
Attitude	Relationship of baby to itself
Lie	Long axis of baby to long axis of mother
Engagement	Biparietal diameter has entered the pelvic inlet
Station	Presenting part's relationship to ischial spine in centimeters. Negative numbers indicate proximal to the ischial spines, zero at the ischial spines, and positive numbers distal to the ischial spines. Numbers range from -5 to 0 to +5.

TABLE 3.6	The Biophysical Profile Score	
	Give 2 points	Give 0 points
Nonstress test	Reactive	<2 accelerations
Amniotic fluid index	One 2 by 2 cm pocket	No pocket seen
Fetal breathing movements	Last over 30 seconds	<30 seconds
Fetal extremity movements	Three or more episodes	<3 episodes
Fetal tone	Extension to flexion; flex at rest	Extended at rest

Intrauterine pressure catheter: placed in the uterus to monitor contraction strength using Montevideo units; a good baseline is 10 to 15 mm Hg; contractions in labor increase the tocodynamometer by 20 to 80 units; calculate the total Montevideo units over a 10-minute window of time to assess adequacy of contractions

Sometimes labor must be induced. Use prostaglandins to initiate cervical dilation; both intravaginal and oral forms are available. After the cervix has dilated and become sufficiently thin (effaced), rupture the membranes and administer oxytocin to stimulate uterine contractions. Generally, this leads to delivery of the baby.

Cesarean section may be considered because of complications in labor or to reduce risks to the mother. Obstetric indications for cesarean section include malpresentation of the baby, such as breech or transverse lie, placenta previa, failure to progress in labor, failed instrument delivery, or maternal complications (e.g., severe maternal bleeding). Cesarean section also may be performed for fetal distress and if the risks of labor and vaginal delivery are considered excessive (e.g., a significantly dilated aortic root or severe left ventricular dysfunction).

In addition to potential benefits, cesarean section has negative consequences for both the mother and the baby. Maternal risks include greater blood loss than with vaginal delivery, bladder injury, risk of infection, higher risk of thromboembolism, and potential complications in future pregnancies. Fetal risks include the potential for laceration and a higher risk of respiratory complications.

Even after delivery, there is a risk of obstetric complications, such as postpartum hemorrhage. Defined as more than 500 cc of blood loss within 2 hours of delivery, postpartum hemorrhage may be caused by retained placenta, uterine atony, or perineal tears. A retained placenta must be removed. Uterine atony is treated with uterotonics, or if this fails, surgically.

Women may be offered genetic screening or genetic testing if a specific condition is suspected. Genetic screening may include the following.

1. First-trimester screen: combination of fetal nuchal translucency measurement on ultrasound and maternal serum protein quantitative measurement (pregnancy-associated plasma protein, HCG, alpha fetoprotein); screens for trisomies 21, 18, and 13 with about 90% sensitivity; this can be offered to all women between 11 0/7–13 6/7 weeks' gestation
2. Maternal cell-free fetal DNA screen (often called noninvasive prenatal testing): screens for trisomies 21, 18, and 13 and monosomy X; can be offered to all women beyond 10 weeks' gestation
3. Maternal serum quad screen: measures levels of maternal serum alpha fetoprotein (msAFP), bHCG, unconjugated estriol, and inhibin A to assess risk for trisomies 21 and 18; can be offered to all women between 15 0/7 and 21 6/7 weeks' gestation with about 85% sensitivity
4. Open neural tube or abdominal wall defects: can test msAFP between 15 0/7 and 21 6/7 weeks' gestation with about 95% sensitivity (best if between 16 and 20 weeks)
5. Maternal serum for carrier status of single-gene disorders (e.g., cystic fibrosis, Tay-Sachs disease); can be offered to all women at any time

Genetic testing options include amniocentesis and chorionic villus sampling, both of which are invasive and involve a risk of fetal loss.

Preimplantation genetic testing samples one of the blastocyst's cells before implantation when a woman is undergoing in vitro fertilization.

Ectopic pregnancy occurs in about 1 in 100 pregnancies. The most common location is in the ampulla of the fallopian tubes, but such pregnancies also can occur in the ovary, cervix, uterine serosa, or peritoneal cavity. Symptoms of ectopic pregnancy include episodic lower abdominal pain and vaginal bleeding caused by inadequate progesterone support. Signs include unilateral tenderness on bimanual examination, palpation of a mass on bimanual examination, and Cullen's sign (periumbilical hematoma). Laboratory evaluation often reveals an inappropriate rise in bHCG. Risk factors for ectopic pregnancy are a history of fallopian tube disease, such as endometriosis or infection; previous fallopian tube surgery; assisted reproductive technologies; and current intrauterine contraceptive devices. Ultrasound examination shows the absence of an intrauterine pregnancy or a small fluid collection (pseudo-sac) within the endometrial cavity. Typically, a complex adnexal mass is identified, as is free fluid or blood in the cul-de-sac or intraperitoneal cavity. If the ectopic pregnancy is caught early enough, when the mass size is less than 4 cm and unruptured, treatment is with methotrexate 50 mg/M^2. Serial bHCG levels are followed 4 and 7 days later. A drop of 15% should occur between days 4 and 7. If the drop is less than 15%, administer a second dose of methotrexate. If the mass is greater than 4 cm, salpingostomy or salpingectomy may be required and can be done laparoscopically if the procedure is nonemergent.

If the membranes rupture before 37 weeks of gestation, the delivery is defined as premature. Causes of premature membrane rupture include intrauterine infection, polyhydramnios, cervical insufficiency, and abruptio placenta. The membranes also may rupture after amniocentesis. The diagnosis of ruptured membranes can be made by visual examination of fluid in the fornices, ferning of fluid on a slide, a positive Nitrazine test result (paper turns blue), or oligohydramnios on an ultrasound examination. In 70% of women, premature rupture of the membranes causes labor within the first week. If the woman is beyond 34 weeks of gestation, expedite delivery. If she is at less than 34 weeks, administer antibiotics, usually ampicillin and azithromycin. At any sign of chorioamnionitis, abruption, active labor, or fetal compromise, patients are typically admitted to the hospital, and delivery is initiated.

Spontaneous abortions are spontaneous deliveries at fewer than 20 weeks of gestation. They occur in 15% to 25% of pregnancies. Sixty percent of spontaneous abortions are associated with a genetic abnormality, the most common being trisomy 16 and monosomy X. Other causes include maternal Mullerian defects, antiphospholipid antibody syndromes, maternal endocrine problems, and luteal phase defects. A threatened abortion is an intrauterine pregnancy with bleeding and a closed cervix; it requires an obstetric visit. A missed abortion is embryonic or fetal death without passage of all products of conception. It is suspected if there are no fetal heart tones by 8 weeks' gestation. An inevitable abortion is diagnosed when the cervix becomes dilated. In such cases, the pregnancy will proceed to either a complete or an incomplete abortion. An incomplete abortion, which occurs when products of conception remain in the uterus, requires medical management or a dilation and curettage. A complete abortion occurs when ultrasound confirms that there is no evidence of retained products of conception. In this situation, it is necessary to follow bHCG until levels reach zero to make sure the patient does not have a gestational trophoblastic neoplasia (molar pregnancy).

Intrauterine growth retardation may occur from many causes, including hypertension, diabetes, renal disease, malnutrition, abnormal placentation, abruption, infections (cytomegalovirus [CMV], toxoplasmosis, and rubella), and multiple gestation. Growth retardation is classified as symmetric if all body parts are affected and asymmetric if the head is spared. Symmetric growth retardation is usually caused by an insult occurring early in pregnancy, such as a viral infection. Doppler velocimetry measurements can help identify the potential cause and time the delivery. Delivery is necessary if there is an abnormal fetal heart tracing or fetal umbilical artery end-diastolic flow that is reversed or absent.

Macrosomia, defined as an estimated fetal weight over the 90th percentile for gestational age, may be caused by maternal diabetes, maternal obesity, or multiparity or if the pregnancy is postterm. It is assessed by fetal ultrasound and followed by repeat ultrasound every 2 weeks. The discovery of macrosomia should lead to reevaluation of the mother for gestational diabetes if it has not been previously diagnosed. Macrosomia places the fetus at increased risk for shoulder dystocia and birth trauma, low Apgar scores, hypoglycemia, polycythemia, hypocalcemia, and jaundice. It is managed by tight control of diabetes, if present. Medical staff should prepare for dystocia. If a woman with macrosomia is over 39 weeks' gestation, labor should be induced. Consider a cesarean delivery if the fetus is larger than 5000 g in the absence of diabetes or more than 4500 g in the setting of diabetes.

Oligohydramnios can be diagnosed on ultrasound by the amniotic fluid index, calculated by dividing the mother's abdomen into four quadrants, measuring the largest pocket of fluid in each, and summing the pocket depths. A value less than 5 cm indicates oligohydramnios. Its most common cause is rupture of the membranes, but it also can be caused by fetal genitourinary abnormalities such as renal agenesis, polycystic kidney disease, renal tract obstruction, or intrauterine growth retardation. For preterm patients, management is hydration with oral intake or hypotonic intravenous fluids; for term patients, delivery should be initiated.

Polyhydramnios also can be diagnosed by the amniotic fluid index. A value greater than 25 cm is considered abnormal, as is a maximal pocket depth of greater than 8 cm. Polyhydramnios occurs in 2% to 3% of pregnancies. It is associated with aneuploidy, hydrops, poorly controlled diabetes, and lack of fetal swallowing caused by obstruction or neurologic injury. Polyhydramnios is monitored by ultrasound, and if severe enough, it may be treated with therapeutic amniocentesis.

Intrauterine fetal demise is another unfortunate situation that may be encountered. The cause may be congenital anomalies, placental abruption, or intrauterine infection, but more often it is unexplained. Intrauterine fetal demise is diagnosed when no fetal cardiac activity can be detected by ultrasound examination. Retained conceptus over 3 to 4 weeks leads to hypofibrinogenemia secondary to the release of thromboplastic substances of the decomposing fetus, and this may lead to disseminated intravascular coagulation in the mother. Therefore, delivery should be accomplished as soon as possible, although it is not an emergency unless there is evidence of disseminated intravascular coagulation. To determine the potential cause, the following workup can be offered: perform an amniocentesis; screen maternal serum for TORCH infections (toxoplasmosis, rubella, CMV, HSV, and syphilis); check maternal hemoglobin bA1c, thyroid-stimulating hormone, and antiphospholipid antibody panel; and send a portion of fetal fascia lata or cord blood for karyotype and microarray.

The Apgar score (Table 3.7) is a way to quickly assess the health of a newborn. It is an acronym for appearance, pulse, grimace, activity, and respiration. Each aspect is scored on a scale of 0 to 2, and the points are summed. The assessment is made 1 to 5 minutes after birth. A score of 3 or less is considered critical. Scores of 7 or above are considered normal.

Abbreviations commonly used in obstetric practice are listed in Box 3.1.

BOX 3.1   Common Obstetric Abbreviations

LMP: last menstrual period
EDC: estimated date of confinement
EDD: estimated date of delivery; EDC and EDD are often used interchangeably
G: gravidity, or total number pregnancies
P: parity, or how many pregnancies have reached 20 0/7 weeks
LEEP: loop electrocautery excision procedure
D&C: dilation and curettage
POCs: products of conception
PROM: premature rupture of membranes
PPROM: preterm premature rupture of membranes
SVD: spontaneous vaginal delivery
LTCS: low transverse cesarean section
RLTCS: repeat LTCS
FAVD: forceps-assisted vaginal delivery
VBAC: vaginal birth after cesarean section
VAVD: vacuum-assisted vaginal delivery
SAB: spontaneous abortion (miscarriage)
EAB: elective abortion
IUFD: intrauterine fetal demise

TABLE 3.7

The Apgar Score Criterion	Score of 0	Score of 1	Score of 2
Appearance	Blue or pale all over	Blue extremities; body pink	Pink all over
Pulse	Absent	<100 beats/min	>100 beats/min
Grimace	No response to stimulation	Grimace on suction or aggressive stimulation	Cry on stimulation
Activity	None	Some flexion	Flexed arms and legs that resist extension
Respiration	Absent	Weak, irregular gasping	Strong, robust cry

BIBLIOGRAPHY

Davies GA, Tessier JL, Woodman MC, Lipson A, Hahn PM. Maternal hemodynamics after oxytocin bolus compared with infusion in the third stage of labour: a randomized controlled trial. *Obstet Gynecol.* 2005;105:294–299.

Hurt JK. *Pocket Obstetrics and Gynecology.* : Wolters Kluwer; 2015.

Thomas Z. *Comprehensive Handbook Obstetrics & Gynecology.* 2nd ed. : Phoenix Medical Press; 2012.

4

Prepregnancy Counseling

William T. Schnettler, MD, FACOG

Pregnant women with heart disease have an increased risk of both maternal and fetal complications. Given that an estimated 1 million women in the United States have underlying congenital heart disease, the likelihood that a health care provider will care for such a patient is increasing. Certain conditions, such as pulmonary hypertension or prior peripartum cardiomyopathy, carry such high risk that they may contraindicate a pregnancy. In the Western world, the most common maternal heart disease is congenital, accounting for about 80% of patients. In the developing world, rheumatic valvular heart disease predominates.

This chapter provides an overview of prepregnancy counseling for women with heart disease, with an emphasis on its advantages for this patient population. We also discuss the scoring systems and tests used to ascertain the risk of maternal and fetal complications for patients hoping to become pregnant.

PREPREGNANCY COUNSELING: AN OVERVIEW

Ideally, risk assessment in patients with heart disease takes place before a woman becomes pregnant to present her with as accurate a prognosis as possible for both herself and her future child. If counseling was not provided before conception, it should be provided as early as possible during pregnancy. Counseling should involve the patient, her spouse or partner, and any other family members or significant individuals she chooses. The health care providers discuss the effect of pregnancy on the maternal cardiovascular system,

whether this risk will change over time or with treatment, and how pregnancy may affect the long-term health of the woman. They also counsel the patient on risks to the fetus and alternative options, such as adoption or surrogacy. Additionally, health care providers may refer women to centers with expertise in adult congenital heart disease and high-risk pregnancy care. Whenever possible, we believe that counseling should involve both cardiologists and fetal-maternal medicine specialists. In most cases when the mother's condition may be inherited, genetics counselors should also be involved. Prepregnancy counseling allows early assessment of the patient's history, exam findings, imaging and electrocardiographic (ECG) studies, and possibly exercise testing before the advent of the physiologic changes inherent with pregnancy. Counseling can help a woman make important decisions regarding surgical repair before pregnancy or to choose the appropriate timing of pregnancy.

Prepregnancy counseling also opens the door to discussions regarding the risks of congenital abnormalities. Genetic counseling should be a major focus in these discussions with specific details regarding the potential inheritance of certain lesions. The background congenital heart disease rate of 0.6% to 2.0% may be altered by an individual's family history, specific type of lesion, and exposure to teratogens. The risk for congenital heart disease in a fetus carried by a mother with congenital heart disease is estimated to be 4% to 6%, with left-sided heart lesions carrying an even higher risk. Diseases such as Marfan syndrome or 22q11 deletions carry a 50% inheritance risk and warrant discussion for in utero genetic testing. Having the opportunity to discuss these risks and the availability of genetic testing options before the start of pregnancy gives women time to discuss and contemplate these often-difficult ethical and personal considerations.

In sum, the prepregnancy counseling session provides women and couples essential information to help plan and determine the appropriate prepregnancy testing, surgical repair, pregnancy timing, and antepartum management strategies that best fit their lives. We strongly encourage all women with underlying cardiovascular disease to take advantage of this option.

RISK-ASSESSMENT SCORING SYSTEMS AND TESTS

Numerous scoring systems and tests can help assess the risk of both maternal and fetal complications in patients with heart disease. These include the CARPREG risk score, the World Health Organization (WHO) risk classification system, the measurement of maternal serum B-type natriuretic peptides (BNPs), and cardiopulmonary exercise testing.

CARPREG Risk Score

Researchers have identified many maternal risk factors and have developed several systems to score such risks. The CARPREG risk score, developed in 2001, includes both congenital and acquired heart disease in pregnancy. Significant predictors for adverse maternal and fetal outcomes include prior episodes of congestive heart failure, transient ischemic attack or stroke, arrhythmias occurring before pregnancy, New York Heart Association (NYHA) class III or IV functional status, cyanosis, and left-sided blood flow obstruction (mitral valve area <2 cm sq, aortic valve area <1.5 cm sq, or peak left ventricular outflow gradient >30 mm Hg). The CARPREG risk score demonstrated that the numeric sum of an individual's historical or current risk factors correlates with the likelihood of a cardiovascular event in a subsequent pregnancy. A woman with zero points on this scale carries a 5% risk for cardiovascular complications in pregnancy, whereas a woman with more than 1 point carries a 75% risk for such complications.

Because the CARPREG system was believed to potentially overestimate risk, a second risk-scoring system was developed focusing solely on congenital heart disease in pregnancy. The ZAHARA risk scoring

system demonstrated a lower rate of overall cardiovascular complications in pregnancy, 7.6% among all 1802 participants. Its investigators found the following to be independent predictors for maternal and neonatal complications: a history of an arrhythmic event, left heart obstruction (peak outflow tract gradient >50 mm Hg), NYHA functional class III or higher, moderate and severe aortic or mitral valvular regurgitation, repaired or unrepaired cyanotic heart lesion, need for cardiac medications before pregnancy, or a mechanical heart valve. Unfortunately, the ZAHARA system aggregated all severities of cardiovascular events into a composite such that prediction of more serious events (e.g., heart failure) could not be determined relative to events that are more benign (e.g., arrhythmia).

The CARPREG 2 study, published in 2018, followed 1938 pregnancies in women with heart disease. Points were assigned based on the following risk factors.
1. Prior cardiac event or arrhythmia: 3
2. Baseline NYHA functional class II or III, or cyanosis: 3
3. Mechanical heart valve: 2
4. At least mild systolic dysfunction: 2
5. Valvular disease causing left ventricular outflow tract obstruction: 2
6. Pulmonary hypertension: 2
7. Coronary artery disease: 2
8. High-risk aortopathy: 2
9. No prior cardiac intervention: 1
10. Late pregnancy assessment: 1

Adverse events occurred in 16% of pregnancies. Maternal cardiac death or cardiac arrest was rare and occurred in 0.6% of pregnancies. For study purposes, patients were divided into two groups. One-third of the group was used to derive the predictors of adverse events (derivation group), and two-thirds of the group were used to validate the predictors (validation group). The results in the validation group (1269 patients) are reported below. The overall risk of complications was
0 or 1 point: 5% (477 pregnancies)
2 points: 10% (222 pregnancies)
3 points: 15% (204 pregnancies)
4 points: 22% (138 pregnancies)
>4 points: 41% (228 pregnancies)

The most common complications were arrhythmias and congestive heart failure. Most complications occurred in the antenatal period, followed by the postpartum period, with the lowest frequency during labor and delivery. Whereas arrhythmias were most likely to present in the second trimester, heart failure most commonly occurred in the third trimester or postpartum.

World Health Organization Risk Classification System

As a result of the differing findings with the CARPREG risk score and because the specific type of cardiac disease is predictive, the WHO developed a useful risk classification system that applies to all forms of congenital and acquired heart disease. In all likelihood, it is the best method for risk estimation when counseling a woman with underlying heart disease who is contemplating pregnancy. The WHO scoring system contains four risk categories as shown in Table 4.1.

The application of both the CARPREG and WHO scoring systems requires a comprehensive history, physical exam, and thorough echocardiographic and ECG studies.

Measurement of Maternal Serum B-Type Natriuretic Peptides

Another potentially useful predictor may be the measurement of maternal serum BNPs. A study of 169 women with underlying cardiac disease found that N terminal pro-brain natriuretic peptide (NT-pro BNP), measured at 20 weeks' gestation, was relatively sensitive (81.3%) and specific (61.8%) with a positive predictive value of 18.3% for predicting cardiovascular complications using a cut-off of less than 128 pg/mL. The negative

TABLE 4.1   **World Health Organization (WHO) Scoring System for Assessing Risk of Adverse Cardiac Events in Pregnancy**

Score	Conditions	Comments
I	Pulmonic stenosis Patent ductus arteriosus Mitral valve prolapse Repaired simple defects, such as ASD or VSD Premature atrial or premature ventricular beats	No increase in maternal mortality; small or no increase in morbidity
II	Unoperated ASD or VSD Repaired tetralogy of Fallot Most arrhythmias Mild left ventricular dysfunction[a] Hypertrophic cardiomyopathy[a] Marfan syndrome without aortic dilation[a] Repaired coarctation[a]	Small increase in maternal mortality or moderate increase in morbidity
III	Mechanical valve Systemic right ventricle Fontan circulation Cyanotic disease unrepaired Other complex congenital disease Aortic dilation (40–45 mm) with Marfan syndrome Aortic dilation (45–50 mm) with a bicuspid valve	Significantly increased risk of maternal mortality or severe morbidity
IV	Pulmonary hypertension Severe left ventricular dysfunction (EF <30% or NYHA class III or IV) Previous peripartum cardiomyopathy Severe mitral stenosis Severe symptomatic aortic stenosis Marfan syndrome with aortic dilation >45 mm Aortic dilation >50 mm with a bicuspid aortic valve Native severe coarctation	High risk of maternal mortality; pregnancy contraindicated

[a]WHO II or III.
ASD, Atrial septal defect; *EF*, ejection fraction; *NYHA*, New York Heart Association; *VSD*, ventricular septal defect.

predictive value for cardiovascular complications was 96.9% when the NT-pro BNP measured at 20 weeks' gestation was less than 128 pg/mL. In normal pregnancies, median BNP values are less than 20 pg/mL and are stable throughout gestation. BNP levels also become elevated in preeclampsia.

Cardiopulmonary Exercise Testing

Performance and heart rate response during cardiopulmonary exercise testing before pregnancy have been shown to correlate with adverse cardiac events in pregnancy. A lower chronotropic index score identifies potential risk (as does chronotropic incompetence (CRI), which is a CRI <0.8), but no single cut-off has been established. The chronotropic index is the ratio of actual maximum heart rate achieved and the maximum predicted heart rate. The maximum predicted heart rate can be calculated by the formula 220 – patient's age.

BIBLIOGRAPHY

Balci A, Sollie Szarynska KM, van der Bijl AG, et al. Prospective validation and assessment of cardiovascular and offspring risk models for pregnant women with congenital heart disease. *Heart.* 2014;100(17):1373–1381.

Cauldwell M, Ghonim S, Uebing A, et al. Preconception counseling, predicting risk and outcomes in women with mWHO 3 and 4 heart disease. *Int J Cardiol.* 2017;234:76–80.

Cauldwell M, Von Klemperer K, Uebing A, et al. A cohort study of women with Fontan circulation undergoing preconception counselling. *Heart.* 2016;102(7):534–540.

Drenthen W, Boersma E, Balci A, et al. Prediction of pregnancy complications in women with congenital heart disease. *Eur Heart J.* 2010;31:2124–2132.

Jastrow N, Meyer P, Khairy P, et al. Prediction of complications in pregnant women with cardiac diseases referred to a tertiary center. *Int J Cardiol.* 2011;151(2):209–213.

Khairy P, Ouyang DW, Fernandes SM, Lee-Parritz A, Economy KE, Landzberg MJ. Pregnancy outcomes in women with congenital heart disease. *Circulation.* 2006;113: 517–524.

Lu CW, Shih JC, Chen SY, et al. Comparison of 3 risk estimation methods for predicting outcomes in pregnant women with congenital heart disease. *Circ J.* 2015;79(7): 1609–1617.

Pijuan-Domènech A, Galian L, Goya M, et al. Cardiac complications during pregnancy are better predicted with the modified WHO risk score. *Int J Cardiol.* 2015;195: 149–154.

Resnik JL, Hong C, Resnik R, et al. Evaluation of B-type natriuretic peptide (BNP) levels in normal and preeclamptic women. *Am J Obstet Gynecol.* 2005;193(2):450–454.

Siu SC, Sermer M, Colman JM, et al. Prospective multicenter study of pregnancy outcomes in women with heart disease. *Circulation.* 2001;104:515–521.

Suwanrath C, Thongphanang P, Pinjaroen S, Suwanugsorn S. Validation of modified World Health Organization classification for pregnant women with heart disease in a tertiary care center in southern Thailand. *Int J Womens Health.* 2018;10:47–53.

5

Cardiac Conditions That May Affect Pregnancy

John H. Wilson, MD, FACC, FHRS

The pathologic changes that occur in women with cardiac disease may have major implications during pregnancy and delivery. This chapter discusses, in general terms, the potential complications that may occur related to cardiovascular pathology and suggests some management strategies.

Between 1990 and 2013, the maternal mortality rate in the United States increased 136%, rising from a rate of 12 maternal deaths per 100,000 live births to 28 maternal deaths per 100,000 live births. During this same period, the rate fell by 38% throughout the rest of the developed world. Various factors contributed to this trend, including an increasing maternal age, body mass index (BMI), and higher prevalence of underlying comorbid conditions. A significant variation in maternal mortality ratios exists between races (the rate is higher among non-Hispanic black women) and age groups (higher among women of advanced maternal age). Cardiomyopathy and hypertensive disorders represent two of the leading causes of maternal mortality. Prompt recognition and treatment of these perinatal complications is one way to reduce overall maternal mortality in the United States.

HYPERTENSION

Hypertension is the most common medical problem encountered in pregnancy, occurring in 2% to 3% of pregnancies. It can be divided into four types:
1. Chronic hypertension
2. Preeclampsia
3. Preeclampsia superimposed on chronic hypertension
4. Gestational hypertension

Traditionally, chronic hypertension in pregnancy has been defined as blood pressure over 140 mm Hg systolic or 90 mm Hg diastolic before pregnancy or before 20 weeks of gestation. The new recommendations from the American College of Cardiology (ACC) and the American Heart Association now classify normal blood pressure as less than 120 mm Hg systolic and 80 mm Hg diastolic and stage 1 hypertension as a systolic pressure of 130 to 139 mm Hg or a diastolic pressure of 80 to 89 mm Hg. The American College of Obstetrics and Gynecology's (ACOG's) latest guidelines state that for a woman classified as having stage 1 hypertension before pregnancy, it is reasonable to treat her as having chronic hypertension. For a pregnant woman without a prior diagnosis of hypertension who presents with a blood pressure in the stage I range, it is unclear what the best option is, and further investigation is warranted. Low-dose aspirin to prevent preeclampsia has not proven beneficial in this group.

The new onset of hypertension after the first 20 weeks of gestation should arouse suspicion of preeclampsia. Preeclampsia is usually defined as pregnancy-induced hypertension combined with proteinuria over 300 mg/24 hours. However, proteinuria is not universally present in preeclampsia. The 2013 ACOG guidelines state that in the absence of proteinuria, preeclampsia is diagnosed as hypertension in association with thrombocytopenia (platelet count <100,000/µL), impaired liver function (elevated blood levels of liver transaminases to twice normal), the new development of renal insufficiency (elevated serum creatinine >1.1 mg/dL or a doubling of serum creatinine in the absence of other renal disease), pulmonary edema, or new-onset cerebral or visual disturbances. Chronic hypertension is a risk factor for preeclampsia, increasing the risk four- to fivefold. Gestational hypertension is characterized by the onset of hypertension after 20 weeks of pregnancy in the absence of proteinuria or other signs of preeclampsia.

Endothelial dysfunction represents one suggested mechanism whereby hypertensive disorders of pregnancy lead to multiple organ failure, including cardiomyopathy, acute kidney disease, pulmonary edema, respiratory collapse, seizures, and death. Serum concentrations of vasodilators such as nitric oxide, prostacyclin, and hyperpolarization factor are shown to decrease among women with hypertensive disorders of pregnancy, and serum concentrations of vasoconstrictors such as endothelin-1 and thromboxane A2 increase. Upstream regulatory changes contributing to the shift in concentration of these vasoactive molecules include a diminishment in proangiogenic factors such as vascular endothelial growth factor and placental-like growth factor and an increase in antiangiogenic factors such as soluble FMS-like tyrosine kinase inhibitor-1, endoglin, and angiotensin II. The effects of these changes include increased capillary permeability and enhanced vascular smooth muscle contractility clinically witnessed as edema, labile elevations in blood pressure, increased systemic vascular resistance, and vasospasm to numerous organs, including the brain, retina, kidneys, liver, and uteroplacental interface. In addition, recent evidence supports an association between the imbalance in these angiogenic factors and the subsequent development of peripartum cardiomyopathy.

Because of these vascular changes, the intravascular volume among women with hypertensive disorders of pregnancy may be altered. Women with preeclampsia often demonstrate a diminished intravascular volume manifested by hemoconcentration, elevated hematocrit, and elevated serum osmolality. Additionally, their intravascular oncotic pressure drops secondary to increased albumin secretion into the urine and interstitial compartment. Decreased intravascular volume may potentiate the already enhanced vascular smooth muscle contractility in an overexaggerated homeostatic attempt to restore perfusion to maternal organs. However, 70% of the intravascular volume lies in venules, which contain little vascular smooth muscle and contractility. As more volume is forced out of the intravascular compartment through dysfunctional endothelial walls by increased hydrostatic pressure and diminished oncotic pressure, the volume within the venules and venous system decreases. These physiologic changes to the maternal vasculature can be assessed by astute clinical examination, laboratory evaluation, and sonography.

Hypertension (blood pressure over 140/90 mm Hg) developing after 20 weeks' gestation mandates an evaluation to exclude preeclampsia. Preeclampsia occurs in an estimated 5% of pregnancies and is twice as common during a woman's first pregnancy.

In mild cases of hypertension (blood pressure <160/100 mm Hg) during pregnancy, treatment has not been found to reduce the incidence of preeclampsia. In many women with preexisting hypertension, it is possible to reduce or eliminate their antihypertensive drugs during pregnancy because the normal decline in blood pressure that occurs with pregnancy also occurs in women with hypertension.

Several options are available for the emergency treatment of patients with severe acute-onset hypertension. These include intravenous (IV) labetalol and IV hydralazine. Oral nifedipine is also an option. Labetalol should be avoided in women with asthma. IV nitroprusside should be used only for the shortest possible time because of concerns of cyanide and thiocyanate toxicity.

For chronic oral therapy during pregnancy, methyldopa, labetalol, and nifedipine are considered acceptable. Methyldopa is often considered the drug of choice because of its historic safety record. It does not alter maternal cardiac output or blood flow to the uterus and kidneys. Labetalol has been shown to be as effective as methyldopa in pregnant women, and it does not alter uterine or renal blood flow. However, its safety record is not as well established as that of methyldopa. Oral hydralazine appears generally safe for fetuses, but a few cases of thrombocytopenia have been reported. It may be combined with methyldopa or labetalol. Hydrochlorothiazide may be considered as a second- or third-line agent.

Vasodilator antihypertensives such as hydralazine, nifedipine, and nitroprusside should be avoided in patients with left heart obstruction (e.g., aortic stenosis or coarctation).

Atenolol should be avoided as it has been associated with growth retardation in the fetus.

Angiotensin-converting enzyme (ACE) inhibitors have been associated with a number of fetal adverse events, including growth retardation, renal failure, persistent patent ductus arteriosus, respiratory distress, hypotension, and prepartum death. They are contraindicated during pregnancy.

Diuretics may be used to treat patients with hypertension, but they reduce maternal plasma volume and may cause electrolyte disturbance. They may be used to treat those with preeclampsia.

Women with chronic hypertension should be considered at risk for preeclampsia, and consideration should be given to initiation of low-dose aspirin (81 mg/day), which should be initiated between weeks 12 and 16.

Recent studies have shown that the development of preeclampsia or gestational hypertension are risk factors for the development of hypertension and adverse cardiac events later in life.

POSTPARTUM HYPERTENSION

Postpartum hypertension may be caused by persistence of gestational hypertension or preeclampsia or arise de novo after delivery. The incidence is unknown, in part because many women do not have their blood pressure checked between the immediate postpartum period and their follow-up at 6 weeks. Of women who are hypertensive during pregnancy, roughly half will continue to have hypertension postpartum.

Etiologies for new-onset postpartum hypertension include delayed mobilization of the increased plasma volume that occurs during normal pregnancy and fluid retention related to the use of nonsteroidal antiinflammatory drugs. The use of ergot alkaloids (to treat uterine atony) also may initiate or exacerbate hypertension.

Patients with chronic hypertension can be expected to have hypertension postpartum.

Preeclampsia may persist or even present postpartum. The majority of postpartum preeclampsia develops within 48 hours after delivery, but it can first manifest as late as 6 weeks postpartum. Preeclampsia is the most common cause for persistent hypertension after delivery.

Studies of women with preeclampsia superimposed on chronic hypertension show that their blood pressures often increase at 3 to 6 days postpartum.

Reversible cerebral vasoconstriction syndrome is a poorly understood angiopathy that develops between days 3 and 14 postpartum. The presenting symptoms are thunderclap headaches and other neurologic manifestations such as seizures and visual disturbance. Hypertension is present in 60% of patients.

Evaluation of a woman with new onset postpartum hypertension should include evaluation for proteinuria to exclude late-onset preeclampsia. Treatment of hypertension is similar to that in pregnant women. Furosemide given to patients who experience antenatal preeclampsia reduces the need for other antihypertensive agents.

A major concern in treating postpartum women with hypertension is to avoids antihypertensive drugs that could be excreted into breast milk and affect a breast-feeding baby.

CONGENITAL HEART DISEASE

Most data regarding cardiac and obstetric risk to women with congenital heart disease (CHD) during pregnancy derive from retrospective case series. Many women with CHD considering pregnancy may have received inconsistent guidance regarding pregnancy risks. Because of these concerns, the ACC has developed guidelines for physicians caring for women with CHD who are considering pregnancy or who are already pregnant. Although many women with CHD tolerate the hemodynamic changes of pregnancy, others may face significant immediate or late risks of pregnancy, including volume overload, arrhythmias, progressive cardiac dysfunction, and death. Cardiac medications may need to be adjusted during pregnancy and counseling provided to discuss the options for and potential impact of these changes. Substitutes must be found for medications they are taking that may be teratogenic (e.g., ACE inhibitors, angiotensin-receptor blockers).

Some specific complications may be more common in women with certain types of CHD, such as hypertension, which is more common in women with coarctation. The offspring of patients with adult congenital heart disease (ACHD) have an increased risk of CHD and other events such as prematurity. All women with CHD should receive appropriate counseling regarding contraception choices. To achieve optimal outcomes, we recommend a multidisciplinary team that includes ACHD specialists and maternal-fetal medicine obstetricians with expertise in caring for women with heart disease.

The ACC guidelines are outlined next along with the anatomic pathologic (AP) classification scheme used by the organization.

1. Women with congenital heart disease should receive prepregnancy counseling with input from an adult congenital cardiologist to determine maternal cardiac, obstetric, and fetal risks, as well as potential long-term risks to the mother.
2. An individualized plan of care that addresses expectations and contingencies should be developed for and with women with CHD who are pregnant or who may become pregnant and shared with the woman and all caregivers.
3. Women with ACHD receiving chronic anticoagulation should be counseled, ideally before conception, on the risks and benefits of specific anticoagulants during pregnancy.

4. Women with ACHD AP classification IB-D, IIA-D, and IIIA-D should be managed collaboratively during pregnancy by ACHD cardiologists, obstetricians, and anesthesiologists experienced in ACHD

5. In collaboration with an adult congenital heart cardiologist to ensure accurate assessment of pregnancy risk, patients at high risk of maternal morbidity or mortality, including women with pulmonary arterial hypertension, Eisenmenger syndrome, severe systemic ventricular dysfunction, severe left-sided obstructive lesions, or ACHD AP classification ID, IID, and IIID, should be counseled against becoming pregnant or be given the option of terminating pregnancy.

6. Men and women of childbearing age with CHD should be counseled on the risk of CHD recurrence in offspring.

7. Exercise testing can be useful for risk assessment in women with ACHD classification IC D, IIA D, and IIID who are considering pregnancy.

The ACHD AP Classification scheme referred to uses anatomy and physiological stage to classify patients with ACHD. The scheme, outlined later, uses three classifications for complexity of anatomy (I, II, III) and four for physiologic stage (A, B, C, D) (Table 5.1).

PULMONARY HYPERTENSION

Pulmonary hypertension is defined as a mean pulmonary arterial pressure greater than 25 mm Hg as assessed by right heart catheterization. Pulmonary hypertension may be caused by cardiac disease with right-to-left shunting of blood (Eisenmenger syndrome), associated with connective tissue disease or idiopathic (primary). It probably would be best to consider patients with pulmonary hypertension as belonging to one of these three distinct groups. Unfortunately, all these conditions are rare, and the number of pregnant patients with them is small, so almost all series mix the three groups. During pregnancy, pulmonary resistance falls in normal women. In patients with pulmonary hypertension, this fall is limited, leading to a rise in pulmonary pressures, which often leads to right heart failure. Shifting of the intraventricular septum caused by the increased right heart pressures also may impair left heart filling, leading to diastolic left-sided impairment, which compromises cardiac output. Women with Eisenmenger syndrome may have increasing right-to-left shunting, which leads to hypoxemia and may lead to increased pulmonary vasoconstriction and worsening right heart failure. Pulmonary hypertension during pregnancy is a high-risk situation for both the mother and the fetus, so pregnancy in women with pulmonary hypertension should be discouraged. The maternal mortality rate has been reported as high as 56% in patients with severe pulmonary hypertension, although more recent studies indicate mortality rates of 17% in patients with idiopathic pulmonary hypertension and 28% in those with CHD. One series from France has reported a mortality rate as low as 5% in a group of women with pulmonary hypertension associated with CHD. One reason for the much lower rate may be the apparent lower mortality rate in women who respond to calcium channel blockers or other therapy. Most cases of death in women with pulmonary hypertension occur in the early postpartum period. Heart failure is the most common cause, but others include sudden death and thromboembolism.

If a woman with pulmonary hypertension does become pregnant, she must be monitored carefully, and if signs of decompensation are detected, early therapeutic abortion should be considered.

Neonatal survival rates are about 90%. The main risks to the fetus are related to maternal hypoxemia and include preterm delivery, growth retardation, and stillbirth.

Many of the drugs used to treat patients with pulmonary hypertension are contraindicated during pregnancy. Endothelin receptor antagonists are category X. Calcium channel blockers are category C. Sildenafil has been used in individual cases and appears to be safe, but experience with the drug is limited. Continuous infusion of prostacyclin (epoprostenol) has been used in select patients with good outcomes reported.

For women with pulmonary hypertension, it is unclear whether vaginal delivery or cesarean section is preferable, but guidelines from the Pulmonary Vascular Research Institute recommend cesarean section. The adverse effects of vaginal delivery include Valsalva maneuver, which increases intrathoracic pressure, labor-induced vagal responses, sympathetic nervous system activation cause by pain, and autotransfusion during uterine contraction. If vaginal delivery is chosen, low-dose epidural analgesia is strongly recommended; if dosed slowly, it has little deleterious effect on hemodynamics. If cesarean section is performed, slowly titrated epidural anesthesia is ideal because it minimizes adverse hemodynamic effects. At least 20 to 30 minutes is required to achieve an adequate block while maintaining stable hemodynamics. General anesthesia

TABLE 5.1   American College of Cardiology Adult Congenital Heart Disease Anatomic and Pathologic Classification Scheme

A. Anatomy

I: Simple
Native disease
Isolated small ASD
Isolated small VSD
Mild isolated pulmonic stenosis
Previously ligated or occluded ductus arteriosus
Repaired conditions
Repaired secundum ASD or sinus venosus defect without significant residual shunt or chamber enlargement
Repaired VSD without significant residual shunt or chamber enlargement

II: Moderate Complexity
Repaired or unrepaired conditions
Aorto-left ventricular fistula
Anomalous pulmonary venous connection, partial or total
Anomalous coronary artery arising from the pulmonary artery
Anomalous aortic origin of a coronary artery from the opposite sinus
AVSD: partial or complete, including primum ASD
Congenital aortic valve disease
Congenital mitral valve disease
Coarctation of the aorta
Ebstein anomaly (disease spectrum includes mild, moderate, and severe variations)
Infundibular right ventricular outflow obstruction
Ostium primum ASD
Moderate and large unrepaired secundum ASD
Moderate and large persistently PDA
Pulmonary valve regurgitation (moderate or greater)
Pulmonary valve stenosis (moderate or greater)
Peripheral pulmonary stenosis
Sinus of Valsalva fistula or aneurysm
Sinus venosus defect
Subvalvar aortic stenosis excluding hypertrophic obstructive cardiomyopathy
Supravalvar aortic stenosis
Straddling atrioventricular valve
Repaired tetralogy of Fallot
VSD with associated abnormality and/or moderate or greater shunt

III: Complex
Cyanotic congenital heart defect (unrepaired or palliated, all forms)
Double-outlet ventricle
Fontan procedure
Interrupted aortic arch
Mitral atresia
Single ventricle (including double inlet left ventricle, tricuspid atresia, hypoplastic left heart, any other anatomic abnormality with a functionally single ventricle)
Pulmonary atresia (all forms)
TGA, both classic (d-TGA) and corrected (l-TGA)
Truncus arteriosus
Other abnormalities of atrioventricular and ventriculoarterial connection (e.g., crisscross heart, isomerism, heterotaxy syndromes, ventricular inversion)

TABLE 5.1 **American College of Cardiology Adult Congenital Heart Disease Anatomic and Pathologic Classification Scheme—Cont'd**

B. Physiological Stage

Stage A
NYHA FC I symptoms
No hemodynamic or anatomic sequelae
No arrhythmias
Normal exercise capacity
Normal renal, hepatic, and pulmonary function

Stage B
NYHA FC II symptoms
Mild hemodynamic sequelae (mild aortic enlargement, mild ventricular enlargement, mild ventricular dysfunction)
Mild valvular disease
Trivial or small shunt (not hemodynamically significant)
Arrhythmia not requiring treatment
Abnormal objective cardiac limitation to exercise

Stage C
NYHA FC III symptoms
Significant (moderate or greater) valvular disease; moderate or greater ventricular dysfunction (systemic, pulmonic, or both)
Moderate aortic enlargement
Venous or arterial stenosis
Mild or moderate hypoxemia or cyanosis
Hemodynamically significant shunt
Arrhythmias controlled with treatment
Pulmonary hypertension (less than severe)
End-organ dysfunction responsive to therapy

Stage D
NYHA FC IV symptoms
Severe aortic enlargement
Arrhythmias refractory to treatment
Severe hypoxemia (almost always associated with cyanosis)
Severe pulmonary hypertension
Eisenmenger syndrome
Refractory end-organ dysfunction

ASD, Atrial septal defect; *AVSD*, atrioventricular septal defect; *FC*, functional class; *NYHA*, New York Heart Association; *PDA*, patent ductus arteriosus; *TGA*, transposition of the great vessels; *VSD*, ventricular septal defect.

and spinal anesthesia can be administered safely but cause more significant hemodynamic disturbance. They require close monitoring (including invasive hemodynamic monitors) and strict attention to fluid status, oxygenation, and ventilation. If general anesthesia is required, intubation, laryngoscopy, and positive-pressure ventilation will likely increase pulmonary pressure. Extracorporeal membrane oxygenation should be available. Delivery in the operating room should be considered.

If necessary, the physician may consider inducing labor; there are cases in which prostaglandin E and oxytocin have been used with good outcome. Prostaglandin E generally reduces pulmonary artery pressure. Oxytocin is a vasodilator and must be used cautiously to avoid hypotension.

It is probably best to avoid direct pulmonary artery pressure monitoring with a Swan-Ganz catheter because there is an increased risk of pulmonary artery rupture and thrombosis in patients with pulmonary hypertension.

The patient's hemodynamics may not return to baseline for 6 months, so monitoring must be continued after delivery. Several weeks of in-hospital monitoring postpartum is usually recommended.

Symptomatic postpartum therapy may include inhaled nitric oxide, inhaled iloprost, or IV epoprostenol.

Thromboembolic risk is high, and generally thromboprophylaxis should be initiated. In women with a history of thromboembolic disease, higher levels of anticoagulation may be needed.

Fluid management is difficult because both hyper- and hypovolemia are detrimental.

Because pregnancy is to be discouraged in patients with pulmonary hypertension, contraception is often prescribed. Estrogen-containing contraceptives are not recommended because of the increased risk of venous thromboembolism and the deleterious effects of estrogen on the pulmonary vasculature. Progesterone-only preparations, such as medroxyprogesterone acetate and etonogestrel, may be used. Intrauterine devices (IUDs) and progestin-only implants are acceptable contraceptive methods for women with pulmonary hypertension. However, on insertion, IUDs and implants may cause vasovagal responses, and such responses may be poorly tolerated in women with pulmonary hypertension.

INCREASED RISK FOR THROMBOSIS

Pregnant women may require anticoagulation for many reasons, including high risk of deep vein thrombosis (DVT), prosthetic heart valves, and atrial fibrillation. In some patients, such as those with pulmonary hypertension or cardiomyopathy, anticoagulation should be considered. Low-molecular-weight heparin (LMWH) and unfractionated heparin are the agents of choice. LMWHs do not reliably prolong the partial thromboplastin time, which may make monitoring difficult.

Pregnancy induces a hypercoagulable state through multiple mechanisms. It increases levels of factors VII, VIII, IX, X, and fibrinogen; reduces levels of proteins S and C; and reduces fibrinolysis. The risk of a thromboembolic event is three to five times higher during pregnancy than in the nonpregnant state. Pregnancy also promotes venous stasis because of progesterone-mediated venous dilation and compression of the vena cava by the uterus. Patients with preeclampsia may develop nephrotic syndrome, which can lead to acquired antithrombin deficiency, further enhancing a hypercoagulable state.

Several groups have proposed scoring systems for assessment of thromboembolic risk in pregnant women. Dargaud et al. proposed the system presented in Table 5.2.

TABLE 5.2   Risk Score for Assessment of Thromboembolic Risk (Dargaud et al.)[a]

		Points
Personal history of VTE	History of VTE antepartum, massive PE or CVT, or VTE at age younger than 16 years	6
	Spontaneous or estrogen-induced PE or proximal DVT	3
	Transient risk factor–induced PE or proximal DVT	2
	Spontaneous or estrogen-induced distal calf DVT	2
	Transient risk factor–induced calf DVT	1
If personal history of VTE	Recurrent VTE	3
	Residual venous thrombi	3
	VTE in the past 2 years	2
Thrombophilia	Homozygous mutations or combined thrombophilia risk factors	3
	Protein C deficiency, protein S deficiency, heterozygous F5 G1691A mutation, heterozygous F2 G20210A mutation	1
	If no hypercoagulability detected, family history of severe or recurrent VTE	1
Other risk factors	Bed rest, immobilization	2
	Twin pregnancy	1
	Age older than 35 years	1
	BMI >30	1

[a]Patients were assigned to one of three prophylaxis strategies based on this score (Table 5.3).
BMI, Body mass index; *CVT,* cerebral venous thrombosis; *DVT,* deep vein thrombosis; *PE* = pulmonary embolus; *VTE,* venous thromboemboli.

They also proposed a prophylactic management strategy based on this protocol. Using this strategy, outlined in Table 5.3, in 286 patients resulted in only three DVTs. One occurred during pregnancy and two in the postpartum period after withdrawal of LMWH. One patient had a serious postpartum hemorrhage.

Investigators from Sweden (Lindgvist et al.) have suggested this point scoring system to address risk of thrombosis in pregnancy. The schema is outlined in Table 5.4.

After adding together all risk factors, a total of 1 point or less indicates that no preventive action is needed. A

total of 2 points indicates that short-term prophylaxis (e.g., with LMWH) should be used. Prophylactic treatment should be started 2 hours after delivery and given 7 days postpartum. A total of 3 points increases the necessary duration of postpartum prophylaxis to 6 weeks. A previous distal DVT indicates a minimum of 12 weeks (3 months) of therapeutic anticoagulation therapy. A previous proximal DVT or pulmonary embolism requires a minimum of 26 weeks (6.5 months) of therapy. If the therapy duration reaches delivery time, the remaining duration may be given after delivery, possibly extending the minimum of 6 weeks of postpartum therapy. In a very high-risk pregnancy, high-dose antepartum prophylaxis should be continued at least 12 weeks after delivery.

Women with antiphospholipid syndrome should have an additional low-dose prophylactic treatment of aspirin.

Coumadin cause teratogenesis. However, warfarin can be used after 12 weeks for patients with prosthetic valves.

When LWMH is used, we recommend checking anti–factor Xa levels after treatment is started and every 1 to 3 months thereafter, keeping levels (checked 4 hours after the dose) at 0.5 to 1.2 U/mL. Patients should be

TABLE 5.3 Prophylactic Strategy Based on Risk Score

Score	Description
<3	No LMWH antepartum; LMWH for at least 6 weeks postpartum
3–5	LMWH in third trimester; LMWH for at least 6 weeks postpartum
≥6	LMWH antepartum throughout pregnancy; LMWH for at least 6 weeks postpartum

LMWH, Low-molecular-weight heparin.

TABLE 5.4 Thrombotic Risk Score (Lindgvist et al.)

Points	Risk Factor
1 minor risk factor	Heterozygous for factor V Leiden mutation
1 minor risk factor	Heterozygous for factor II mutation
1 minor risk factor	Overweight, in this case defined as a BMI >28 at early pregnancy
1 minor risk factor	Cesarean section
1 minor risk factor	DVT: heredity in a first-degree relative
1 minor risk factor	Age older than 40 years
1 minor risk factor	Preeclampsia
1 minor risk factor	Hyperhomocysteinemia
2 points: intermediate risk factors	Protein S or protein C deficiency
2 points: intermediate risk factors	Immobilization (after, e.g., bone fracture or prolonged bed rest)
3 points: intermediate risk factors	Homozygous for factor V Leiden mutation
3 points: intermediate risk factors	Homozygous for factor II mutation
4 points: severe risk factors	Previous DVT
4 points: severe risk factors	Antiphospholipid syndrome without previous DVT
	Lupus anticoagulant
Very high risk	Artificial heart valves
Very high risk	Antithrombin III deficiency
Very high risk	Multiple previous thromboses
Very high risk	Antiphospholipid syndrome with previous DVT
Very high risk	Previous PE

BMI, Body mass index; *DVT,* deep vein thrombosis; *PE,* pulmonary embolus.

monitored for heparin-induced thrombocytopenia, although it appears rare in pregnancy.

LEFT VENTRICULAR DYSFUNCTION

Left ventricular (LV) dysfunction is usually divided into two types, systolic and diastolic. Systolic dysfunction is pump failure, which leads to pulmonary congestion and, if severe enough, to fluid retention, right ventricular (RV) overload, and edema. Diastolic dysfunction is failure of ventricular relaxation, which leads to increased end diastolic pressure, which is reflected in increased left atrial pressure. Increased left atrial pressure inhibits pulmonary venous return and may lead to pulmonary congestion and dyspnea.

Systolic Dysfunction

It may be difficult to recognize systolic heart failure in pregnant patients because some of the clinical signs and symptoms also may be present in pregnant women without heart failure. These include dyspnea, exercise intolerance, and edema. For this reason, echocardiography should be used early if LV systolic dysfunction is suspected.

Treatment of pregnant women with LV dysfunction is similar to treatment in the nonpregnant state. Beta blockers can be continued or initiated. ACE inhibitors should not be used because of the risk of oligohydramnios and renal failure in the fetus. If ACE inhibitors were being given before pregnancy, consider using hydralazine and long-acting nitrates instead. Digitalis is safe during pregnancy. Furosemide can be used to help relieve symptoms.

Diastolic Dysfunction

Diastolic heart failure may occur in isolation or in combination with systolic failure. When it occurs in isolation, it is usually because of LV hypertrophy. Diastolic dysfunction in pregnancy may occur because of preexisting heart disease or preeclampsia. It has been reported that as many as 20% of women with preeclampsia demonstrate diastolic dysfunction. There is no good treatment, but diuretics can relieve symptoms. Patients are sometimes treated with long-acting nitrates or calcium channel blockers, such as verapamil, all of which may be used in pregnancy.

RIGHT VENTRICULAR DYSFUNCTION

Right ventricular dysfunction usually leads to edema. There is no good treatment for patients with RV dysfunction per se. It is unclear that beta blockers, ACE inhibitors, hydralazine nitrate combinations, or digitalis can improve RV function. If the RV dysfunction is caused by pulmonary hypertension, that condition can be treated as outlined in the section on pulmonary hypertension. Diuretics can relieve edema.

CYANOTIC CONGENITAL HEART DISEASE

Cyanotic CHD comprises a mixed group of patients, including some who have right-to-left shunts, some who have had partial surgical repairs, and some who did not undergo intervention. The more common etiologies are tetralogy of Fallot, Ebstein's anomaly with an atrial septal defect, pulmonary atresia, and tricuspid atresia. If pulmonary hypertension develops such that right-sided pressures approximate left-sided pressures, a persistent right-to-left or bidirectional shunt will occur, a condition known as Eisenmenger syndrome.

All women with cyanotic CHD have an increased maternal and fetal risk during pregnancy. Women with Eisenmenger syndrome have a particularly high risk.

Women with cyanosis tend to have erythrocytosis, which predisposes them to thrombotic events. Anticoagulants must be used judiciously, as these patients are also predisposed to bleeding complications. Compression stockings are often recommended to prevent DVT. Diuresis can aggravate the thrombotic tendency, so diuretics must be used cautiously. These women also appear to be at risk for congestive heart failure and endocarditis. Fetal risk is also increased. The worse the cyanosis, the higher the risk of spontaneous abortion. Fetuses that do survive are at increased risk of premature birth and low birth weight.

The prognosis for pregnant women with Eisenmenger syndrome is very bleak. In one study, over half of the women died as a consequence of their pregnancy. Women with Eisenmenger syndrome should be counseled against pregnancy. If they do become pregnant, termination of the pregnancy should be considered. If pregnancy is continued, patients should be treated as are others with pulmonary hypertension.

VALVULAR LESIONS

Aortic Stenosis

A bicuspid valve is the most common cause of aortic stenosis in women of childbearing age. Patients with bicuspid valves have an increased risk of concomitant aortopathy. Aortic dilation, aneurysms, or a coarctation may be present; any of these increases the risk of aortic dissection. All pregnant women with a bicuspid valve should undergo an evaluation of the aorta.

Mild and moderate degrees of aortic stenosis may be well tolerated during pregnancy, but pregnant women with severe aortic stenosis are susceptible to pulmonary edema. The best method for assessing the severity of aortic stenosis is the calculated valve area. A normal valve area is 2.0 to 4.0 cm². Aortic stenosis is considered severe if the valve area is less than 1.0 cm². In clinical practice, the mean gradient is commonly used to estimate the severity of aortic stenosis. Pregnant women with a mean transvalvular gradient that remains less than 50 mm Hg usually tolerate pregnancy without major adverse consequences.

For those patients with significant aortic stenosis, the already limited valve orifice cannot accommodate the dramatic blood volume expansion and increased cardiac output of pregnancy. A significant increase in the transvalvular gradient may lead to pulmonary edema. The time of greatest risk begins in the second trimester, when increases in cardiac output are greatest, and it persists until several days postpartum, when blood volume and cardiac output begin to return to prepregnancy levels. In the immediate postpartum period, relief of vena caval compression and the autotransfusion from the placenta add to the volume overload state.

Oxytocin is a vasodilator and must be used cautiously because it may decrease blood pressure significantly in patients with severe aortic stenosis.

Aortic Regurgitation

Chronic regurgitant lesions are often well tolerated during pregnancy. Although the increase in blood volume tends to increase the regurgitant volume, other mechanisms, such as the increase in heart rate and the decrease in vascular resistance, partially compensate. Acute aortic regurgitation is poorly tolerated.

Mitral Stenosis

Pregnant women with mitral stenosis do not tolerate well the increased blood volume and increased cardiac output of pregnancy. A stenotic valve cannot accommodate the increased flow, and the transmitral gradient increases, putting the patient at risk for pulmonary edema. Another detrimental effect

of pregnancy is that the heart rate tends to increase, leading to a shortening of the diastolic filling period, which further impairs forward flow across the stenotic valve. The time of greatest risk begins in the second trimester, when increases in cardiac output are greatest, and it persists until several days postpartum, when blood volume and cardiac output begin to return to prepregnancy levels. In the immediate postpartum period, relief of vena caval compression and the autotransfusion from the placenta add to the volume overload state. Patients with mitral stenosis are at risk for atrial fibrillation, and if it occurs during pregnancy, it is poorly tolerated. In patients with mitral stenosis, the tachycardia and loss of atrial contraction further impede antegrade flow.

Although the maternal mortality rate is low in the presence of mitral stenosis, the risk to the fetus is considerable. Fetal growth retardation and premature delivery rates are approximately 14% in mild mitral stenosis, 28% in moderate stenosis, and 33% in severe cases.

Consideration should be given to relieving mitral stenosis before a woman becomes pregnant. If the mitral stenosis is severe and is first discovered after the woman becomes pregnant, consider a performing percutaneous commissurotomy during the pregnancy. Medical therapy is with beta blockers to slow the heart rate, and diuretics. Anticoagulation is necessary if atrial fibrillation occurs.

Mitral Regurgitation

Chronic regurgitant lesions are often well tolerated during pregnancy. Although the increase in blood volume tends to increase the regurgitant volume, other mechanisms, such as the increase in heart rate and the decrease in vascular resistance, partially compensate. Acute mitral regurgitation, such as might be seen with rupture of chordae, is not well tolerated.

MORBID OBESITY

Morbid obesity (BMI >40) has been shown to increase the risk to both the mother and the baby. It is associated with a fivefold increase in risk of stillbirth, a threefold increase in the risk of cesarean delivery, and a 34% increase in the use of instrumental delivery. Morbid obesity is also associated with both early and late deliveries. The risk of overweight babies is increased by a factor of 4. The risk of fetal distress or low Apgar scores is doubled.

Other complications associated with obesity include an increased risk of gestational diabetes, preeclampsia, postpartum hemorrhage, genital and urinary tract infections, and postpartum wound infection. The risks increase with the degree of obesity, and they persist even after accounting for confounding demographic factors.

PULMONIC STENOSIS

Pulmonic stenosis is well tolerated during pregnancy. Because of impairment of right-sided forward flow, the increase in blood volume may lead to peripheral edema. Depending on its severity, peripheral edema can be treated with leg elevation, compression stockings, diuretics, or a combination of these.

PULMONIC REGURGITATION

Chronic pulmonic regurgitation, like other regurgitant lesions, is generally well tolerated during pregnancy. Although the increase in blood volume tends to increase the regurgitant volume, other mechanisms, such as the increase in heart rate and the decrease in pulmonary vascular resistance, partially compensate.

Severe pulmonary regurgitation, particularly if associated with RV dysfunction, has been shown to be an independent predictor of maternal complications. In these patients, pregnancy sometimes causes severe RV dilation and dysfunction, which may persist after delivery. Patients who have severe pulmonary regurgitation and reduced RV function may be considered for pulmonic valve replacement before pregnancy.

TRICUSPID STENOSIS

Tricuspid stenosis causes obstruction to right-sided forward flow, and if severe, it may cause peripheral edema, which is exacerbated by the increase in blood volume during pregnancy. Depending on its severity, peripheral edema can be treated with leg elevation, compression stockings, diuretics, or a combination of these.

TRICUSPID REGURGITATION

Chronic tricuspid regurgitation is well tolerated during pregnancy. Although the increase in blood volume tends to increase the regurgitant volume, other mechanisms, such as the increase in heart rate and the

decrease in pulmonary vascular resistance, partially compensate.

MIXED VALVULAR DISEASE

Mixed valvular disease is most often seen in patients who have had rheumatic fever. The worst combination for pregnant patients is a combination of mitral stenosis and aortic stenosis because both lesions have additive effects on impairing forward flow. With the increase in blood volume and cardiac output of pregnancy, the valvular gradients increase, leading to pulmonary congestion. If mitral stenosis is present, the increased heart rates often seen in pregnancy limit diastolic filling time and are an additional burden. Because regurgitant lesions are fairly well tolerated during pregnancy, in patients with a combination of stenotic and regurgitant lesions, the prognosis will be determined primarily by the severity of the stenotic lesions. For patients with aortic or mitral stenosis combined with right-sided obstructing lesions (tricuspid or pulmonic stenosis, which are well tolerated), the prognosis will be determined primarily by the severity of the left-sided lesions.

PROSTHETIC HEART VALVES

Normally functioning tissue prosthetic valves are of little concern during pregnancy. If a tissue prosthesis is stenotic or regurgitant, the prognosis and management will be the same as for a native valve lesion of similar severity. In patients with mechanical prosthetic valves, anticoagulation must be maintained, and this is a difficult proposition during pregnancy. For this reason, young women requiring valve replacement are often advised to have a tissue rather than a mechanical valve.

Warfarin is the only acceptable method of chronic anticoagulation for patients with mechanical prosthetic valves. Unfortunately, warfarin is not well tolerated by fetuses. The fetal liver produces only small amounts of the vitamin K–dependent clotting factors, so the appropriate dose for the mother is an overdose for the fetus. Warfarin used during pregnancy can lead to fetal malformations known as warfarin embryopathy; these include nasal hypoplasia, stippled epiphyses, and, less commonly, central nervous system and eye abnormalities. The risk of warfarin embryopathy is greatest during the first trimester. It is generally agreed that as soon as pregnancy is discovered in a woman with a prosthetic valve, warfarin should be stopped, and therapy with heparin should be initiated. The gold standard of treatment is therapy with IV heparin. How long this therapy should be continued is unclear, but it is probably at least 9 to 12 weeks. Alternate strategies, such as subcutaneous heparin or LMWH are unproven. Even so, the subcutaneous administration of LMWH is increasing because of its convenience.

A recent literature review suggested that continuation of warfarin throughout pregnancy in patients with mechanical heart valves is safest for the mother, and that if the dose of warfarin is kept below 5 mg/day, the risk to the fetus is minimal.

BAFFLES, SHUNTS, AND CONDUITS

Baffles are most commonly encountered in patients who have had a reparative operation for transposition of the great vessels. These baffles are in the atrium and serve to direct blood flow from the superior and inferior vena cavae to the physiologic right ventricle and pulmonary venous blood to the physiologic left ventricle. This type of procedure is called a Mustard repair. As long as they are functioning normally, baffles should create no problem in pregnancy. Patients with transposition and Mustard repair do run the risk of failure of the physiologic left ventricle, which is morphologically a right ventricle required to generate systemic pressures. The function of the physiologic left ventricle should be assessed and monitored during pregnancy.

Conduits are encountered in patients who have had a Rastelli repair, usually for transposition of the great vessels with pulmonic stenosis. These conduits connect the right ventricle to the pulmonary artery. Patients with such repairs tolerate pregnancy well assuming there is no conduit stenosis and RV function is adequate.

Rhythm Management Devices

One may encounter three basic types of rhythm management devices in pregnant patients: implantable loop recorders, pacemakers, and defibrillators. The devices themselves should not create problems during pregnancy, and the prognosis depends on the original indications for the device.

Loop recorders are diagnostic recording devices and do not affect cardiac function. They are not affected by diagnostic x-rays, nor are they affected by magnetic resonance imaging (MRI) scans, but they may record an MRI artifact and should be cleared before an MRI scan in the event they lose stored data. Loop recorders also are not affected by remote electrocautery, but they may record an artifact.

Pacemakers may be single-chamber, dual-chamber, or biventricular devices. Single-chamber pacemakers are used only in patients with bradycardia and permanent atrial fibrillation. Dual-chamber pacemakers are used to treat patients with heart block and sinus node dysfunction and are most likely to be encountered during pregnancy. Biventricular pacemakers are used to treat certain patients with systolic heart failure. In younger patients with LV dysfunction and a reasonable life expectancy, it is likely a defibrillator with biventricular pacing capabilities would be used, so it is highly unlikely that a pregnant patient would have a biventricular pacemaker. Pacemakers are not affected by diagnostic x-rays. Newer pacemakers may be MRI compatible, allowing patients to have MRI scans, although special programming is usually required. In patients with older, non–MRI-compatible devices, MRI scans can be done with reasonable safety, but in many centers it is difficult to find a radiologist willing to perform the study. It is unlikely that cautery used during an obstetric procedure will affect a pacemaker, but it is not impossible. In the unlikely event that cautery affected the pacemaker, the effect would be temporary inhibition of the pacemaker while cautery was on. Simply stopping cautery would allow the pacemaker to resume normal function. If a patient is pacemaker dependent, one can program the pacemaker to a nonsensing mode while cautery is used. In some (but not all) pacemakers, a magnet will cause asynchronous pacing.

Whenever a patient with a pacemaker is to undergo a procedure, it is best to have the device clinic (or company representative, if local device clinic personnel are unavailable) interrogate the device, so that all providers know how it is programmed and contingencies for emergencies are preplanned.

Implantable cardioverter defibrillators (ICDs) could be single-chamber, dual-chamber, or biventricular devices. Defibrillators will have all functions of a bradycardia pacemaker, as well as the ability to treat life-threatening ventricular arrhythmias with antitachycardia pacing, as well as with cardioverting or defibrillating shocks. Biventricular defibrillators are used to treat certain patients with systolic heart failure. If a pregnant woman presents with a biventricular device, it is important to assess and monitor LV function because she has, or had, significant LV dysfunction. Some patients receiving these devices have dramatic improvement in LV function. It is expected that if such improvement occurred, it will be maintained with pregnancy. Defibrillators are not affected by diagnostic x-rays. Newer defibrillators may be MRI compatible, allowing patients to have MRI scans, although special programming is usually required. In patients with older, non–MRI-compatible devices, MRI scans can be done with reasonable safety, but in many centers it is difficult to find a radiologist willing to perform the study. It is unlikely that cautery used during an obstetric procedure will affect a defibrillator, but it is not impossible. In the unlikely event that cautery affects the defibrillator, either of two effects could occur. The first is temporary inhibition of the pacemaker function of the device while cautery is on. Simply stopping cautery would allow the pacemaker to resume normal function. The second possible effect is that the cautery signals would be detected and interpreted as ventricular fibrillation, causing an inappropriate shock to be delivered. If a patient is pacemaker dependent, one can program the pacemaker to a nonsensing mode while cautery is used. In some (but not all) defibrillators, a magnet placed over the device will suspend detection and prevent all shocks. Magnets do not affect the pacing functions of defibrillators.

Whenever a patient with an ICD is to undergo a procedure, it is best to have the device clinic (or company representative, if local device clinic personnel are unavailable) interrogate the device, so that all providers know how it is programmed, and contingencies for emergencies are preplanned.

BIBLIOGRAPHY

Hypertension

ACOG Committee Opinion No. 743. Low-dose aspirin use during pregnancy. American College of Obstetricians and Gynecologists. *Obstet Gynecol*. 2018;132:e44–e52.

ACOG Practice Bulletin Number 202. Chronic hypertension in pregnancy. *Obstet Gynecol*. 2019;1331:e1–e25.

ACOG Practice Bulletin Number 203. Gestational hypertension and preeclampsia. *Obstet Gynecol*. 2019;1331: e26–e44.

American College of Obstetricians and Gynecologists Task Force on Hypertension in Pregnancy. 2013.

Bouta A, et al. Manifestations of metabolic syndrome after hypertensive pregnancy. *Hypertension*. 2004;43:825–831.

Brown MA, Buddle MI. What's in a name: Problems with the classification of hypertension in pregnancy. *J Hypertens*. 1997;15:1049–1054.

Brown MA, et al. Randomized trial of management of hypertensive pregnancies by Korortkoff phase IV or phase V. *Lancet*. 1998;352:777–781.

Building U.S. Capacity to review and prevent maternal deaths. (2017). *Report from maternal mortality review committees: a view into their critical role*. https://www.cdcfoundation.org/sites/default/files/upload/pdf/MMR-IAReport.pdf

Carson M. Hypertension and Pregnancy. Medscape; updated 2016.

Forest JC, et al. Pregnancy complications and maternal risk of ischaemic heat disease: a retrospective study of 129,290 births. *Lancet*. 2001;357:2002–2006.

Harper MA, et al. Phaechromocytoma in pregnancy. Five cases and a review of the literature. *Br J Obstet Gynaecol*. 1989;96:594–606.

Higgins JR, de Swiet M. Blood pressure measurement and classification in pregnancy. *Lancet*. 2001;357:131–135.

Jones DC, Hayslett JP. Outcome of pregnancy in women with moderate or severe renal insufficiency. *N Engl J Med*. 1996;335:226–232.

Jungers P, et al. Pregnancy in women with ipaired renal function. *Clin Nephrol*. 1997;47:281–288.

Lamming GD, et al. Phaechromocytoma in pregnancy; still a cause of matenal death. *Clin Exp Hypertens*. 1990;9: 57–68.

Levine RJ, Maynard SE, Qian C, et al. Circulating angiogenic factors and the risk of preeclampsia. *N Engl J Med*. 2004;350(7):672–683.

Maynard SE, Min JY, Merchan J, et al. Excess placental soluble fms-like tyrosine kinase 1 (sFlt1) may contribute to endotheial dysfunction, hypertension, and proteinuria in preeclampsia. *J Clin Invest*. 2003;111:649–658.

National high blood pressure education program woring group. Report on high blood pressure in pregnancy. *Am J Obstet Gyenecol* 2000;181:5S1-S22.

Patten IS, Rana S, Shahul S, et al. Cardiac angiogenic imbalance leads to peripartum car diomyopathy. *Nature*. 2012;485(7398):333–338.

Say L, Chou D, Gemmill A, et al. Global causes of maternal death: a WHO systematic analysis. *Lancet Glob Health*. 2014;2(6):e323.

Shennan A, et al. Lack of reproducibility in pregnancy of Korotkoff phase IV as measured by mercury sphygmomanometry. *Lancet*. 1996;347:139–142.

Siddiqi T, et al. Hypertension during pregnancy in insulin dependent diabetic women. *Obstet Gynecol*. 1991;77:514–519.

Morbid obesity

Cedergreen MI. Maternal morbid obesity and the risk of adverse pregnancy outcome. *Obstet Gynecol.* 2004;103(2):219–224.

Kumari AS. Pregnancy outcome in women with morbid obesity. *Int J Obstet Gynecol.* 2001;73(2):101–107.

NJ Maternal obesity and pregnancy outcome: a study of 287,213 pregnancies in London. *Int J Obesity.* 2001;25:1175–1182.

Post-partum hypertension

August P, Malha L. Postpartum hypertension "It ain't over til' it's over". .*Circulation.* 2015;132:1690–1692.

Magee L, Sadeghi S. Prevention and treatment of postpartum hypertension. *Cochrane Database Syst Rev.* 2005 CD004351.

Sibai B. Etiology and management of postpartum hypertension-preeclampsia. *Am J Obstet Gynecol.* 2012;206(6):470–475.

Tan LK, de Swiet M. The management of postpartum hypertension. *Bjog.* 2002;109:733–736.

Walters BN, Thompson ME, Lee A, de Swiet M. Blood pressure in the puerperium. *Clin Sci (Lond).* 1986;71:589–594.

Congenital heart disease

Levine GN, et al. 2018 ACHD guidline: Executive summary. *JACC.* 2019;73(12):1494–1563.

Pulmonary hypertension

Ladouceur M, et al. Pregnancy outcomes in patients with pulmonary arterial hypertension associated with congenital heart disease. *Heart.* 2017;103:287–292.

Hemnes AR, et al. Statement on pregnancy in pulmonary hypertension from the Pulmonary Vascular Research Institute. *Pulm Circ.* 2015;5(3):435–465.

Risk of thrombosis

Abdul Sultan A, West J, Tata LJ, Fleming KM, Nelson-Piercy C, Grainge MJ. Risk of first venous thromboembolism in pregnant women in hospital: Population based cohort study from England. *BMJ.* 2013;347:f6099.

Dargaud Y, et al. A risk score for the management of pregnant women with increased risk of venous thromboembolism: a multicenter prospective study. *Br J Hametology.* 2009;145(6):825–835.

de Boer K, ten Cate JW, Sturk A, Borm JJ, Treffers PE. Enhanced thrombin generation in normal and hypertensive pregnancy. *Am J Obstet Gynecol.* 1989;160(1):95–100.

De Jong PG, Goddijn M, Middeldorp S. Antithrombotic therapy for pregnancy loss. *Hum Reprod Update.* 2013;19(6):656–673.

Eichinger S, Evers JLH, Glasier A, et al. Venous thromboembolism in women: A specific reproductive health risk. *Hum Reprod Update.* 2013;19(5):471–482.

James AH, Grotegut CA, Brancazio LR, Brown H. Thromboembolism in pregnancy: recurrence and its prevention. *Semin Perinatol.* 2007;31(3):167–175.

Lindqvist PG, et al. Postpartum thromboembolism: Severe events might be preventable using a new risk score mode. *Vasc Health Risk Manag.* 2008;4(5):1081–1087.

Schaefer C, Hannemann D, Meister R, et al. Vitamin K antagonists and pregnancy outcome. A multi-centre prospective study. *Thromb Haemost.* 2006;95(6):949–957.

Diastolic dysfunction

Muthyala T, et al. Maternal cardiac diastolic dysfunction by Doppler echocardiography in women with preeclampsia. *J Clin Diagn Res.* 2016;10(8):QC01–QC03.

Peripartum Heart Failure Caused by Left ventricular diastolic dysfunction. *J Am Osteopathic Association* 2010; 110:87-90

Schannwell CM, Zimmerman T. Left ventricular hypertrophy and diastolic dysfunction in healthy pregnant women. *Cardiology.* 2002;97(2):73–78.

Wells GL, Little WC. Peripartum cardiomyopathy presenting as diastolic heart failure. *Congest Heart Fail.* 2008;14(1):52–54.

Right ventricular dysfunction

Zengin E, et al. Right heart failure in pregnant women with cyanotic congenital heart disease – the good, the bad, and the ugly. *Int J Cardiol.* 2016;202:773–775.

Cyanotic congenital heart disease

Patrizia P, et al. Pregnancy in cyanotic congenital ehart disease outcome of the mother and fetus. *Circulation.* 1994;89:2673–2676.

Valvular heart disease

Elkayam U, Bitar F. Valvular Heart Disease and Pregnancy. *JACC.* 2005;46(2).

Nanna M, Stergiopoules K. Pregnancy complicated by valvular heart disease: An update. *J Am Heart Assoc.* 2014;3(3):e000712.

Silwa K, et al. Management of valvular disease in pregnancy: a global perspective. *Eur Heart J* 201536(18):1078-1089.

Stout KK, Otto CM. Pregnancy in women with valvular heart disease. *Heart.* 2007;93(5):552–558.

Valvular Heart Disease Pregnancy complicated by valvular heart disease: an update. *JAHA* 2014;3:e000712

Prosthetic heart valves

Badduke ER, et al. Pregnancy and childbearing in a population with biologic valvular prosthesis. *J thorac Cardiovasc Surg.* 1991;102:179–186.

Bartoloti U, et al. Pregnancy in patients with a porcine vale bioprosthesis. *Am J Cardiol.* 1982;50:1051–1054.

Ben Ismail M, et al. Cardiac valve prostheses, and anticoagulation and pregnancy. *Br Heart J.* 1986;55:101–105.

Bennett GG, Oakley CM. Pregnancy in a patient with mitral valve prosthesis. *Lancet*. 1968;291:616–619.

Born D, et al. Pregnancy in patients with prosthetic heart valves: the effects of anticoagulation on mother,, fetus, and neonate. *Am Heart J*. 1992;124:413–417.

Chen WWC, et al. Pregnancy in patients with prosthetic heart valves: an experience with 45 pregnancies. *Q J Med*. 1982;51:358–365.

Cotrulo M, et al. Coumadin anticoagulation during pregnancy in patients with mechanical valve prostheses. *Eur J Cardiothorac Surg*. 1991;5(6):300–305.

Ginsberg JS, Barron WM. Pregnancy and prosthetic heart valves. *Lancet*. 1994;344:1170–1172.

Ginsberg JS, Chan WS, Bates SM, Kaatz S. Anticoagulation of pregnant women with mechanical heart valves). *Arch Intern Med*. 2003;163(6):694–698.

Hanania G, et al. Pregnancy in patients with valvular prostheses – retrospective cooperative study in France (155 cases). *J Arch Mal Coeur Vaiss*. 1994;87:429–437.

Hung I, Rahimtoola SH. Prosthetic heart valves and pregnancy. *Circulation*. 2003;107:1240–1246.

Hurbe-Alessio I, et al. Risks of anticoagulant therapy in pregnant women with artificial heart valves. *N Engl J Med*. 1986;315:1390–1393.

Idir M, et al. Collapse and massive pulmonary edema secondary to thrombosis of a mitral mecchanical heart valve prostesis during low-moleular weight heparin therapy. *J Heart Valve Dis*. 1999;8:303–304.

Iturbe-Alessio I, Fonseca MC, Mutchinik O, Santos MA, Zajarías A, Salazar E. Risks of anticoagulant therapy in pregnant women with artificial heart valves. *N Engl J Med*. 1986;315(22):1390–1393.

Jaimeson WRF, et al. Pregnancy and bioprosthethesis: influence on structural valve deteriation. *Ann Thorac Surg*. 1995;60:S282–S287.

Kim BJ, An SJ, Shim SS, et al. Pregnancy outcomes in women with mechanical heart valves. *J Reprod Med*. 2006;51(8):649–654.

Larrea JL, et al. Pregnancy and mechanical valve prosthesis: a high risk situation for the mother and the fetus. *Ann Throac Surg*. 1983;36:459–463.

Pavunkuar P, et al. Pregnancy in patients with prosthetic cardiac valve: a ten year eperience. *Scand J Thorac Cardiovasc Surg*. 1988;22:9–22.

Salaar F, et al. The problem of cardiac valve prostheses, anticoagulation, and pregnancy. *Circulation*. 1984;70(suppl 1):169–177.

Salazar E, et al. Failure of adjusted doses of subcutaneous heparin to prevent throb-embolic phenomena in pregnant patients with mechanical cardiac valve prosthesis. *J Am Coll Cardiol*. 1996;27:1698–1705.

Salazar E, Izaguirre R, Verdejo J, Mutchinick O. Failure of adjusted doses of subcutaneous heparin to prevent thromboembolic phenomena in pregnant patients with mechanical cardiac valve prostheses. *J Am Coll Cardiol*. 1996;27(7):1698–1703.

Sharouni F, et al. Outcome of pregnancy in women with valve prosthesis. *Br Heart J*. 1994;71:196–201.

Steinberg Maternal and fetal outcomes of anticoagulation in pregnant women with mechanical heart valves. *JACC*. 2017;69(22):2681–2691.

Baffels, shunts, and conduits

Canobbio MM, et al. Pregnancy Outcomes after atrial repair for transposition of the great arteries. *Am J Card*. 2006;98:668–672.

Clarkson PM, et al. Outoe of pregnancy after thee mustard operation for transposition of the great arteries with intact ventricular septum. *JACC*. 1994;24(1):190–193.

Drenthen W, et al. Risk of complications during pregnancy after Senning or Mustard (atrial) repair of complete transposition of the Great arteries. *Eur Heart J*. 2005;26(23):2588–2595.

Pacemakers

Grover S, et al. Management of cardiac pacemakers in a pregnant patient. *Open J Obstet Gynecol*. 2015;5:60–69.

Natale A, et al. Implantable cardioverter-defibrillators and Pregnancy A safe combination? *Circulation*. 1997;96:2808–2812.

Piper JM, Berkus M, Ridgway LE. Pregnancy complicated by chronic cardiomyopathy and an implantable cardioverter defibrillator. *Am J Obstet Gynecol*. 1992;167:506–507.

6

Obstetric Events That Affect Cardiac Patients

William T. Schnettler, MD, FACOG

Pregnancy dramatically increases the demands on a woman's heart. Both stroke volume and cardiac output increase significantly in response to a number of factors, including increased oxygen demands by the growing fetus, the enlarging breasts, and the enlarging uterus; increased work by the mother because of weight gain; and the placental bed acting like an arteriovenous fistula. This chapter reviews the events that affect (or that may affect) cardiac patients, including changes that occur during the antenatal, peripartum, and postpartum periods; analgesia and anesthesia; assisted delivery; cesarean delivery; deep vein thrombosis (DVT); multiple-gestation pregnancies; preeclampsia and eclampsia; HELLP (hemolysis, elevated liver enzymes, and low platelet counts) syndrome; induction of labor; postpartum hemorrhage; premature labor; and pulmonary embolus.

ANTENATAL PERIOD

In the antenatal period, circulating blood volume increases by 50% to 70%. Systemic vascular resistance falls starting at about 5 weeks and continues until about week 32, when it begins to rise. This is caused by circulating prostacyclin (PGI$_2$) and shifting of blood to the low-resistance placental circulation. Pulmonary vascular resistance also drops significantly. Cardiac output typically increases 30% to 50%. Women who are unable to increase their cardiac output or who require increased filling pressures to do so may develop heart failure. Heart rate typically increases by 20 to 30 beats/min above prepregnancy levels. Oxygen consumption typically rises 20% to 30%, which may lead to myocardial ischemia in women with coronary artery disease.

PERIPARTUM PERIOD

The first stage of labor involves uterine contractions, which expel up to 500 cc of blood into the circulation. This phenomenon is sometimes called the autotransfusion effect. Increased catecholamine levels during labor cause increases in heart rate, blood pressure, and cardiac output; the latter increases about 10% during labor. Immediately after delivery and when the vena cava is no longer obstructed, cardiac output may increase as much as 80% above prepregnancy levels. It returns to normal about 60 minutes after delivery.

POSTPARTUM PERIOD

Complete resolution of the hemodynamic changes of pregnancy may take 3 to 6 months. Blood volume decreases by 10% within 3 days postdelivery. Blood pressure initially falls and then increases from day 3 to day 7 postpartum, and then it returns to prepregnancy levels by 6 weeks. Systemic vascular resistance increases over the 2-week postpartum period and achieves values about 30% over that at delivery. Heart rate decreases to baseline in about 2 weeks. Cardiac output increases as much as 80% in the first few hours after delivery and then gradually declines to baseline over the next 6 months.

ANALGESIA AND ANESTHESIA

The method of anesthesia used during labor and delivery may have profound effects on hemodynamics. Regional anesthesia using epidural or spinal anesthesia blunts the stress response, resulting in less catecholamine release, which results in less tachycardia and hypertension. The denser neural blockade required for cesarean section is associated with greater autonomic blockade, which can lead to vasodilation and hypotension. Regional anesthesia cannot be used safely in the presence of a coagulopathy or in the presence of active anticoagulation therapy.

General anesthesia also significantly reduces catecholamine release, resulting in less tachycardia and hypotension. It may depress respiration in the newborn. There is an increased risk of blood loss in cesarean section performed under general anesthesia because volatile anesthetics relax the uterus.

ASSISTED DELIVERY

Assisted delivery is the use of instruments such as forceps or ventouse. It is performed most often when patients fail to progress during the second stage of labor, but it also may be performed to avoid the adverse effects of pushing in a cardiac patient. Both pushing and the stress of nonassisted delivery cause significant increases in peripheral vascular resistance, which may be harmful to women with significantly dilated aortas or severe left ventricular dysfunction.

CESAREAN DELIVERY

Cesarean delivery avoids the fluctuations in blood pressure associated with vaginal delivery, but the anesthesia it requires does cause blood pressure to fluctuate. Spinal anesthesia blocks the sympathetic nerves, causing vasodilation and hypotension. Rarely, general anesthesia may be required. General anesthesia also may cause hypotension. The blood loss with cesarean delivery is double that with vaginal delivery. Moreover, with cesarean delivery, there is an increased risk of wound and uterine infection and an increased risk of thromboembolic complications.

DEEP VEIN THROMBOSIS

Pregnancy is a hypercoagulable state, and the compression of the pelvic veins by the expanding uterus creates stasis; both of these (the hypercoagulable state and stasis) predispose the patient to DVT. The risk of venous thromboembolism is fivefold higher in pregnant women than nonpregnant women. Puerperium is the time of greatest risk, with an up to 20 times greater relative risk. Approximately 80% of events occur in the first 3 weeks after delivery. DVT in pregnancy is more commonly left

sided and is most likely to involve the iliofemoral veins. It can present with various combinations of pain and swelling in the leg, lower abdominal pain, low-grade fever, and an elevated white count.

Many (>50%) women who present with symptoms suggesting DVT do not actually have it, so it is imperative to confirm the diagnosis with objective testing. Duplex scanning is the usual first-line test. If the test result is negative but clinical suspicion is high, it is usually recommended to treat for 1 week and then repeat the duplex scan. If the scan result is again negative, treatment is stopped unless clinical suspicion remains high. In that case, either magnetic resonance venography or conventional venography may be considered.

D-dimer measurements may be unreliable in the diagnosis of DVT during pregnancy. D-dimer levels increase during normal pregnancy and increase with complications such as preeclampsia and placental abruption. Furthermore, false-negative D-dimer results have been reported during pregnancy.

The standard treatment for DVT in pregnancy is low-molecular-weight heparin (LMWH). Treatment should be provided for a minimum of 3 months and for at least 6 weeks postpartum. Usually, leg elevation and early mobilization with compression stockings also are recommended.

Pregnant women who develop DVT should be screened for a hypercoagulable state. It is difficult to evaluate coagulation parameters during pregnancy, so only a limited screening, for antithrombin deficiency and antiphospholipid antibodies, is recommended.

MULTIPLE-GESTATION PREGNANCIES

Multiple-gestation pregnancies are associated with significantly higher maternal complication rates than singleton pregnancies. The risks of hypertensive disorders, heart failure, and myocardial infarction are increased. The risks of other pregnancy-related complications, such as premature rupture of the membranes, abruptio placenta, and postpartum hemorrhage, are increased as well.

Multiple-gestation births also are associated with an increased risk for the fetuses, including premature birth, low birth weight, and intrauterine growth restriction.

In women pregnant with twins, the size of the uterus is roughly the same as for singletons until about 18 weeks of gestation, when it rapidly enlarges so that it is twice normal size by 35 weeks.

Weight gain in the mother is greater with multiple-gestation pregnancies. The increase in amniotic fluid is greater, as are the increases in cardiac output and maternal blood volume.

PREECLAMPSIA AND ECLAMPSIA

Preeclampsia is a disease that occurs in pregnant women and is characterized by hypertension and proteinuria. It is diagnosed when a woman who was not hypertensive before pregnancy develops hypertension (blood pressure >140/90 mm Hg) after 20 weeks of pregnancy and proteinuria of at least 0.3 g/24 hours. In recent years, it has been recognized that proteinuria is not universally present in patients with preeclampsia. The 2013 American College of Obstetricians and Gynecologists guidelines state that in the absence of proteinuria, preeclampsia is diagnosed as hypertension in association with thrombocytopenia (platelet count <100, 000/μL), impaired liver function (elevated blood levels of liver transaminases to twice normal), the new development of renal insufficiency (elevated serum creatinine >1.1 mg/dL or a doubling of serum creatinine in the absence of other renal disease), pulmonary edema, or new-onset cerebral or visual disturbances. Preeclampsia, which occurs in 1% to 3% of pregnancies, is a leading cause of maternal death and is responsible for about half of all preterm deliveries. In the following paragraphs, we summarize available information about its etiology, risk factors, maternal and fetal effects, diagnosis, management, and treatment.

Etiology

The precise cause of preeclampsia is unknown, but it is thought to occur when reduced placental perfusion causes a harmful maternal inflammatory response, resulting in widespread oxidative damage and endothelial dysfunction. Endothelial damage leads to capillary leakage, which may lead to peripheral edema, pulmonary edema, or both. The hypertension is primarily caused by arterial vasospasm. Women with preeclampsia show an increased hyperresponsiveness to vasoactive peptides such as epinephrine. Methyldopa has been shown to reduce this arterial stiffness.

Risk Factors

Risk factors for the development of preeclampsia include maternal age younger than 18 years or older than 35 years, preexisting hypertension, previous personal or family history, first pregnancy, obesity, and others. It is more common in Blacks than in Whites or Hispanics.

Maternal and Fetal Effects

Preeclampsia causes both a maternal and a fetal syndrome. The maternal syndrome may manifest as eclampsia (cerebral edema, seizures, or both), HELLP syndrome, renal impairment, pulmonary edema, disseminated intravascular coagulation, or abruption of the placenta. The fetal syndrome may manifest as fetal growth restriction, premature delivery (usually iatrogenic), or death.

Diagnosis

There is no way to predict the development of preeclampsia, so monitoring blood pressure is the best way to make an early diagnosis. Approximately one-third of women who develop hypertension after 20 weeks of gestation will develop preeclampsia. Symptoms include visual disturbances, including scotoma, headaches, and sometimes right-upper-quadrant abdominal discomfort caused by liver swelling. Edema is often, but not invariably, present.

Management

The management of patients with preeclampsia involves treatment of hypertension and careful monitoring of the fetus. Often, bed rest or restricted activity is prescribed, but there is little evidence that this is beneficial. Ideally, the baby will not be delivered before 34 weeks, after which time the fetal lungs should be mature. The only real treatment for preeclampsia and eclampsia is delivery.

Treatment

The treatment of patients with hypertension is the same as for other causes of hypertension in pregnancy. For the emergency treatment of severe, acute-onset hypertension, several options are available, including intravenous (IV) labetalol, IV hydralazine, and oral nifedipine. Labetalol should be avoided in women with asthma. IV nitroprusside should be used only for the shortest possible time because of concerns of cyanide and thiocyanate toxicity.

For chronic oral therapy during pregnancy, methyldopa, labetalol, and nifedipine are considered acceptable. Methyldopa is often considered the drug of choice because of its historic safety record. It does not alter maternal cardiac output or blood flow to the uterus and kidneys. However, it is not an extremely potent antihypertensive, and it is slow in onset. Labetalol has been shown to be as effective as methyldopa in pregnant women, and it does not alter uterine or renal blood flow. However, it does not have a safety record as well established as methyldopa. Oral hydralazine appears generally safe for the fetus, but a few cases of thrombocytopenia have been reported. It may be combined with methyldopa or labetalol.

Atenolol should be avoided as it has been associated with growth restriction in fetuses. Similarly, angiotensin-converting-enzyme inhibitors have been associated with a number of fetal adverse events, including growth restriction, renal failure, persistent patent ductus arteriosus, respiratory distress, hypotension, and prepartum death. They are contraindicated during the second and third trimesters, as are angiotensin-receptor blockers.

Diuretics may be used to treat preeclampsia if patients develop signs of either cerebral or pulmonary edema. In severe cases, magnesium sulfate ($MgSO_4$) is given to prevent seizures.

Thromboprophylaxis should be considered. Preeclampsia is a risk factor for thrombosis, particularly in association with other risk factors, such as a body mass index greater than 30, age older than 35 years, multiparity, or antenatal bed rest for more than 4 days. Thromboprophylaxis also should be considered after cesarean section for eclampsia.

Indications for delivery include uncontrolled hypertension in spite of treatment, development of HELLP syndrome, renal impairment, eclampsia, pulmonary edema, coagulopathy, and fetal distress.

During the third stage of labor in patients with preeclampsia or eclampsia, oxytocin can be used, but ergometrine should be avoided.

It is possible for preeclampsia, or pregnancy-related hypertension, to first manifest in the postpartum period.

The recurrence rate with repeat pregnancies is about 10%. Low-dose aspirin (81 mg/day) may be helpful in preventing recurrences. The development of preeclampsia predicts a lifetime increased risk for hypertension, ischemic heart disease, and stroke.

Hellp Syndrome

HELLP syndrome is a manifestation of preeclampsia. It is diagnosed when liver enzymes become elevated and platelet counts drop. It is treated with delivery.

Induction of Labor

Induction of labor involves the use of various drugs to cause thinning and dilation of the cervix, followed by other drugs to induce uterine contractions. Prostaglandin E_2 (PGE_2; dinoprostone) or a PGE_1 analog (misoprostol) is used to dilate the cervix. They can be given intravaginally, orally, or both. There do not appear to be any cardiac or hemodynamic effects. Syntocinon is used to induce uterine contraction.

Induction of labor in women with heart disease seems to be safe for both the mother and baby. Women with heart disease undergoing induction of labor have the same rate of cesarean delivery as those without heart disease undergoing induction. The risk of complications in women with heart disease is the same whether they undergo induction of labor or not.

Postpartum Hemorrhage

Postpartum hemorrhage is defined as the loss of more than 500 cc of blood within the first 24 hours after delivery. Causes include retained placenta, which must be removed, and uterine atony, which may be treated medically or surgically with various techniques. The medications used to increase uterine tone include methylergonovine, ergonovine malate, carboprost (prostaglandin similar to F2-α), oxytocin, and Cytotec (synthetic prostaglandin E1 analog).

Premature Labor

If a fetus is thought to be viable and labor has initiated prematurely, it is common practice to try and prevent premature delivery or to delay delivery and initiate drugs to help mature the fetus's lungs.

The drugs that inhibit uterine contraction and delay delivery are called tocolytics. Over the years, many drugs, including IV ethanol, have been tried, but they have been shown to be ineffective. Drugs currently in use and their potential cardiac side effects are shown in Table 6.1.

Typically, tocolysis is effective only for up to 7 days. However, this may be sufficient time to transfer a patient to a specialized center with capabilities to manage preterm deliveries (if they are not already at one) or to administer steroids to enhance fetal lung maturity. The potential risk of steroid administration to the mother is fluid retention.

Pulmonary Embolus

Pulmonary embolus is often difficult to diagnose, but it is associated with significant mortality. Therefore, it is

TABLE 6.1 Common Medications Used for Tocolysis or Preterm Prevention, Highlighting Their Mechanisms of Action and Maternal, Fetal, and Neonatal Effects

Drug	Mechanism	Maternal Side Effects	Fetal and Neonatal Effects
Terbutaline	B₂ agonist	Arrhythmias, pulmonary edema, myocardial ischemia, hypertension, tachycardia	Constriction of ductus arteriosus, pulmonary hypertension (reversible), decreased renal function, oligohydramnios, intraventricular hemorrhage, hyperbilirubinemia, necrotizing enterocolitis
Nifedipine	Calcium channel blocker	Hypotension. Calcium channel blockers given with magnesium may cause cardiovascular collapse	None known
Atosiban	Oxytocin receptor antagonist		
Indomethacin	Nonsteroidal ant-inflammatory	Renal impairment, hepatic impairment	Constriction of ductus arteriosus, pulmonary hypertension (reversible), decreased renal function, oligohydramnios, intraventricular hemorrhage, hyperbilirubinemia, necrotizing enterocolitis
Sulindac	Nonsteroidal antiinflammatory	Coagulation disorders, thrombocytopenia, asthma	

critical to have a high index of suspicion when patients present with shortness of breath or sudden-onset pleuritic chest pain. Patients also may present with hemoptysis or syncope. Patients usually will have tachycardia and tachypnea and may have leg swelling suggesting a DVT, which is the usual source of the embolus. Typically, their oxygen saturation will be low.

The differential diagnosis includes pulmonary infection, so typically, a chest x-ray examination should be performed. This should not be withheld because of pregnancy, because the radiation dose to the fetus is quite low (<10 Gy; 50, 000 Gy is the dose needed to put fetus at significant risk). In pulmonary embolus patients, the chest radiograph is usually normal or shows nonspecific findings.

Typically, an electrocardiogram (ECG) to exclude myocardial infarction is performed. Virtually always, the ECG will show sinus tachycardia if a pulmonary embolus has occurred. Other findings on the ECG can suggest pulmonary embolus and are caused by the acute elevation of right-sided pressures. These findings include right-axis deviation; right bundle branch block; peaked p waves; and the S1, Q3, T3 pattern (S wave in lead I, a Q wave in lead III, and an inverted T wave in lead III).

The D-dimer test is not helpful in pregnancy.

Depending on the patient's clinical status and whether or not an aortic dissection is being considered in the differential diagnosis, computed tomography angiography (CTA) of the chest may be ordered. The radiation dose to the fetus is estimated at less than 500 Gy (again, 50,000 Gy is needed to put the fetus at significant risk). If CTA is not performed and the patient is stable, it may be reasonable to proceed with duplex scanning of the legs. If DVT is detected, then treatment with LMWH should be started, and no further diagnostic testing is needed. If the duplex scan result is normal, additional investigation to look for a pulmonary embolus will be necessary. This could be either a CTA (fetus exposed to <500 Gy) or a ventilation perfusion scan (estimated fetal exposure 350–500 Gy).

There are several treatment options for massive pulmonary emboli. One is thrombolysis with recombinant tissue plasminogen activator or streptokinase. A risk is maternal bleeding around the access site or placenta, which occurs 1% to 5% of the time. Thrombolysis can be given intravenously or can be catheter directed. Another option is thrombectomy, which can be done surgically or can be catheter based. Various combinations of thrombolysis, embolectomy, and clot fragmentation may be performed with catheter-based procedures. A third option is to start IV unfractionated heparin to prevent clot recurrence and propagation. The patient's stability and local expertise dictate which of these options is chosen.

If the embolus is smaller and the patient is hemodynamically stable, treatment with LMWH is appropriate. Because only about 5% of women presenting with signs and symptoms of pulmonary embolus actually have one, it is imperative to confirm the diagnosis before treatment. The recommended dosages of enoxaparin are 1.0 mg/kg twice a day both antenatally and postnatally.

Inferior vena cava filters should be considered only in cases of recurrent emboli on adequate doses of anticoagulant.

Pregnant women developing a pulmonary embolus should be screened for a hypercoagulable state. It is difficult to evaluate coagulation parameters during pregnancy, so only a limited screening, for antithrombin deficiency and antiphospholipid antibodies, is recommended.

BIBLIOGRAPHY

Antenatal

Sanghavi M, Rutherford JD. Cardiovascular physiology of pregnancy. *Circulation*. 2014;130:1003–1008.

Thornburg KL, Jacobson SL, Giraud GD, Morton MJ. Hemodynamic changes in pregnancy. *Semin Perinatol*. 2000;24: 11–14.

Peripartum

Pritchard JA, Rowland RC. Blood volume changes in pregnancy and the puerperium III. Whole body and large vessel hematocrits in pregnant and nonpregnant women. *Am J Obstet Gynaecol*. 1964;88:391–395.

Rovinsky JJ, Jaffin H. Cardiovascular hemodynamics in pregnancy. I. Blood and plasma volumes in multiple pregnancy. *Am J Obstet Gynaecol*. 1965;93:1–15.

Postpartum

San-Frutos L, Engels V, Zapardiel I, et al. Hemodynamic changes during pregnancy and postpartum: a prospective study using thoracic electrical bioimpedance. *J Matern Fetal Neonatal Med*. 2011;11:1333–1340.

Anesthesia

Fernandes SM, Arendt KW, Landzberg MJ, Economy KE, Khairy P. Pregnant women with congenital heart disease: cardiac anesthetic and obstetrical implications. *Expert Rev Cardiovasc Ther*. 2010;8:439–448.

Hands ME, Johnson MD, Saltzman DH, Rutherford JD. The cardiac, obstetric, and anesthetic management of pregnancy complicated by acute myocardial infarction. *J Clin Anesth*. 1990;4:258–268.

Sukhminder JSB, Sukhminder KB. Anaesthetic challenges and management during pregnancy: strategies revisited. *Anesth Essays Res*. 2013;7:160–167.

Assisted Delivery

Midwall J., Jaffin H., Herman M.V., Kupersmith J. Shunt flow and pulmonary hemodynamics during labor and delivery in the Eisenmenger syndrome. *Am J Cardiol*. 198;42(2):299–303.

Cesarean Section

Langesaeter M, Roos-Hesselink JW, Pijuan-Domènech A, et al. Regional anaesthesia for a Cesarean section in women with cardiac disease: a prospective study. *Acta Anaesthesiol Scand*. 2010;54:4–54.

Ruys TP, Roos-Hesselink JW, Pijuan-Domènech A, et al. Is planned cesarean section in women with cardiac disease beneficial? *Heart*. 2014;101:530–536.

Deep Venous Thrombosis in Pregnancy

Anderson BS, et al. The cumulative incidence of venous thromboembolism during pregnancy and puerperium—an 11 year Danish population based study of 63,000 pregnancies. *Acta Obstet Gyenaecol Scand*. 1998;77:170–173.

Carr MH, Towers CV, Eastenson AR, Pircon RA, Iriye BK, Adashek JA. Prolonged bed rest during pregnancy: does the risk of deep vein thrombosis warrant the use of routine heparin prophylaxis? *J Matern Fetal Med*. 1997;6: 264–267.

Danilenko-Dixon DR, Heit JA, Silverstein MD, et al. Risk factors for deep vein thrombosis and pulmonary embolus during pregnancy or post partum: a population based, case-control study. *Am J Obstet Gynecol*. 2001;184: 104–110.

Hirsh DR, Mikkola KM, Marks PW, et al. Pulmonary embolism and dep venous thrombosis during pregnancy or oral contraceptive use: prevalence of factor V Leiden. *Am Heart J*. 1996;131:1145–1148.

Jacobsen AF, Dragsund M, Rosseland LA. *Am J Obstet Gynecol*. 2008;198:233–234.

Lindqvist P, Dahlbäck B, Maršál K. Thrombotic risk during pregnancy: a population study. *Obstet Gynecol.* 1999;94: 595–599.

Peek MJ, Nelson-Piercy C, Manning RA, de Swiet M, Letsky EA. Activated protein C resistance in normal pregnancy. *Br J Obstet Gynaecol.* 1997;104:1084–1086.

Rutherford S, et al. Thromboembolic disease associated with pregnancy: an 11 year review. *Am J Obstet Gynecol.* 1991;164(suppl):286.

Toglia MR, Weg JG. Venous thromboembolism during pregnancy. *N Engl J Med.* 1996;355:108–113.

Multiple Gestation

Dera A, et al. Twin pregnancy—physiology, complications and the mode of delivery. *Arch Perinat Med.* 2007;13(3): 7–16.

Preeclampsia

Altman D, Carroli G, Duley L, et al. Do women with pre-eclampsia, and their babies benefit from magnesium sulfate? The MAGIC trial: a randomized placebo controlled trial. *Lancet.* 2002;359:1877 1890.

CLASP a randomized trial of low dose aspirin for the prevention and treatment of pre-eclampsia among 9364 pregnant women. CLASP collaborative group. *Lancet.* 1994;343: 619–629.

Duley L, Gülmezoglu AM, Henderson-Smart DJ, Chou D. Magnesium sulfate and other anticonvulsants for women with pre-eclampsia. *Cochrane Database Syst Rev.* 2010;11

Duley L, Henderson-Smart D, Knight M, King J. Antiplatelet drugs for prevention of pre-eclampsia and its consequences: systematic review. *BMJ.* 2001;322:329–333.

Männistö T, Mendola P, Vääräsmäki M, et al. Elevated blood pressure in pregnancy and future cardiovascular risk. *Circulation.* 2013;127:681–690.

Melchiorre K, Sutherland GR, Liberati M, Thilaganathan B. Preeclampsia is associated with persistent postpartum cardiovascular impairment. *Hypertension.* 2011;58:709–715.

Shahul S, Rhee J, Hacker MR, et al. Subclinical left ventricular dysfunction in preeclamptic women with preserved left ventricular ejection fraction: a 2D speckle-tracking imaging study. *Circ Cardiovasc Imaging.* 2012;5:734–739.

Shennan A, et al. Oscillometric blood pressure measurements in severe pre-eclampsia: validation of the Space lab90207. *Br J Obstet Gynaecol.* 1996;103:171–173.

Walker JJ. Pre-eclampsia. *Lancet.* 2000;356:1260–1265.

Induction of Labor

Oron G, Hirsch R, Ben-Haroush A, et al. Pregnancy outcomes in women with heart disease undergoing induction of labour. *BJOG.* 2004;111:669–675.

Rush RW, Mabin T, Bennett MJ. Induction of labour in pregnancy complicated by heart disease. *S Afr Med J.* 1983;64 (19):736–738.

Sau AK, Vasishta K, Dhar KK, Khunnu B. Induction of labour in pregnancy complicated by heart disease. *Aust N Z J Obstet Gynaecol.* 1993;33(1):37–39.

Postpartum Hemorrhage

Sheiner E, Sarid L, Levy A, Seidman DS, Hallak M. Obstetric risk factors and outcome of pregnancies complicated with early postpartum hemorrhage: a population-based study. *J Matern Fetal Neonatal Med.* 2005;18:149–154.

Premature Labor

Tocolytics for preterm labor in cardiac patients. *BMJ.* 2003;327:604.

Pulmonary Embolus

Chan WS, Ray JG, Murray S, Coady GE, Coates G, Ginsberg JS. Suspected pulmonary embolism in pregnancy. *Arch Intern Med.* 2002;162:1170–1175.

Ramsay R, Byrd L, Tower C, James J, Prescott M, Thachil J. The problem of pulmonary embolism diagnosis in pregnancy. *Br J Haematol.* 2015;170(5):727–728.

Simcox LE, Ormesher L, Tower C, Greer IA. Pulmonary thrombo-embolism in pregnancy: diagnosis and management. *Breathe.* 2015;11(4):282–289.

7

Managing Specific Cardiac Conditions During Pregnancy, Labor, and Delivery

William T. Schnettler, MD, FACOG

AORTIC DISSECTION

For the expectant mother, there is an increased risk of aortic dissection because of the histologic and hemodynamic changes that occur during pregnancy. Histologic changes in the aortic wall include fragmentation of the reticulum fibers, diminished mucopolysaccharides, and loss of corrugation of the elastic fibers. Hemodynamic changes include increased stroke volume and blood volume.

In patients with Marfan syndrome, who are predisposed to aortic dissection, there is an approximately 1% risk of aortic rupture during pregnancy. As reflected in various guidelines, pregnant women with Marfan syndrome and a dilated aorta (>4.5 cm) are at increased risk of aortic dissection.

Treatment of type A dissection, involving the ascending aorta, is surgical. Treatment of type B dissection, limited to the descending aorta, is medical, with surgery reserved for complications, such as leakage, rupture, or continuing expansion. When surgery is undertaken for type A dissection, two lives must be considered. If the fetus is at less than 28 weeks' gestation, surgery with the fetus in situ is recommended. If the fetus is viable and over 32 weeks' gestation, cesarean delivery followed immediately with aortic repair is recommended. If the fetus is between 28 and 32 weeks' gestation, a decision about the best option must be made.

AORTIC REGURGITATION

Aortic regurgitation is generally well tolerated during pregnancy. If it is severe or associated with preexisting left ventricular (LV) dysfunction, congestive heart failure may occur and should be treated as systolic left-sided failure is treated in other conditions.

AORTIC STENOSIS

Mild and moderate degrees of aortic stenosis may be well tolerated during pregnancy, but women with severe aortic stenosis have a significant risk of complications during pregnancy. Patients of concern are those with a valve area less than 1.0 cm^2 or a mean gradient over 50 mm Hg. In such patients, the already limited valve orifice cannot accommodate the dramatic blood volume expansion and increased cardiac output of pregnancy. The result is a significant increase in the transvalvular gradient, which may lead to pulmonary edema. The time of greatest risk begins in the second trimester, when increases in cardiac output are greatest, and persists until several days postpartum, when blood volume and cardiac output begin to return to prepregnancy levels. In the immediate postpartum period, relief of vena caval compression and the autotransfusion from the placenta add to the volume overload state. The main risk is that patients will develop left-sided congestive heart failure. Therapy should include diuretics and beta blockers; the latter may be particularly helpful because they slow the heart rate, which is beneficial for patients with aortic stenosis. Digitalis is generally not useful except in the presence of concomitant severe LV systolic failure. A patient with symptomatic severe aortic stenosis without significant aortic regurgitation may be a candidate for an aortic balloon valvuloplasty. This procedure can reduce the degree of stenosis and help the patient get through the pregnancy.

Vasodilators are contraindicated in aortic stenosis. Oxytocin is a vasodilator and must be used cautiously because it may decrease blood pressure significantly. Epidural and spinal anesthesia should be titrated slowly and cautiously because of vasodilation and hypotension, which may worsen valvular gradients.

ARRHYTHMOGENIC RIGHT VENTRICULAR CARDIOMYOPATHY

Arrhythmogenic right ventricular (RV) cardiomyopathy is a rare inherited type of cardiomyopathy that is caused by genetic mutations coding for the desmosomal proteins. The prevalence is estimated at 1 in 5000. This disorder is estimated to be responsible for 20% of sudden deaths in young people. Inheritance is autosomal dominant. These defects lead to RV dysfunction, fibrofatty infiltration of the right ventricle, and life-threatening arrhythmias usually originating in the right ventricle. Because arrhythmias often develop during exercise-induced catecholamine increases, patients are usually advised to limit exercise. The left ventricle is often involved as well. Generally, implantable cardioverter defibrillators are used in patients who have had ventricular arrhythmias or aborted sudden cardiac death. The number of reported cases of pregnancy in women with this disorder is small, but they seem to do well. Bauce et al. (2006) reported on six women, all of whom did well. Two had vaginal deliveries and four had cesarean sections. The fetuses had no negative consequences.

ATRIAL SEPTAL DEFECT

There are three types of atrial septal defects (ASDs): ostium primum, ostium secundum, and sinus venosus. The ostium primum type is usually part of an atrioventricular (AV) canal defect (see later discussion). Ostium secundum defects are in the fossa ovalis, and sinus venosus defects are higher in the atrium near the junction of the superior vena cava.

In the absence of pulmonary hypertension, most patients with ASDs tolerate pregnancy well. There is an increased risk of atrial arrhythmias, such as atrial fibrillation.

Patients with ASDs who do not have pulmonary hypertension have left-to-right shunting of blood through the ASD. The increased blood volume of pregnancy tends to increase the shunt, but the decreased peripheral resistance tends to reduce the shunt, so the net change is usually minimal. Postpartum hemorrhage, with the sudden onset of vasoconstriction, coupled with reduced venous return, may lead to a dramatic increase in the atrial shunt. Patients with a repaired ASD (either surgical or transcatheter device closure) without long-term sequelae are at low risk of cardiac complications during pregnancy.

ATRIOVENTRICULAR CANAL DEFECTS

Atrioventricular canal (also called AV septal) defects refer to a spectrum of defects with abnormalities of the AV valves, atrial septum, and ventricular septum. A complete AV canal defect constitutes a primum ASD, an inlet ventricular septal defect (VSD), and a common five-leaflet AV valve. Surgical repair involves closing the septal defects and separating the common AV valve into left and right AV valves. Incomplete or partial AV canal defects typically have a primum ASD with a cleft mitral valve. Despite surgical repair, there may be variable degrees of regurgitation. AV canal defects are associated with Down syndrome. Most patients with Down syndrome are unable to become pregnant. Complete AV canal defects are usually repaired in infancy. If a patient has partial defects, it is possible that they will have escaped detection or be unrepaired at the time of pregnancy.

The hemodynamic effects of these lesions depend on the size of the septal defect and the degree of shunting, as well as the degree of mitral and tricuspid regurgitation. Pulmonary hypertension, if present, dramatically increases the risk of pregnancy.

Patients with residual shunts are at increased risk of endocarditis.

The incidence of congenital heart disease in children of women with AV canal defects may be higher than with other maternal congenital heart conditions.

COARCTATION OF THE AORTA

Most women with a history of coarctation of the aorta have had a surgical repair before they become pregnant. The risk of coarctation during pregnancy depends on the presence of residual obstruction, aneurysm at the coarctation repair site, and associated lesions, such as a bicuspid aortic valve or aortopathy. Noncontrast magnetic resonance imaging should be considered during pregnancy for patients with repaired coarctation who have never had cross-sectional imaging. It will allow for detection of residual arch narrowing, aneurysm at the repair site, and accurate measurement of the thoracic aorta. Patients with a coarctation repaired with Dacron-patch aortoplasty are at particularly high risk of aneurysm formation and aortic rupture during pregnancy.

Patients with coarctation may also have berry aneurysms in the brain.

A potential hazard during pregnancy is severe hypertension, which is difficult to treat. Patients with a history of coarctation also have an increased risk of preeclampsia. Patients with coarctation have abnormal aortic walls and are prone to aortic dissection, a risk that increases during pregnancy. Vaginal delivery is preferred, but it is important to limit the second stage of labor in high-risk patients so as to minimize aortic stress. The risk of endocarditis is increased in patients with a bicuspid aortic valve.

Mothers with a history of coarctation have a higher-than-expected (3%) risk of having a baby with congenital heart defects.

COR PULMONALE AND LUNG DISEASE

In general, pregnancy stresses the cardiovascular system more than the respiratory system, and the pulmonary hypertension associated with pulmonary disease presents a greater hazard to the pregnant woman than the lung disease itself.

Conditions Resulting in Reduced Lung Volumes

Women with reduced lung volumes, even prior pneumonectomy, usually tolerate pregnancy well. Dyspnea at rest, however, should be a cause for concern. Emphysema caused by α_1-antitrypsin has been associated with a good pregnancy outcome (in a single case).

Cystic Fibrosis

Women with cystic fibrosis have reduced fertility rates, but if they do become pregnant, the outlook is not necessarily bleak. Data reported in 2001 from the United Kingdom cystic fibrosis registry included information on 1143 pregnancies. Seventy-four percent of the women carried the baby to term, 17% delivered prematurely, and 8% had spontaneous abortions. A US registry study reported no increase in mortality rate nor any decline in lung function in women who became pregnant versus those who did not. Whereas women with a forced expiratory volume in 1 second (FEV_1) over 75% of predicted can expect an uncomplicated pregnancy, those with an FEV_1 less than 60% of predicted are at risk for a preterm delivery. An FEV_1 less than 50% is considered a relative contraindication to pregnancy. Women with pulmonary hypertension are at high risk and should be discouraged from attempting pregnancy.

Women who have had lung transplantation may be able to have a successful pregnancy, but it is recommended that they wait at least 2 years after transplant.

Pleural Effusion

Although it has been little studied, asymptomatic pleural effusion seems to be a common occurrence postpartum. In one series, bilateral pleural effusions were detected by ultrasound examination in 21% of women; the effusion was not associated with any clinical feature of the pregnancy. There appears to be little or no clinical consequence, but it is important to be aware of this phenomenon so as not to assume that a woman with a postpartum pleural effusion has pathology.

Pulmonary Arteriovenous Malformations

Pulmonary arteriovenous malformations (PAVMs) present a serious risk to pregnant women and their babies, even if they are asymptomatic. The biggest risk is massive hemoptysis. Pulmonary arteriovenous fistulas may be asymptomatic and may not have been identified before pregnancy. About 90% occur as a part of hereditary hemorrhagic telangiectasia syndrome, so they may be picked up on the basis of personal or family history of severe recurrent gastrointestinal or nose bleeds.

Ideally, all PAVMs will have been treated with embolization before pregnancy. If not, they are likely to grow during pregnancy. Pregnant patients with PAVMs are at risk for massive and possibly fatal hemorrhages. Any hemoptysis in these women should be regarded as a medical emergency and patients considered for embolization, early delivery, or both.

Neuromuscular Disease

A variety of neuromuscular diseases may cause respiratory compromise: the muscular dystrophy syndromes, primary alveolar hypoventilation syndrome, spinal muscular atrophy, and various types of sleep apnea. Although data are limited, successful pregnancies have been achieved in patients with most of these disorders, with the proviso that respiratory function was carefully monitored and, when necessary, supported.

Scoliosis

Severe scoliosis may compromise lung function and cause pulmonary hypertension or cor pulmonale.

Whatever its cause, pulmonary hypertension greatly increases the risk of pregnancy, but in its absence, most women with scoliosis tolerate pregnancy well. Women with adolescent-onset scoliosis are generally at low risk for respiratory compromise during pregnancy. If a woman whose thoracic scoliosis is less than 50% becomes pregnant, a good outcome can be expected. Women with respiratory compromise and a vital capacity less than 1 L may be at risk for pregnancy complications and should be monitored carefully. Monitoring for nocturnal hypoxemia is especially important as respiration during REM sleep depends on diaphragmatic movement, which may be compromised.

It has been reported that pregnancy can cause the progression of scoliosis. However, surgical correction before pregnancy has been associated with increased severe back pain during pregnancy, and depending on the location of prior instrumentation, it may not be considered safe to proceed with regional anesthesia during delivery. If regional anesthesia is performed, it may not be as effective as it is in those patients who have not had back surgery.

CORONARY ARTERY DISEASE

Pregnant women presenting with angina are evaluated in much the same way as nonpregnant women. Generally, stress testing is the first step. If the resting electrocardiogram (ECG) shows normal stress test (ST) segments, a plain ECG treadmill test may suffice. If the ST segments are not normal at rest, then stress echocardiography is appropriate because nuclear studies should not be performed during pregnancy. If results of stress testing are positive, the appropriate course is coronary angiography with angioplasty and stenting, if needed, at the same setting. If possible, angiography should be delayed until after the third trimester. The uterus should be shielded. Because of the hypercoagulable state during pregnancy, drug-eluting stents are preferred. Aspirin and clopidogrel can be used during pregnancy.

For medical treatment of angina, metoprolol is considered safer than atenolol based on a study showing lower birthweights in women treated with atenolol. There is no information on the effects of statin drugs on fetal development, so these drugs probably should not be used.

Pregnancy can be safely undertaken by women who have had a prior coronary artery bypass grafting procedure.

DILATED CARDIOMYOPATHY PRECEDING PREGNANCY

There is virtually no information regarding how to manage patients with preexisting dilated cardiomyopathy as distinct from peripartum cardiomyopathy. It is unknown whether patients with this disorder will undergo worsening of LV function associated with pregnancy, as do many patients with peripartum cardiomyopathy. Management is the same as it would be for patients with LV dysfunction of any etiology. Beta blockers can be continued or initiated. Angiotensin-converting enzyme (ACE) inhibitors should not be used because of the risk of oligohydramnios and renal failure in the fetus. If ACE inhibitors were being given before pregnancy, consider substituting hydralazine and long-acting nitrates instead. Digitalis is safe during pregnancy. Furosemide can be used to help relieve symptoms.

DOUBLE-OUTLET RIGHT VENTRICLE

Double-outlet right ventricle describes a heterogeneous group of anomalies with the common feature of both great vessels originating from the morphologic right ventricle. It may be associated with a relatively normal left ventricle connected to the right ventricle by a VSD or a hypoplastic left ventricle. In some cases, there is also transposition of the great arteries (TGA). For pregnant women with double-outlet right ventricle, the prognosis depends on their specific anatomy and what type of surgical repair was performed; it is impossible to make generalizations.

EBSTEIN'S ANOMALY

In Ebstein's anomaly, the tricuspid valve is displaced toward the cardiac apex. The displacement results in varying degrees of tricuspid regurgitation and enlargement of the right atrium, which will have a ventricularized portion. Ebstein's anomaly is associated with accessory AV bypass tracts and atrial arrhythmias. The degree of tricuspid regurgitation and RV dysfunction can vary widely, depehnding on the degree of tricuspid displacement. Roughly 50% of patients have an ASD or a patent foramen ovale (PFO). Some patients with right-to-left shunts are cyanotic.

There have been a number of reports on small series of patients with Ebstein's anomaly undergoing pregnancy. In the largest, 44 women had 111 pregnancies. The live birth rate was 75%. There were seven therapeutic terminations and 19 spontaneous abortions. Most of the spontaneous abortions (13 of 19) occurred in the patients with an ASD or PFO. There were no maternal deaths and two neonatal deaths.

Pregnancy after tricuspid valve repair or replacement is well tolerated. Women with cyanosis considering pregnancy are often candidates for surgical repair and may want to consider this before pregnancy.

EHLERS-DANLOS TYPE IV (VASCULAR TYPE)

Ehlers-Danlos syndromes are a group of connective tissue disorders characterized by hypermobile joints. A number of different types have been described. Of concern during pregnancy is the vascular type (type IV), which can be associated with a variety of complications, including uterine rupture. These patients also are susceptible to rupture of the aorta, with a risk estimated at 25% of pregnancies. In patients with vascular-type Ehlers-Danlos syndrome, arterial dissections may be difficult to repair because of tissue fragility. A report of 183 pregnancies in 81 women showed that 12 women died within 2 weeks of delivery. Five died from uterine rupture, and 7 died because of a rupture of a major blood vessel. Pregnancy in these women should be considered high risk. It is not known if cesarean section can improve the outcome. The vascular type of Ehlers-Danlos syndrome is autosomal dominant, so women have a 50% chance of passing it on to their children.

HYPERTROPHIC CARDIOMYOPATHY

Women with hypertrophic cardiomyopathy (HOCM) generally tolerate pregnancy well. Diastolic dysfunction is common. Late in the disease, systolic dysfunction may develop in some patients. Patients usually have some mitral regurgitation. Theoretically, the increased intravascular volume of pregnancy, which leads to ventricular dilation, should be beneficial in reducing the subaortic obstruction. However, this effect is offset by the increase in cardiac output, and subaortic gradients tend to increase as pregnancy progresses. The increased heart rate of pregnancy exacerbates diastolic dysfunction.

Tachycardia caused by the pain and stress of delivery and the blood loss related to delivery may increase the degree of obstruction and increase the risk of pulmonary edema.

Patients with any degree of systolic dysfunction and those with severe gradients appear to be at greater risk during pregnancy. Peak gradients over 30 mm Hg should trigger increased vigilance.

Patients with HOCM are at risk for arrhythmias including ventricular tachycardia and atrial fibrillation. Pregnancy does not seem to worsen arrhythmic burden, but data are limited. Atrial fibrillation is poorly tolerated by patients with HOCM, and if it occurs, early cardioversion should be undertaken.

In patients with HOCM, beta blockers should be continued during pregnancy. Metoprolol is preferred. There are concerns about atenolol causing fetal growth restriction. Verapamil can be used but has been associated with heart block in fetuses.

Vaginal delivery is preferred; cesarean section should be reserved for obstetric indications.

Epidural and spinal anesthesia should be titrated slowly and cautiously because of vasodilation and hypotension, which may worsen subvalvular gradients.

Oxytocin should be used carefully to avoid hypotension, tachycardia, and arrhythmia. Administer only a slow intravenous (IV) infusion.

Blood loss should be replaced, but excessive fluid could put the patient at risk for pulmonary edema.

INAPPROPRIATE SINUS TACHYCARDIA

Inappropriate sinus tachycardia is a condition that is relatively common and predominantly seen in young women. It is defined as a syndrome in which the resting daytime heart rate exceeds 100 beats/min and the average 24-hour heart rate is over 90 beats/min. The tachycardia also must produce symptoms and have no identifiable cause. Postural changes in blood pressure must be excluded. Symptoms include palpitations, dizziness, lightheadedness, and near syncope. The etiology is uncertain. Inappropriate sinus tachycardia should be distinguished from both orthostatic hypotension and postural orthostatic tachycardia syndrome (POTS), in which the tachycardia occurs predominantly or only on standing. Often, it is associated with other types of autonomic dysfunction and psychiatric issues.

Beta blockers are the mainstay of therapy; if they fail, ivabradine (a relatively new drug that specifically targets the sinus node) has been successful in a few cases.

However, ivabradine is not recommended for use during pregnancy because of findings of embryofetal toxicity in animal studies. Physical training is helpful, but it is often difficult to get patients to exercise as they dislike the associated increase in heart rate. Often, compression garments and drugs, such as fludrocortisone, are used to increase intravascular volume, but these therapies are unproven. Fludrocortisone should not be used in pregnant women because teratogenicity has been demonstrated in animal studies. In refractory cases, catheter or surgical ablation of the sinus node is sometimes undertaken, but ablation can lead to complications, such as the need for a pacemaker; symptoms can recur even in procedures that initially appear successful.

The prevalence of inappropriate sinus tachycardia is uncertain, but one European study found a prevalence of 1% in middle-aged participants. Despite the fact that this is a relatively common condition, reports of cases in pregnant women are very limited, suggesting that the physiologic changes in the cardiovascular system and the fluid retention of pregnancy may have a beneficial effect. The few case reports of pregnant women with inappropriate sinus tachycardia suggest that it is generally benign. At least one case of rate-related cardiomyopathy in pregnancy has been reported.

KAWASAKI DISEASE

Kawasaki disease is a systemic febrile illness of childhood characterized by diffuse vasculitis. There is no definitive test, and the diagnosis is made on clinical grounds. Typical features include abrupt onset of high fever, polymorphous exanthem, pharyngeal erythema, cracked fissured lips, a strawberry tongue, bilateral conjunctival injection, cervical lymphedema, extremity changes (edema, palmar, and sole erythema), and periungual desquamation in the convalescent phase. The most serious manifestation is coronary arteritis, which can lead to the formation of a coronary aneurysm in 20% to 25% of untreated patients. Treatment with aspirin and IV immunoglobulin can reduce this risk to about 5%. About half of the coronary aneurysms in patients with Kawasaki disease will regress. Those that persist may lead to ischemic heart disease, myocardial infarction (MI), and death. The aneurysms virtually never rupture but are prone to thrombosis. Most women will have had their coronary artery disease

addressed by the time they are of childbearing age and may not require extensive further evaluation. Persistent aneurysms pose an ongoing risk of thrombosis, and those greater than 8 mm seem to be especially high risk. Because pregnancy is a hypercoagulable state, the concern is that it may trigger aneurysm thrombosis. Although the numbers are small, virtually all reported cases of pregnancy in women with Kawasaki disease have resulted in good outcomes for both the mother and the baby. Treatment with low-dose aspirin (81 mg/day) seems sufficient to prevent aneurysm thrombosis in pregnant women. However, the 2017 Kawasaki disease guidelines recommend that those with medium to large coronary artery aneurysms should be supervised by a multidisciplinary team, including a cardiologist, to aid in thromboprophylaxis management during pregnancy and delivery.

LEFT VENTRICULAR NONCOMPACTION

Left ventricular noncompaction is a rare cardiomyopathy characterized by deep trabeculations in the LV myocardium. The degree of LV dysfunction is variable. Some individuals present with overt heart failure, fatal arrhythmias, and thromboembolic events; others remain asymptomatic. Echocardiographic criteria to help identify and assess noncompaction rely on the presence of LV myocardial trabeculations and a two-layer distinction between compacted and noncompacted myocardium. One must be careful of making an initial diagnosis in a pregnant woman because an increase in the degree of LV trabeculation in pregnancy has been reported to occur in as many as 25% of women. In 8% of pregnant women, the trabeculations are pronounced enough to meet the criteria for making a diagnosis of LV noncompaction. During a postpartum follow-up period of 24 ± 3 months, 73% of women demonstrated complete resolution of trabeculations, and 5% showed a marked reduction in the trabeculated layer.

If the diagnosis of LV noncompaction is made before pregnancy, the potential risk during pregnancy depends on the degree of LV dysfunction. It is uncertain if the usual medical therapy for LV dysfunction benefits patients with noncompaction. Successful pregnancies in women with noncompaction have been reported. In one case report, the woman had an uncomplicated course, but the baby also had noncompaction and died of heart failure shortly after birth.

LOEYS-DIETZ SYNDROME

Loeys-Dietz is a genetic syndrome with clinical features similar to Marfan syndrome, including an aorta susceptible to aneurysms and dissection, hypertelorism, and a cleft palate. Congenital heart defects, such as ASDs, bicuspid aortic valves, and patent ductus arteriosus (PDA), are sometimes present. The concern during pregnancy is that the aorta might rupture, and patients should be managed accordingly. Hypertension, if present, should be treated aggressively. Beta blockers may be considered, and the second stage of labor should be curtailed.

MARFAN SYNDROME

Patients with Marfan syndrome are predisposed to aortic dissection. They have an approximately 1% risk of aortic rupture. If aortic dissection occurs, surgery is the treatment of choice for type A dissection. Medical therapy with beta blockers is the treatment of choice for type B dissections.

As reflected in various guidelines, women with Marfan syndrome and a dilated aorta, larger than 4.5 cm, are probably at increased risk and should undergo surgical repair before pregnancy.

Women with Marfan syndrome should be kept on beta blockers throughout pregnancy. Labetalol is probably the agent of choice because it has a history of extensive use in pregnancy. Metoprolol is a reasonable alternative. When given early in pregnancy, atenolol has been associated with fetal growth restriction and thus should be avoided altogether.

Women with Marfan syndrome have an increased risk of spontaneous abortion and premature delivery, likely because of connective tissue abnormalities in the uterus, which occur in some patients with Marfan syndrome.

Cesarean section should be considered to avoid the blood pressure fluctuations associated with vaginal delivery.

MITRAL REGURGITATION

Mitral regurgitation is generally well tolerated during pregnancy. If it is severe or if it is associated with pre-existing LV dysfunction, congestive heart failure may occur and should be treated as systolic left-sided failure is treated in patients with other conditions.

MITRAL STENOSIS

Mitral stenosis is poorly tolerated during pregnancy. Ideally, it will be detected and treated before pregnancy. Medical treatment can be with beta blockers to prolong diastolic filling time. For younger women with rheumatic mitral stenosis who become pregnant, percutaneous valvuloplasty can be considered.

Patients who do have mitral stenosis and become pregnant typically develop symptoms during the second trimester, when heart rate and cardiac output increase significantly. The usual symptom is dyspnea; occasionally, atrial fibrillation occurs. If the stenosis is severe, pulmonary edema may occur.

The best way to estimate the degree of stenosis is with a valve area. A normal value is 4.0 to 6.0 cm^2. Severe stenosis is indicated by a valve area of 1.5 cm^2 or less.

MYOCARDIAL INFARCTION

Myocardial infarction is a rare complication of pregnancy, with an incidence of 1 in 10,000 pregnancies. The most common cause of MI in pregnancy is probably coronary dissection, and although data are virtually nonexistent, the risk of recurrence during subsequent pregnancies is believed to be high. Other causes include coronary atherosclerosis, thrombosis, and cocaine abuse. About 80% of MIs occur in the peripartum period. Older literature suggests that MI during pregnancy most commonly involves the left anterior descending artery.

The diagnosis of MI in pregnant women is made as it is in patients who are not expecting: a clinical history of typical chest pain, ECG changes of ST-segment elevation or Q waves, and elevation of cardiac enzymes. In the postpartum period, creatine kinase isoenzyme MB (CKMB) levels rise because they are released from the myometrium. Troponin levels should not be affected by pregnancy.

Pregnant women with MI should be investigated with coronary angiography. Angioplasty should be undertaken urgently for appropriate cases with thrombotic or embolic etiologies. Dissection in pregnancy usually involves most of the length of the affected coronary artery and therefore must be treated surgically. Delivery is deferred until the interventions for the MI have been completed. The mortality rate is high.

PERICARDIAL DISEASE

About 40% of women develop a benign hydropericardium by the third trimester, but the development of pericarditis is unusual. When pericardial disease does develop, it may take the form of idiopathic pericarditis, pericarditis associated with connective tissue disease, constrictive pericarditis, or tamponade.

Idiopathic Pericarditis

Idiopathic pericarditis, the most common type of pericardial disease seen in the general population, is thought to be caused by a viral infection. It is often treated with antiinflammatory drugs to relieve symptoms. Aspirin and nonsteroidal antiinflammatory drugs (NSAIDs) are commonly used. Colchicine and steroids also are used. There is no predilection for the development of pericarditis during pregnancy, but sporadic cases occur.

Aspirin is the drug of choice for pregnant patients requiring treatment of acute pericarditis. NSAIDs are relatively contraindicated in pregnancy because of their potential associated effects, such as closing of the ductus or adversely affecting fetal renal function. However, they may be used safely before 32 weeks of gestation. Steroids may be considered for use at any time during pregnancy but are probably best reserved for resistant cases or those associated with connective tissue disease. Colchicine is a category C (US Food and Drug Administration) drug because animal reproduction studies have shown adverse effects on fetuses. However, reports of several hundred women taking colchicine during pregnancy have not shown adverse effects on either mother or baby.

A report of idiopathic pericarditis in six pregnancies treated with aspirin 800 mg three times a day and prednisone 2.5 to 25.0 mg/day found that both the women and the babies did well. One woman developed HELLP (hemolysis, elevated liver enzymes, and low platelet counts) syndrome, probably unrelated to the pericarditis. One mother had a recurrence of pericarditis 12 months later.

Rarely, pericarditis is caused by infections other than a virus, such as tuberculosis, and may require treatment with antibiotics. Treatment would be the same as in a nonpregnant patient. Unusual causes of pericarditis, such as those associated with cancer, cardiac trauma, or uremia, may be encountered rarely in pregnancy. Treatment is unchanged by pregnancy.

Pericarditis Associated with Connective Tissue Disease

Many connective tissue diseases can cause pericarditis, and when this happens, most cases are treated in the same way as idiopathic pericarditis. Often, steroids are used earlier, particularly if there are other signs of disease flare. If indicated, steroids can be used at any time during pregnancy.

Constrictive Pericarditis

In most cases, constrictive pericarditis does not require treatment during pregnancy, but several cases of pericardiectomy during pregnancy have been reported, with good outcomes for both the mother and baby.

Tamponade

Cardiac tamponade is immediately life threatening and must be treated by removing pericardial fluid, either by needle drainage or a surgical drainage. It occurs only rarely in pregnancy, but it must be recognized and treated in the same way as if the woman was not pregnant, that is, by urgent drainage. To limit exposing the fetus to radiation, ultrasound guidance is preferable to fluoroscopic guidance.

PERIPARTUM CARDIOMYOPATHY

Peripartum cardiomyopathy is defined as the development of systolic heart failure in the last month of pregnancy or within 5 months after delivery without identifiable etiology. Risk factors include maternal age older than 30 years, gestational hypertension, and twin pregnancies.

Treatment is the same as for systolic heart failure of any cause. Beta blockers, such as carvedilol, are the mainstay of therapy for systolic heart failure in nonpregnant patients, and there is no reason to think they should not be effective during pregnancy, but they have not been studied extensively. ACE inhibitors can be used postpartum, but they are contraindicated during pregnancy. Hydralazine and nitrates may be used during pregnancy. Diuretics are used for relief of congestion.

Patients with severe LV dysfunction are at risk for the development of mural thrombi; anticoagulation should be considered. In patients with persistent LV dysfunction, the mortality rate may be as high as 20% with subsequent pregnancies.

In about 50% of patients, normalization of LV function occurs within 6 months of delivery.

PERIPHERAL EDEMA

Peripheral edema is very common, occurring in up to 80% of normal pregnancies. Typically, it manifests late in the second trimester or in the third trimester; the development of edema earlier than this may indicate a pathologic situation. In general, there is no recommended treatment for peripheral edema during pregnancy. Sodium restriction is ineffective. In the absence of pulmonary edema, diuretics generally should be avoided because of the potential adverse effects on hemodynamics and electrolyte concentrations. For comfort, women should avoid standing for prolonged periods or sitting with the legs dependent; frequent leg movement is appropriate. Lying on the side also may be helpful because it avoids vena cava compression. In cases of severe leg edema, wearing compression stockings or wrapping the legs with elastic wraps can be helpful; reportedly, a figure-8 wrap is more effective than a spiral wrap.

PATENT DUCTUS ARTERRIOSUS

The outcome of pregnant patients with a PDA is usually favorable, but clinical deterioration and heart failure have been reported. A large, nonrestrictive PDA would be expected to cause pulmonary hypertension before reaching childbearing age. In these cases, pregnancy is contraindicated. In patients with pulmonary hypertension, reversal of the shunt can occur secondary to hypotension and can be prevented with vasopressors. Patients with a history of a patent ductus that has been ligated or a small hemodynamically insignificant PDA, are expected to do well in pregnancy with a low risk of cardiac complications.

POSTURAL ORTHOSTATIC TACHYCARDIA SYNDROME

Postural orthostatic tachycardia syndrome is a syndrome in which the heart rate increases with standing but blood pressure does not drop, which distinguishes it from orthostatic hypotension. The diagnosis of POTS is made based on a 30-beats/min increase in heart rate with a change from sitting to standing and with a less-than-20-mm-Hg drop in systolic blood pressure and the development of symptoms.

Treatment includes drugs, such as beta blockers and ivabradine, to slow the heart rate and compression garments and fludrocortisone to increase intravascular volume. Vasoconstrictors, such as ProAmatine, are often used; another common therapy is serotonin reuptake inhibitors.

POTS does not seem to contribute to pregnancy-related complications.

About half of women with POTS report improvement of symptoms with pregnancy. About one-third report worsening of symptoms, and the rest have unchanged symptoms. Postpartum, about half of women report improved or stable symptoms.

PULMONARY ATRESIA

Pulmonary atresia with a VSD is generally considered an extreme form of tetralogy of Fallot, in which there is congenital atresia of the RV outlet. In pulmonary atresia with VSD, the anatomy and size of the main and branch pulmonary arteries dictate surgical options. In the most severe form, there is an absence of a main pulmonary artery and an absence or severe hypoplasia of the branch pulmonary arteries; the lungs receive their blood flow from collateral arteries extending from the aorta (major aortopulmonary collateral arteries). In such cases, patients rarely survive to adulthood without surgical intervention. There is one report of 14 patients who had 24 pregnancies. Two were unoperated. There were no maternal deaths and one neonatal death. The miscarriage rate was 50%.

Pulmonary atresia with intact ventricular septum is a condition in which, by definition, there is no VSD, and the only outflow from the right atrium is across an ASD. Surgical repair is based on the size of the right ventricle and tricuspid valve. In cases in which the tricuspid valve and right ventricle are markedly hypoplastic, patients undergo surgical palliation as a single ventricle (see later discussion). In patients with an adequate tricuspid valve and right ventricle, their management and pregnancy outcomes are similar to patients with tetralogy of Fallot.

PULMONARY HYPERTENSION

Pulmonary hypertension is defined as a mean pulmonary artery pressure greater than 25 mm Hg as assessed by right heart catheterization. Pulmonary hypertension is classified into five main types based on etiology: (1)

pulmonary arterial hypertension, which can be idiopathic or associated with other conditions, such as systemic sclerosis or congenital heart disease; (2) pulmonary hypertension associated with left-heart disease; (3) pulmonary hypertension associated with lung disease; (4) chronic thromboembolic pulmonary hypertension; and (5) an idiopathic group. Surgical procedures are recommended for those with the chronic thromboembolic type; surgery could be considered before pregnancy. It would be best to consider patients with pulmonary hypertension as five distinct groups, but because all these conditions are rare and the number of pregnant patients with them is small, almost all series mix etiologic groups.

Improved medical care for patients with pulmonary hypertension has increased their life expectancy, resulting in more women with pulmonary hypertension considering pregnancy or becoming pregnant. Pulmonary hypertension during pregnancy is a high-risk situation for both the mother and the fetus, and thus, pregnancy in women with pulmonary hypertension should be discouraged. The maternal mortality rate has been reported as high as 56% in patients with severe pulmonary hypertension, although, as for all patients with pulmonary hypertension, the prognosis for pregnant women with the disorder has been improving. More recent studies indicate mortality rates of 17% in patients with idiopathic pulmonary hypertension and 28% in those with congenital heart disease, and most recently, a group from France has reported a 5% maternal mortality rate in a group of women with pulmonary hypertension related to congenital heart disease. The reduced mortality rate may be due, in part, to the apparent lower mortality in women who respond to calcium channel blockers or other therapy. Most cases of death occur in the early postpartum period. Heart failure is most common, but sudden death and thromboembolism also contribute.

During pregnancy, pulmonary resistance decreases in normal women. In patients with pulmonary hypertension, this decrease is limited, leading to a rise in pulmonary pressures, which often leads to right heart failure. Shifting of the intraventricular septum caused by the increased right heart pressures also may impair left heart filling, leading to diastolic left-sided impairment, which compromises cardiac output. Women with Eisenmenger syndrome may have increasing right-to-left shunting, which leads to hypoxemia, and may lead to increased pulmonary vasoconstriction and worsening right heart failure.

A retrospective review of pregnant women with pulmonary hypertension was conducted at four academic tertiary care institutions from 2001-2015 and detailed the use of advanced therapies such as pulmonary vasodilators, extracorporeal membrane oxygenation, inotropes, and vasopressors. Women with primary pulmonary arterial hypertension (type 1) or chronic thromboembolic pulmonary hypertension (type 4) were more likely require advanced therapies and dual therapy than women with other types of pulmonary hypertension. Use of anticoagulation varied by site with incomplete data from all institutions. Intrapartum pulmonary artery catheterization was utilized in nearly 30% of the women in labor, and no adverse events were reported to have occurred following placement or use of the pulmonary artery catheters.[1]

When mothers have pulmonary hypertension, neonatal survival rates are about 90%. The main risks to the fetus are related to maternal hypoxemia and include preterm delivery, growth restriction, and stillbirth.

If a woman with pulmonary hypertension does become pregnant, she must be monitored carefully, and if signs of decompensation are detected, early therapeutic abortion should be considered. Deterioration of pulmonary hypertension during pregnancy occurs most often between weeks 20 and 24, by which time most of the pregnancy-associated hemodynamic changes have occurred. In women who decompensate during this time period, therapeutic abortion is recommended. A second period of high risk occurs postpartum. If a woman with pulmonary hypertension deteriorates, vasodilator therapy should be started immediately because outcomes are poor in cases in which therapy is delayed.

Many of the drugs used to treat pulmonary hypertension are contraindicated during pregnancy (Table 7.1). Endothelin receptor antagonists are category X. Treatment options for pregnant women with pulmonary hypertension include calcium channel blockers (category C), epoprostenol, iloprost, phosphodiesterase type 5 (PDE5) inhibitors, oxygen, nitric oxide, and others. Combination therapy—often used in nonpregnant patients—also may be necessary in pregnant patients.

Calcium Channel Blockers

Calcium channel blockers in high doses are used to treat patients deemed vasoreactive. Vasoreactivity is defined

TABLE 7.1   **Pulmonary Hypertension Therapies**

Class	Drug	Administration	Cons
Calcium channel blockers	Diltiazem, amlodipine, nifedipine	Oral	Only works in 10% of patients
PDE5 inhibitor	Tadalafil	Oral	
PDE5 inhibitor	Sildenafil	Oral	
ERA	Bosentan	Oral	Potential teratogenicity
ERA	Sitaxsentan	Oral	Potential teratogenicity
ERA	Ambrisentan	Oral	Potential teratogenicity
Prostanoid	Epoprostenol	IV	IV
Prostanoid	Iloprost	IV	IV
Prostanoid	Iloprost nebulized	inhaled	
Prostanoid	Treprostinil	SC, oral, inhaled	
Stimulates nitric oxide production	Soluble guanylate cyclase stimulator	Oral	Not believed to be safe in pregnancy

ERA, endothelin receptor antagonist; *PDE5*, phosphodiesterase type 5 inhibitor; *IV*, intravenous; *SC*, subcutaneous.

at right heart catherization by measuring the response to a pulmonary vasodilating drug such as nitrous oxide. Ideally, this will have been determined before pregnancy. The daily doses that have shown efficacy are 120 to 240 mg for nifedipine, 240 to 720 mg for diltiazem, and 20 mg for amlodipine. The dose is usually titrated upward cautiously. The limiting factor is most often systemic hypotension. Women taking these medications before pregnancy should be continued on them after they become pregnant. Newly diagnosed women with severe pulmonary hypertension are likely better off with other therapies.

Epoprostenol

Epoprostenol is a prostaglandin and vasodilator; continuous infusion of epoprostenol has been used in select cases with good outcomes reported. It has been demonstrated to improve hemodynamics, symptoms, exercise capacity, and mortality rate in nonpregnant patients. It is a pregnancy category B drug. Administered intravenously in an initial dose of 2 to 4 ng/kg/min, it is then titrated upward. The usual optimal dose is between 20 and 40 ng/kg/min. Epoprostenol may cause platelet inhibition, which is of concern during epidural placement. It is considered the best therapy for cases of severe pulmonary hypertension.

Iloprost

Iloprost is a prostacyclin analogue that reduces vascular resistance and arterial pressure. It is a pregnancy category C drug administered by inhalation. Other prostacyclin analogues are under evaluation.

Phosphodiesterase Type 5 Inhibitors

Drugs that inhibit PDE5 are now used frequently to treat patients with pulmonary hypertension. Tadalafil, vardenafil, and sildenafil were originally marketed to treat erectile dysfunction, but they are also potent pulmonary vasodilators. Sildenafil has been used in individual cases and appears to be safe, but experience with this drug is limited. Sildenafil causes vasodilation of both the pulmonary and systemic circulation. It is a pregnancy category B drug; the usual dose is 20 mg three times a day.

Oxygen

Although oxygen is a vasodilator, there are no studies that support its long-term use in improving the prognosis even in patients with Eisenmenger syndrome. It should be used only if hypoxemia is present. Continuous oxygen therapy is recommended for patients with a pO_2 less than 60 mm Hg. If iron deficiency or anemia is present, these should be corrected also.

Nitric Oxide

Breathing low concentrations of nitric oxide produces selective pulmonary vasodilation and increases exercise capacity in patients with pulmonary hypertension. Continuous or intermittent nitrous oxide inhalation has been proposed as a chronic pulmonary vasodilator therapy; however, many patients with pulmonary hypertension do not have a vasodilator response to inhaled nitrous oxide, and in patients who do respond, the duration of vasodilation after cessation is brief. It probably has little place in treatment of pregnant patients with pulmonary hypertension.

Other Therapies

Digoxin is of no proven benefit; neither are beta blockers. For patients who decompensate, the treatment team may need to consider the use of venoarterial extracorporeal membrane oxygenation, right heart assist devices, and heart–lung or double-lung transplant.

In women with pulmonary hypertension, it is unclear whether vaginal delivery or cesarean section is preferable. Guidelines from the Pulmonary Vascular Research Institute recommend the latter, but data from the European registry of pregnancy and cardiac disease found that planned cesarean section offered no advantage for the mother and was associated with an increased risk for the fetus. However, if hemodynamic deterioration occurs, cesarean section is indicated. If vaginal delivery is chosen, low-dose epidural analgesia is best. It has no significant deleterious effect on hemodynamics, and it decreases the adverse hemodynamic consequences of labor. The adverse effects of vaginal delivery include Valsalva maneuver, which increases intrathoracic pressure; labor-induced vagal responses; sympathetic nervous system activation caused by pain; and autotransfusion during uterine contraction. If cesarean section is performed, slowly titrated epidural anesthesia is ideal because it minimizes adverse hemodynamic effects while providing surgical anesthesia. At least 20 to 30 minutes is required to achieve an adequate block while maintaining stable hemodynamics. General anesthesia and spinal anesthesia may be safely administered but cause more significant hemodynamic disturbance. They require close monitoring (including invasive hemodynamic monitors) and strict attention to fluid status, oxygenation, and ventilation. If cesarean section is performed, both general anesthesia and spinal anesthesia may have significant hemodynamic consequences. In women with pulmonary hypertension, careful monitoring and attention to hemodynamics are imperative. Intubation, laryngoscopy, and positive-pressure ventilation may increase pulmonary arterial pressure. A slowly titrated epidural or a low-dose-combined spinal epidural can provide surgical anesthesia with less hemodynamic consequences and may be an ideal option in planned cesarean section. During general anesthesia, it has been reported that laryngoscopy and intubation

lead to increases in pulmonary artery pressure. There also may be a deleterious effect of positive-pressure ventilation on venous return.

If necessary, the physician may consider inducing labor; there are cases when oxytocin and prostaglandin E have been used with good outcome. Prostaglandin E generally reduces pulmonary artery pressure. Oxytocin is a vasodilator and must be used cautiously to avoid hypotension.

It is probably best to avoid direct pulmonary artery pressure monitoring with a Swan-Ganz catheter because there is an increased risk of pulmonary artery rupture and thrombosis in patients with pulmonary hypertension.

The postpartum period is the most critical period to monitor for acute decompensation. If oxytocin is used, it must be infused slowly because large doses can be fatal in patients with unstable hemodynamics. A patient's hemodynamics may not return to baseline for 6 months after delivery, but the majority of changes occur in weeks 2 to 4 postpartum. Monitoring must be continued after delivery, and several weeks of in-hospital monitoring is usually recommended. Therapy for symptomatic women may include nitric oxide, inhaled iloprost, or IV epoprostenol.

Thromboembolic risk is high in pregnant women with pulmonary hypertension, and generally, thromboprophylaxis should be initiated. In women with a history of thromboembolic disease, higher levels of anticoagulation may be needed.

Fluid management is difficult as both hyper- and hypovolemia are detrimental.

Because pregnancy is to be discouraged in patients with pulmonary hypertension, contraception is often prescribed. Estrogen-containing contraceptives are not recommended because of the increased risk of venous thromboembolism and deleterious effects of estrogen on the pulmonary vasculature. Progesterone-only preparations, such as medroxyprogesterone acetate and etonogestrel, may be used. Intrauterine devices and progestin-only implants also are acceptable. On insertion, these may elicit vasovagal responses, which may be poorly tolerated in women with pulmonary hypertension.

PULMONARY VALVE REGURGITATION

Chronic pulmonic regurgitation, like other regurgitant lesions, is well tolerated during pregnancy. Although the increase in blood volume tends to increase the regurgitant volume, the latter is partially compensated for by other mechanisms, such as the increase in heart rate and the decrease in pulmonary vascular resistance.

PULMONIC STENOSIS

Pulmonic stenosis is well tolerated during pregnancy. Because of impairment of right-sided forward flow, the increase in blood volume during pregnancy may lead to peripheral edema, which can be treated with leg elevation, compression stockings, diuretics, or a combination of these, depending on its severity.

SINGLE VENTRICLE

A single ventricle or univentricular–AV connection may present with several varieties, including tricuspid atresia, hypoplastic left heart syndrome, double-inlet left ventricle, unbalanced AV canal, or pulmonary atresia with intact ventricular septum. In all these cases, there is either a severely hypoplastic ventricle (right or left), a hypoplastic or atretic AV valve, or both. Tricuspid atresia is a common single ventricle lesion, in which a single AV valve connecting to a single left ventricle is present. Conversely, in hypoplastic left heart syndrome, there is a single AV valve connected to a single right ventricle. There also may be two AV valves connecting to a single ventricle, which is called a double inlet ventricle. Few patients with single ventricles survive to childbearing age unless a surgical intervention has been performed. Surgical repair can consist of the creation of shunts or a complete palliative repair, a Fontan procedure. A Fontan procedure involves connecting the superior and inferior vena cavae directly to the pulmonary arteries such that pulmonary blood flow is passive without a subpulmonary pump. This circulation causes chronic elevation of the central venous pressure, and the degree of this elevation is the main determinant of the risks of pregnancy.

In patients who have not undergone the Fontan procedure who have pulmonic stenosis that has prevented the development of severe pulmonary hypertension, pregnancy is possible, but it is associated with increased risk for both the mother and the fetus. There are only a few case reports of successful pregnancy in single-ventricle patients who have not had a Fontan procedure. There is greater experience with pregnancy in women who have

had a Fontan procedure. One study of 28 pregnancies in 11 women who had had a Fontan repair reported a live birth rate of 43%. There is a high rate of spontaneous abortion, which may be partly attributed to the fact that many women with a Fontan repair are taking chronic anticoagulation medications. Risks to the mother include atrial arrhythmia, reported to occur in as many as 50% of pregnancies. Mothers also may be at risk for heart failure, reported in almost 10% of pregnancies. Ventricular function typically returns to baseline after delivery.

Thromboembolic complications are also a concern in patients post-Fontan repair, particularly those with a severely dilated right atrium with stasis.

SYSTEMIC LUPUS ERYTHEMATOSUS

Systemic lupus erythematosus (SLE) is a disease that can affect many organ systems, including the reproductive system and the heart. In fact, frequent miscarriage is listed as one of the clinical diagnostic features of SLE. Cardiac manifestations may include pericarditis, myocarditis, valvular heart disease, and coronary thrombosis, as well as systemic and pulmonary hypertension.

Systemic lupus in the mother is believed to be the cause of the majority of cases of congenital heart block. The heart block is usually complete and caused by passive autoimmunity developing in the fetus. It occurs in the offspring of mothers with anti-Ro and anti-La antibodies, which cross the placenta and gain access to the fetal circulation during weeks 16 to 30 of gestation. Patients with lupus who are positive for these antibodies should undergo monitoring to detect the presence of fetal heart block, which may undergo partial reversibility with steroid therapy. Women who have had a baby with congenital complete heart block are at high risk for this to recur during subsequent pregnancies.

About 40% of systemic lupus patients have antiphospholipid antibodies, including anticardiolipin antibodies, and lupus anticoagulant; these are associated with recurrent thrombosis and obstetric complications, such as premature delivery and miscarriage. Systemic lupus patients with anticardiolipin antibodies are also prone to developing valvular heart disease, particularly aortic and mitral regurgitation.

Patients with lupus often have an exacerbation of their disease during or immediately after pregnancy.

TAKOTSUBO CARDIOMYOPATHY

Takotsubo cardiomyopathy is a condition that mimics an acute MI. It is characterized by chest pain, elevated cardiac enzymes, and ST elevation on the ECG. It is associated with a specific pattern of myocardial injury involving the cardiac apex, and it is typically diagnosed when cardiac catheterization reveals normal coronary arteries, with apical dysfunction of the left ventricle. The Mayo clinic has published a list of diagnostic criteria:

1. Transient hypokinesis, dyskinesis, or akinesis of the LV midsegments, with or without apical involvement; the regional wall motion abnormalities extend beyond a single epicardial vascular distribution, and a stressful trigger is often, but not always, present
2. Absence of obstructive coronary disease or angiographic evidence of acute plaque rupture
3. New ECG abnormalities (either ST segment elevation or T-wave inversion) or modest elevation in the cardiac troponin level
4. Absence of pheochromocytoma or myocarditis

Takotsubo cardiomyopathy is most common in females; women account for about 90% of cases. The pathophysiology is thought to involve excess levels of catecholamines. It is often associated with a traumatic event and is sometimes called "broken heart syndrome." Although serious complications—such as cardiac rupture, ventricular fibrillation, and death—can occur, complete recovery of LV function in a few months is the rule. Takotsubo cardiomyopathy has been reported in pregnancy and seems to follow the usual course. Treatment is directed at treating the LV dysfunction with beta blockers. ACE inhibitors may be used postpartum but generally should not be used in pregnancy.

TETRALOGY OF FALLOT

Tetralogy of Fallot consists of a combination of congenital defects, including a VSD just below the aortic valve, an overriding aorta, and some degree of obstruction to RV outflow. Unrepaired, this combination leads to RV hypertrophy, the classical fourth component of the tetralogy. Patients with mild, unrepaired tetralogy may survive until adulthood.

During pregnancy, systemic vascular resistance falls, and this generally causes an increase in the degree of right-to-left shunting in patients with unrepaired tetralogy. After delivery, the degree of right-to-left shunting will likely increase again because of blood loss and hypotension.

Unrepaired tetralogy is often associated with aortic regurgitation, which may further complicate pregnancy. A series of 21 patients with 46 pregnancies who had either unrepaired tetralogy or pulmonary atresia with aortopulmonary collateral reported 15 live births (33%). Nine babies were born prematurely. Eight mothers experienced cardiovascular complications, including two cases of endocarditis.

After repair, the prognosis for pregnancy is much improved. A series from the Netherlands reported on 26 women who had 50 successful pregnancies. Complications occurred in 19% of patients and included symptomatic right heart failure and arrhythmias. Both patients who developed right heart failure had pulmonic regurgitation, which is a common residual after surgical repair.

The risk of congenital heart defects in offspring of a parent with tetralogy has been reported to be 2.5% to 8.3%.

TRANSPOSITON OF THE GREAT ARTERIES

In the following paragraphs, we discuss congenitally corrected L-TGA and D-TGA.

Congenitally Corrected L-Transposition of the Great Arteries

In this condition, systemic venous blood enters the right atrium, which is connected to the mitral valve, and a right-sided morphologic left ventricle that pumps blood to the systemic circulation. Therefore, the morphologic right ventricle is supporting the systemic circulation, and the increased volume load during pregnancy may lead to heart failure. Several series of patients with congenitally corrected transposition have been presented. Unfortunately, the series contain small numbers of patients, and some had other cardiac lesions, so it is difficult to draw firm conclusions; however, in the absence of associated lesions, patients seem to do well. The risks of heart failure were 1 in 22 in one series and 3 in 19 in a second. Both studies were retrospective and involved multiple pregnancies in each group of women. A total of 75 live births were reported; only 1 of the live births had congenital heart disease. There were no maternal deaths.

D-Transposition of the Great Arteries

In this anomaly, the aorta arises from the morphologic right ventricle, and the pulmonary artery arises from the morphologic left ventricle, leading to parallel circulations and causing severe, neonatal cyanosis. There is usually a communication between the two circulations with an ASD, a VSD, or a patent ductus that provide some degree of mixing. Unoperated, patients do not survive until adulthood. With surgical repair, most women will survive to childbearing age. Historically, this defect was repaired with the atrial switch (a Mustard or Senning procedure). These surgeries involve placement of an atrial baffle, which directs pulmonary venous return to the right ventricle and the transposed aorta, and systemic venous return to the left ventricle and pulmonary artery. Similar to those with congenitally corrected transposition, the morphologic right ventricle is supporting the systemic circulation, and the increased volume load during pregnancy may lead to heart failure. RV dysfunction can occur during pregnancy and in some cases does not recover after pregnancy. Given the multiple atrial suture lines, atrial arrhythmias and sinus node dysfunction are common. There is also a high risk of preterm birth—50% in one series involving 25 pregnancies.

Since the late 1980s, the most common operation for D-TGA has been the arterial switch operation. This surgery switches the aorta and pulmonary artery above the valves and makes the left ventricle the systemic ventricle. There are few data on pregnancy outcomes after an arterial switch operation because the early surgical successes are just now reaching childbearing age. In patients with preserved ventricular function without outflow obstruction, pregnancy is expected to be well tolerated.

TRICUSPID ATRESIA

Tricuspid atresia most often results in a single ventricle type of anomaly. Few patients with a single ventricle survive to childbearing age unless a surgical intervention has been performed. Surgical repair can consist of the creation of shunts or a definitive repair, which is a Fontan procedure. The presence or absence of pulmonary hypertension is the main determinant of the risks of pregnancy. The ventricular function is also important in determining the risk of pregnancy. If there is pulmonic stenosis that has prevented the development of severe pulmonary hypertension, pregnancy is possible, but it is associated with increased risk for both the mother and the fetus. There are only a few case reports of successful pregnancy in single-ventricle patients who have not had a Fontan repair. There is a greater experience with pregnancy in women who have had a Fontan repair. One study of 28 pregnancies in 11 women who had had a Fontan repair reported a live birth rate of 43%. There is a high spontaneous abortion rate, which partly caused by to the fact that many women with a Fontan repair are on chronic anticoagulation. Risks to the mother include atrial arrhythmia, which has been reported to occur in as many as 50% of pregnancies. Mothers also may be at risk for heart failure, reported in almost 10% of pregnancies. Ventricular function typically returns to baseline after delivery.

TRICUSPID REGURGITATION

Chronic tricuspid regurgitation is well tolerated during pregnancy. Although the increase in blood volume tends to increase the regurgitant volume, the latter is partially compensated for by other mechanisms, such as the increase in heart rate and the decrease in pulmonary vascular resistance. Tricuspid regurgitation caused by Ebstein anomaly has the associated risk of atrial arrhythmias.

TRICUSPID STENOSIS

Tricuspid stenosis causes obstruction to right-sided forward flow, and if it is severe, the stenosis may cause peripheral edema. The increase in blood volume during pregnancy exacerbates this tendency for edema. Depending on its severity, peripheral edema can be treated with leg elevation, compression stockings, diuretics, or a combination of these.

VASOVAGAL SYNCOPE

Vasovagal syncope, or neurally mediated syncope, is a type of reflex syncope (brief loss of consciousness) caused by a neurologically mediated decrease in blood pressure, heart rate, or both. It may be initiated by a stressor or an event that stimulates the vagus nerve, such as nausea and vomiting. These reflexes can be triggered in virtually anyone if the stimulus is strong enough. Individuals prone to vasovagal syncope may have frequent events that may be triggered easily or for no obvious reason. Intravascular volume depletion is an exacerbating factor.

Treatment to prevent spells includes avoiding triggers such as volume depletion, heat, and drug-induced vasodilation. In addition, hydration and measures to increase intravascular volume, such as salt loading or fludrocortisone, are often used. Vasoconstrictors, such as ProAmatine, also may be helpful. Repetitive tilt or tilt training may be beneficial as well. In rare cases, pacemakers are used to prevent bradycardia, and some can be programmed to pace at faster-than-normal rates with onset of the spell in an attempt to prevent syncope. If pacing is used, a pacemaker with a closed loop rate responsive sensor is likely the most effective type.

There are few reports of vasovagal syncope in pregnancy, suggesting it is uncommon or perhaps not worthy of reporting. Presumably, the increased blood volume of pregnancy is helpful in preventing episodes. Young women with vasovagal episodes usually have a benign prognosis, including during pregnancy. However, there are a few case reports of adverse events attributed to vasovagal syncope in pregnant women. These include abruptio placenta, hypoxic brain injury to the fetus because of prolonged hypotension, and cardiac arrest.

The treatment of vasovagal syncope in pregnancy is the same as in nonpregnant patients.

VENTRICULAR SEPTAL DEFECTS

Patients with small VSDs generally tolerate pregnancy well if pulmonary pressures are normal and the degree of shunting is not significantly altered by pregnancy. Patients with large VSDs may develop pulmonary vascular disease with eventual reversal of shunt, Eisenmenger syndrome, with poor pregnancy outcomes as described earlier. Large VSDs should be closed before pregnancy is considered. In small- to moderate-sized unrepaired VSDs, occasional cases of left-sided congestive heart failure have been reported. In patients who have undergone surgical closure of a VSD, in the absence of pulmonary hypertension, the risk of pregnancy after VSD closure is the same as in patients without heart disease. If residual pulmonary hypertension is present, and the pulmonary pressures are 75% or more of systemic, the risk of pregnancy is high (30%–50% mortality rate). For a child of a woman with a VSD, the risk that the child also will have one is 4% to 11%.

BIBLIOGRAPHY

Aortic Dissection
Anderson RA, Fineron FW. Aortic dissection in pregnancy: importance of pregnancy induced changes in the vessel wall and bicuspid aortic valve in pathogenesis. *Br J Obstet Gynaecol*. 1994;101(12):1085–1088.
Immer FF, Bansi AG, Immer-Bansi AS, et al. Aortic dissection in pregnancy: analysis of risk factors and outcome. *Ann Thorac Surg*. 2003;76:309–314.
Kinney-Hamm L. Acute aortic dissection in third trimester pregnancy without risk factors. *West J Emerg Med*. 2011;12 (4):571–574.
Papatsonis DN, Heetkamp A, van den Hombergh C, et al. Acute type A artic dissection complicating pregnancy at 32 weeks: surgical repair after cesarean section. *Am J Perinatol*. 2009;26:153–157.
Shihata M, Pretorius V, MacArthur R. Repair of an acute type A aortic dissection combined with an emergency cesarean section in a pregnant woman. *Interact Cardiovasc Thorac Surg*. 2008;7:938–940.
Stout CL, Scott EC, Stokes GK, Panneton JM. Successful repair of a ruptured Stanford type B aortic dissection during pregnancy. *J Vasc Surg*. 2010;51:990–992.
Zeebregts CJ, Schepens MA, Hameeteman TM, Morshuis WJ, de la Rivière AB. Acute aortic dissection complicating pregnancy. *Ann Thorac Surg*. 1997;64:1345–1348.

Aortic Regurgitation
Silwa K, Johnson MR, Zilla P, Roos-Hesselink JW. Management of valvular disease in pregnancy. *Eur Heart J*. 2015;36(8):1078–1089.

Aortic Stenosis
Silwa K, Johnson MR, Zilla P, Roos-Hesselink JW. Management of valvular disease in pregnancy. *Eur Heart J*. 2015;36(8):1078–1089.

Arrhythmogenic Right Ventricular Cardiomyopathy
Pregnancy in women with arrhythmogenic right ventricular cardiomyopathy/dysplasia. *Eur J Obstet Gynecol*. 2006;127(2):186-189.

Atrial Septal Defects
Yap SC, Drenthen W, Meijboom FJ, et al. Comparison of pregnancy outcomes in women with repaired versus unrepaired atrial septal defect. *BJOG*. 2009;116(12):1593–1601.

Autoimmune Disease
Gordon C. Pregnancy and autoimmune disease. *Best Pract Res Clin Rheumatol*. 2004;18:359–379.

Atrioventricular Canal Defects
Emanuel R, et al. Evidence of congenital heart disease in the offspring of parents with atrioventricular defects. *Br Heart J*. 1983;49(2):144–147.

Coarctation of the Aorta

Beauchesne LM, Connolly HM, Ammash NM, Warnes CA. Coarctation of the aorta: outcome of pregnancy. *J Am Coll Cardiol*. 2001;38(6):1728–1733.

Deal K, Wooley CF. Coarctation of the aorta and pregnancy. *Ann Intern Med*. 1973;78:706–710.

Parks WJ, Ngo TD, Plauth Jr WH, et al. Incidence of aneurysm formation after Dacron patch aortoplasty repair for coarctation of the aorta: long-term results and assessment using magnetic resonance angiography with three-dimensional surface rendering. *J Am Coll Cardiol*. 1995;26(1):266–271.

Venning S, Freeman LJ, Stanley K. Two cases of pregnancy with coarctation of the aorta. *J R Soc Med*. 2003;96(5):234–236.

Cocaine

Liu SS, Forrester RM, Murphy GS, Chen K, Glassenberg R. Anesthetic management of a parturient with myocardial infarction related to cocaine use. *Can J Anaesth*. 1992;83:347–350.

Livingston JC, Mabie BC, Ramanathan J. Crack cocaine, myocardial infarction and troponin I levels at the time of caesarean delivery. *Eur Heart J*. 1986;7:904–909.

Congenital Heart Disease: General

Khairy DW, Ouyang DW, Fernandes SM, Lee-Parritz A, Economy KE, Landzberg MJ. Pregnancy outcomes in women with congenital heart disease. *Circulation*. 2006;113:517–524.

Uebing A, Steer PJ, Yentis SM, Gatzoulis MA. Pregnancy and congenital heart disease. *BMJ*. 2006;332:401–406.

Cor Pulmonale and Lung Disease

Al-Mobeireek AF, Almutawa J, Alsatli RA. The nineteenth pregnancy in a patient with cor pulmonale and severe pulmonary hypertension: a management challenge. *Acta Obstet Gynecol Scand*. 2003;82(7):676–678.

Mendelson CL. Acute cor pulmonale and pregnancy. Acute cor pulmonale and pregnancy. *Clin Obstet Gynecol*. 1968;11(4):992–1009.

$_1$-Antitrypsin Deficiency

Giesler CF. Alpha 1-antitrypsin deficiency. Severe obstructive disease and pregnancy. *Obstet Gynecol*. 1977;49:31–34.

Alveolar Hypoventilation

Pieters TH, Amy JJ, Burrini D, Aubert G, Rodenstein DO, Collard P. Normal pregnancy in primary alveolar hypoventilation. *Eur Respir J*. 1995;8:1424–1427.

Cystic Fibrosis

Edenborrough FP, et al. The outcome of 75 pregnancies in 55 women with cystic fibrosis in the United Kingdom 1977-1996. *Br J Obstet Gynaecol*. 2000;107:254–261.

Goss CH, Rubenfeld GD, Otto K, Aitken ML. The effect of pregnancy on survival in women with cystic fibrosis. *Chest*. 2003;124:1460–1468.

Scoliosis

Berman AT, Cohen DL, Schwentker EP. The effects of pregnancy on idiopathic scoliosis: a preliminary report on eight cases and a review of the literature. *Spine (Phila Pa 1976)*. 1982;7(1):76–77.

Betz RR, Bunnell WP, Lambrecht-Mulier E, MacEwen GD. Scoliosis and pregnancy. *J Bone Jt Surg*. 1987;69(suppl A):90–95.

Blount WP, Mellencamp DD. The effect of pregnancy on idiopathic scoliosis. *J Bone Jt Surg*. 1986;62(suppl A):1083–1087.

Falick-Michaeli T, Schroeder JE, Barzilay Y, Luria M, Itzchayek E, Kaplan L. Adolescent idiopathic scoliosis and pregnancy: an unsolved paradigm. *Glob Spine J*. 2015;5:179–184.

Kopenhager T, Kopenhager T. A review of 50 pregnant patients with kyphoscoliosis. *Br J Obstet Gynaecol*. 1977;84:585–587.

Phelan JP, Dainer MJ, Cowherd DW. Pregnancy complicated by thoracolumbar scoliosis. *South Ed J*. 1978;71:76–78.

Sawicka EH, Spencer GT, Branthwaite MA. Management of respiratory failure complicating pregnancy in severe kyphoscoliosis: a new use for an old technique? *Br J Dis Chest*. 1986;80:191–196.

Siegler D, Zorah PA. Pregnancy in thoracic scoliosis. *Br J Dis Chest*. 1981;75:367–370.

To WW, Wong MW. Kyphoscoliosis complicating pregnancy. *Int J Gynecol Obstet*. 1996;55(2):123–128.

Pulmonary Arteriovenous Malformation

Anin SR, Ogunnoiki W, Sabharwal T, Harrison-Phipps K. Pulmonary arteriovenous malformation unmasked in pregnancy: a case report. *Obstet Med*. 2013;6(4):179–181.

Esplin MS, Varner MW. Progression of pulmonary arteriovenous malformation during pregnancy: a case report and review of the literature. *Obstet Gynecol Surv*. 1997;52:248–253.

Freixinet J, Sanchez-Palacios M, Guerrero D, et al. Pulmonary arteriovenous fistula ruptured to a pleural cavity in pregnancy. *Scand J Thorac Cardiovasc Surg*. 1995;29(1):39–41.

Shovlin CL, Sodhi V, McCarthy A, Lasjaunias P, Jackson JE, Sheppard MN. Estimates of maternal risk of pregnancy for women with hereditary haemorrhagic telangiectasia (Osler-Weber-Rendu syndrome): suggested approach for obstetric services. *BJOG*. 2008;115(9):1108–1115.

Restrictive Lung Disease

King TE. Restrictive lung disease in pregnancy. *Clin Chest Med*. 1992;13:607–622.

Sleep-Disordered Breathing

Charbonneau M, Falcone T, Cosio MG, Levy RD. Obstructive sleep apnea during pregnancy. Therapy and implications for fetal health. *Am Rev Respir Dis.* 1991;144:461–463.

Cheun JK, Choi KT. Arterial oxygen desaturation rate following obstructive apnea in parturients. *J Korean Med Sc.* 1992;7:6–10.

Edwards N, Middleton PG, Blyton DM, Sullivan CE. Sleep disordered breathing and pregnancy. *Thorax.* 2002;57:555–558.

Ventilator Patients

Bach JR. Successful pregnancies for ventilator users. *Am J Phys Med.* 2003;82:226–229.

Pleural Effusion

Gourgoulianis KI, et al. Benign postpartum pleural effusion. *Eur Respir J.* 1995;8:1748–1750.

Cardiomyopathy, Doxorubicin Induced

Pan P, Moore CH. Doxorubicin-induced cardiomyopathy during pregnancy: three case reports of anesthetic management for cesarean and vaginal delivery in two kyphoscoliotic patients. *Anesthesiology.* 2002;97:513–515.

Coronary Artery Disease

Bauer TW, Moore GW, Hutchins GM. Morphologic evidence for coronary artery spasm in eclampsia. *Circulation.* 1982;65:255–259.

Burchill LJ, Lameijer H, Roos-Hesselink JW, et al. Pregnancy risks in women with pre-existing coronary artery disease or following acute coronary syndrome. *Heart.* 2015;101:525–529.

Burlew BS. Managing the pregnant patient with heart disease. *Clin Cardiol.* 1990;13:757.

Cuthill JA, Young S, Greer IA, Oldroyd K. Anesthetic considerations in a parturient with critical coronary artery disease and a drug-eluting stent presenting for Caesarean section. *Int J Obstet Anesth.* 2005;14:167–171.

Eickman FM. Acute coronary artery angioplasty during pregnancy. *Cathet Cardiovasc Diagn.* 1996;38:369–372.

Klinzing P, Markert UR, Liesaus K, Peiker G. Case report: successful pregnancy and delivery after myocardial infarction and essential thrombocythemia treated with clopidogrel. *Clin Exp Obstet Gynecol.* 2001;28:215–216.

Leonhardt G, Gaul C, Nietsch HH, Buerke M, Schleussner E. Thrombolytic therapy in pregnancy. *J Thromb Thrombolysis.* 2006;21:271–276.

Shade Jr GH, Ross G, Bever FN, Uddin Z, Devireddy L, Gardin JM. Troponin I in the diagnosis of acute myocardial infarction in pregnancy, labor, and post-partum. *Am J Obstet Gynecol.* 2002;187:719–720.

Smith GC, Pell JP, Walsh D, et al. Pregnancy complication and the maternal risk of ischaemic heart disease: a retrospective cohort study of 129,290 live births. *Lancet.* 2001;357:2002–2006.

Tsuda E, Ishihara Y, Kawamata K, et al. Pregnancy and delivery in patients with coronary artery lesions caused by Kawasaki disease. *Heart.* 2005;91:1481–1482.

Turrentine MA, Braems G, Eamirez MM. Use of thrombolytics for the treatment of thromboembolic disease during pregnancy. *Obstet Gynecol Surv.* 1995;50:534–541.

Wilson AM, Boyle AJ, Fox P. Management of ischaemic heart disease in women of child-bearing age. *Intern Med J.* 2004;34:694–697.

Coronary Artery Dissection

Klutstein MW, Tzivoni D, Bitran D, Mendzelevski B, Ilan M, Almagor Y. Treatment of spontaneous coronary artery dissection: report of three cases. *Cathet Cardiovasc Diagn.* 1997;40:372–376.

Togni M, Amann FW, Follath F. Spontaneous multivessel coronary artery dissection in a pregnant woman treated successfully with stent implantation. *Am J Med.* 1999;107:407–408.

Coronary Vasculitis

Rallings P, Exner T, Abraham R. Coronary artery vasculitis and myocardial infarction associated with antiphospholipid antibodies in a pregnant woman. *Aust N Z Med.* 1989;19:347–350.

Cyanotic Heart Disease

Presbitro P, Somerville J, Stone S, Aruta E, Spiegelhalter D, Rabajoli F. Pregnancy in cyanotic congenital heart disease. *Outcome mother fetus Circulation.* 1994;89:2673–2676.

Dilated Cardiomyopathy (Primary)

Yacoub A, Martel MJ. Pregnancy in a patient with primary dilated cardiomyopathy. *Obstet Gynecol.* 2002;99:928–930.

Double-Outlet Right Ventricle

Ito M, Takagi N, Sugimoto S, Oosawa H, Abe T. Pregnancy after undergoing the Fontan procedure for a double outlet right ventricle: report of a case. *Surg Today.* 2002;32:63–65.

Ebstein's Anomaly

Connolly HM, Warnes CA. Ebstein's anomaly: outcome of pregnancy. *J Am Coll Cardiol.* 1994;23(5):1194–1198.

Donnelly JE, Brown JM, Radford DJ. Pregnancy outcome and Ebstein's anomaly. *Br Heart J.* 1991;66(5):368–371.

Katsuragi S, Kamiya C, Yamanaka K, et al. Risk factors for maternal and fetal outcome in pregnancy complicated by Ebstein anomaly. *Am J Obstet Gynecol.* 2013;209:452.e1–452.e6.

Ehlers-Danlos, Vascular Type

Pregnancy and delivery in Ehlers-Danlos syndrome (hypermobility type): review of the literature. *Obstet Gynecol Int* 2011;2011:306413.

Murray ML, Pepin M, Peterson S, Byers PH. Pregnancy-related deaths and complications in women with vascular Ehlers-Danlos syndrome. *Genet Med*. 2014;16(12): 874–880.

Eisenmenger's Syndrome

Arias F. Maternal death in a patient with Eisenmenger's syndrome. *Obstet Gynecol*. 1977;50(1 suppl):76S–80S.

Avila WS, et al. Maternal and fetal outcome in pregnant women with Eisenmenger's syndrome. *Eur Heart J*. 1995;16: 460–464.

Bitsch M, Johansen C, Wennevold A, Osler M. Eisenmenger's syndrome and pregnancy. *Eur J Obstet Gynecol Reprod Biol*. 1988;28:69–74.

Gleicher N, Midwall J, Hochberger D, Jaffin H. Eisenmenger's syndrome and pregnancy. *Obstet Gynecol Surv*. 1979;34: 721–741.

Godwinn TM. Favorable response of Eisenmenger syndrome to inhaled nitric oxide during pregnancy. *Am J Obstet Gynecol*. 1999;180(1 Pt 3):S208–S213.

Heytens L, Alexander JP. Maternal and neonatal death associated with Eisenmenger's syndrome. *Acta Anaesthesiol Belg*. 1986:3745–3751.

Lacassic HJ, Germain AM, Valdés G, Fernández MS, Allamand F, López H. Management of Eisenmenger syndrome in pregnancy with sildenafil and L-arginine. *Eur Heart J*. 1995;16(4):460–464.

Lieber S, Dewilde P, Huyghens L, Traey E, Gepts E. Eisenmenger's syndrome and pregnancy. *Acta Cardiol*. 1985;40:421–424.

Lust KM, Boots RJ, Dooris M, Wilson J. Management of labour in Eisenmenger syndrome with inhaled nitric oxide. *Am J Obstet Gynecol*. 1999;181:419–423.

Midwall J, Jaffin H, Herman MV, Kupersmith J. Shunt flow and pulmonary hemodynamics during labour and delivery in Eisenmenger's syndrome. *Am J Cardiol*. 1978;42: 299–303.

Neilson G, Galea EG, Blunt A. Eisenmenger's syndrome and pregnancy. *Med J Aust*. 1971;1:432–434.

Pitts JA, Crosby WM, Basta LL. Eisenmenger's syndrome in pregnancy: does heparin prophylaxis improve the maternal mortality rate? *Am Heart J*. 1977;93:321–326.

Fontan Repair

Canobbio M, Mair DD, van der Velde M, Koos BJ. Pregnancy outcome after the Fontan repair. *J Am Coll Cardiol*. 1996;28(3):763–767.

Hypertrophic Cardiomyopathy

Autore C, Conte MR, Piccininno M, et al. Risk associated with pregnancy in hypertropic cardiomyopathy. *J Am Coll Cardiol*. 2002;40:1864–1869.

Autore C, Conte MR, Piccininno M, et al. Risks associated with pregnancy in hypertrophic cardiomyopathy. *J Am Coll Cardiol*. 2002;40(10):1864–1869.

Benitez RM. Hypertrophic cardiomyopathy and pregnancy: maternal and fetal outcomes. *J Matern-Fetal Invest*. 1996;6: 51–55.

Oakley GD, McGarry K, Limb DG, Oakley CM. Management of pregnancy in patients with hypertrophic cardiomyopathy. *Br Med J*. 1979;1:1749–1750.

Peliccia F, Cianfrocca C, Gaudio C, Reale A. Sudden death during pregnancy in hypertrophic cardiomyopathy. *Eur Heart J*. 1992;13:421–423.

Shah DM, Sunderji SG. Hypertrophic cardiomyopathy and pregnancy: report of a maternal mortality and review of literature. *Obstet Gynecol Surv*. 1985;40:444–448.

Thaman AV, Varnava A, Hamid MS, et al. Pregnancy related complications in women with hypertrophic cardiomyopathy. *Heart*. 2003;89:752–756.

Turner GM, Oakley CM, Dixon HG. Management of pregnancy complicated by hypertrophic cardiomyopathy. *Br Med J*. 1968;4:281–284.

Idiopathic Inflammatory Myopathy

Silva CA, Sultan SM, Isenberg DA. Pregnancy outcome in adult-onset idiopathic inflammatory myopathy. *Rheumatolgy*. 2003;42:1168–1172.

Inappropriate Sinus Tachycardia

Belham M, Patient C, Pickett J. Inappropriate sinus tachycardia in pregnancy: a benign phenomena? *BMJ Case Rep*. 2017:2016–2017.

Inappropriate sinus tachycardia presenting with palpitations and syncope during pregnancy, successful treatment with metoprolol. *Heart Lung Circ*. 2017;26(suppl 2):S167-S168.

Olshansky BO, Sullivan RM. Inappropriate sinus tachycardia. *J Am Coll Cardiol*. 2013;61:8.

Sağ S, Çoşkun H, Baran İ, Güllülü S, Aydınlar A. Inappropriate sinus tachycardia-induced cardiomyopathy during pregnancy and successful treatment with ivabradine. *Anatol J Cardiol*. 2016;16(3):212–213.

Sheldon RS, Grubb 2nd BP, Olshansky B, et al. 2015 Heart Rhythm Society expert consensus statement on the diagnosis and treatment of postural tachycardia syndrome, inappropriate sinus tachycardia, and vasovagal syncope. *Heart Rhythm*. 2015;12(6):e41–e63.

Still AM, Raatikainen P, Ylitalo A, et al. Prevalence, characteristics and natural course of inappropriate sinus tachycardia. *Europace*. 2005;7(2):95–103.

Kawasaki's Disease

Gordon CT, Jimenez-Fernandez S, Daniels LB, et al. Pregnancy in women with a history of Kawasaki disease: management and outcomes. *BJOG.* 2014;121:1431–1437.

McCrindle BW, Rowley AH, Newburger JW, et al. Diagnosis, treatment, and long-term management of Kawasaki disease: a scientific statement for professionals from the American Heart Association. *Circulation.* 2017;135(17): e927–e999.

Nolan TE, Savage RW. Peripartum myocardial infarction from presumed Kawasaki's disease. *South Med J.* 1990;83: 1360–1361.

Shear R, Leduc L. Successful pregnancy following Kawasaki disease. *Obstet Gynecol.* 1999;94(5 part 2):841–845.

Tsudu E, Ishihara Y, Kawamata K, et al. Pregnancy and delivery in patients with coronary artery lesions caused by Kawasaki disease. *Heart.* 2005;91:1431–1432.

Left Ventricular Noncompaction

Gati S, Papadakis M, Papamichael ND, et al. Reversible de novo left ventricular trabeculations in pregnant women: implications for the diagnosis of left ventricular noncompaction in low-risk populations. *Circulation.* 2014;130(6): 475–483.

Kitao K, Ohara N, Funakoshi T, et al. Noncompaction of the left ventricular myocardium diagnosed in pregnant woman and neonate. *J Perinat Med.* 2004;32(6):527–531.

Munehisa Y, Watanabe H, Kosaka T, Kimura A, Ito H. Successful outcome in a pregnant woman with isolated noncompaction of the left ventricular myocardium. *Intern Med.* 2007;46(6):285–289.

Loeys-Dietz Syndrome

Cauldwell M, Patel RR, Uebing A, Gatzoulis MA, Swan L. Loeys Dietz Syndrome and pregnancy: a case report with literature review and a proposed focused management protocol. *Int J Cardiol.* 2016;214:491–492.

Frise CJ, Pitcher A, Mackillop L. Loeys-Dietz syndrome and pregnancy: the first ten years. *Int J Cardiol.* 2017;226: 21–25.

Marfan Syndrome

Carboni S, Capucci R, Pivato E, Poggi A, Patella A. Marfan's syndrome and pregnancy; a good maternal and fetal outcome. *J Prenat Med.* 2013;7(2):21–24.

Donnelly RT, Pinto NM, Kocolas I, Yetman AT. The immediate and long-term impact of pregnancy on aortic growth rate and mortality in women with Marfan syndrome. *J Am Coll Cardiol.* 2012;60:224–229.

Goland S, Elkayam U. Cardiovascular problems in pregnant women with Marfan syndrome. *Circulation.* 2009;119: 619–623.

Lind J, Wallenburg HC. The Marfan syndrome and pregnancy: a retrospective study in a Dutch population. *Eur J Obstet Gynecol Reprod Biol.* 2001;220:514–518.

Lipscomb KJ, Smith JC, Clarke B, Donnai P, Harris R. Outcome of pregnancy in women with Marfan syndrome. *Br J Obstet Gynaecol.* 1997;104:201–206.

Lipscomb KJ, Smith JC, Clarke B, Donnai P, Harris R. Outcome of pregnancy in women with Marfan's syndrome. *Br J Obstet Gynecol.* 1997;104:201–206.

Meijboom LJ, Drenthen W, Pieper PG, et al. Obstetric complications in Marfan syndrome. *Int J Cardiol.* 2006;110: 53–59.

Meijboom LJ, Vos FE, Timmermans J, Boers GH, Zwinderman AH, Mulder BJ. Pregnancy and aortic root growth in the Marfan syndrome: a prospective study. *Eur Heart J.* 2005;26:914–920.

Meijboom LJ, Vos FE, Timmermans J, Boers GH, Zwinderman AH, Mulder BJ. Pregnancy and aortic growth in the Marfan syndrome: a prospective study. *Eur Heart J.* 2005;26:914–920.

Mulder BJM, Meijboom LJ. Pregnancy and Marfan syndrome an ongoing discussion. *J Am Coll Cardiol.* 2012;60: 230–231.

Pyeritz RE. Maternal and fetal complications of pregnancy in the Marfan syndrome. *Am J Med.* 1981;71:784–790.

Rossiter JP, Repke JT, Morales AJ, Murphy EA, Pyeritz RE. A prospective longitudinal evaluation of pregnancy in the Marfan syndrome. *Am J Obstet Gynecol.* 1995;173: 1599–1606.

Mitral Regurgitation

Hagay ZJ, Weissman A, Geva D, Snir E, Caspi A. Labour and delivery complicated by acute mitral regurgitation due to ruptured chordae tendineae. *Am J Perinatol.* 1995;12: 111–112.

Khanlou H, Khanlou N, Eiger G. Relationship between mitral valve regurgitant flow and peripartum change in systemic vascular resistance. *South Med J.* 2003;96(3):308–309.

Silwa K, Johnson MR, Zilla P, Roos-Hesselink JW. Management of valvular disease in pregnancy. *Eur Heart J.* 2015;36(8):1078–1089.

Tsiaras S, Poppas A. Mitral valve disease in pregnancy: outcomes and management. *Obstetric Med.* 2009;2(1):6–10.

Mitral Stenosis

al Kasab SM, Sabag T, al Zaibag M, et al. Beta-adrenergic receptor blockade in the management of pregnant women with mitral stenosis. *Am J Obstet Gynecol.* 1990;163:37–40.

Barbaos PJB, Lopes AA, Feitosa GS, et al. Prognostic factors of rheumatic mitral stenosis during pregnancy and puerperium. *Arq Bras Cardiol.* 2000;75(3):215–224.

Bryg RJ, Gordon PR, Kudesia VS, Bhatia RK. Effect of pregnancy on pressure gradient in mitral stenosis. *Am J Cardiol.* 1989;63:384–386.

Clark S, Phelan JP, Greenspoon J, Aldahl D, Horenstein J. Labour and deliver in the presence of mitral stenosis: central hemodynamic observation. *Am J Obstet Gynecol.* 1985;152: 984–988.

Norrad RS, Salehian O. Management of severe mitral stenosis during pregnancy. *Circulation.* 2011;124:2756–2760.

Silversides CK, Colman JM, Sermer M, Siu SC. Cardiac risk in pregnant women with rheumatic mitral stenosis. *Am J Cardiol.* 2003;91:1382–1385.

Sliwa K, Johnson MR, Zilla P, Roos-Hesselink JW. Management of valvular disease in pregnancy. *Eur Heart J.* 2015;36(8):1078–1089.

Mitral Valve Prolapse

Haas JH. The effect of pregnancy n the midsystolic click and murmur of the prolapsing posterior leaflet of the mitral valve. *Am Heart J.* 1976;92:407–408.

Mixed Connective Tissue Disease

Kitridou RC. Pregnancy in mixed connective tissue disease. *Rheum Dis Clin North Am.* 2005;31:359–379.

Muscular Dystrophy

Gamzu R, Shenhav M, Fainaru O, Almog B, Kupferminc M, Lessing JB. Impact of pregnancy on respiratory capacity in women with muscular dystrophy and kyphoscoliosis. *J Reprod Med.* 2002;47:53–56.

Myocardial Infarction

Box LC, Hanak V, Arciniegas JG. Dual coronary emboli in peripartum cardiomyopathy. *Tex Heart Inst J.* 2004;31:442–444.

Bredy PL, Singh P, Frishman WH. Acute inferior wall myocardial infarction and percutaneous coronary intervention of the right coronary during active labour. *Cardiol Rev.* 2008;16:260–268.

Chemnitz G, Nevermann L, Schmidt E, Schmidt FW, Lobers J. Creatine kinase (EC-No.2.7.3.2) and creatine kinase isoenzymes during pregnancy and labor and in the cord blood. *Clin Biochem.* 1979;12(6):277–281.

Dufour P, Berard J, Vinatier D, et al. Pregnancy after myocardial infarction and a coronary artery bypass graft. *Arch Gynecol Obstet.* 1997;259:209–213.

Foading Deffo B. Myocardial infarction and pregnancy. *Acta Cardiol.* 2007;62:303–308.

Fujiwara Y, Yamanaka O, Nakamura T, Yokoi H, Yamaguchi H. Acute myocardial infarction induced by ergonovine administration for artificially induced abortion. *Jpn Heart J.* 1993;34:803–808.

Garry D, Leikin E, Fleisher AG, Tejani N. Acute myocardial infarction in pregnancy with subsequent medical and surgical management. *Obstet Gynecol.* 1996;87:802–824.

Hankins GD, Wendel Jr GD, Leveno KJ, Stoneham J. Myocardial infarction during pregnancy: a review. *Obstet Gynecol.* 1985;65:139–146.

Hayashi Y, Ibe T, Kawato H, et al. Post-partum acute myocardial infarction induced by ergonovine administration. *Intern Med.* 2003;42:983–986.

Hu CL, Li YB, Zou YG, et al. Troponin T measurement can predict persistent left ventricular dysfunction in peripartum cardiomyopathy. *Heart.* 2007;93(4):488–490.

James AH, Jamison MG, Biswas MS, Brancazio LR, Swamy GK, Myers ER. Acute myocardial infarction in pregnancy: a United States population-based study. *Circulation.* 2006;113:1564–1571.

James AH, Jamison MG, Biswas MS, Brancazio LR, Swamy GK, Myers ER. Acute myocardial infarction in pregnancy: a United States population-based study. *Circulation.* 2006;113:1564–1571.

Ladner B. Acute myocardial infarction in pregnancy and the puerperium: a population-based study. *Obstet Gynecol.* 2005;105:480–484.

Liao JK, Cockrill BA, Yurchak PM. Acute myocardial infarction after ergonovine administration. *Am J Cardiol.* 1991;68:823–824.

Maeder M, Ammann P, Angehrn W, Rickli H. Idiopathic spontaneous coronary artery dissection: incidence, diagnosis, and treatment. *Int J Cardiol.* 2005;101:363–369.

Mahon NG, Maree A, McKenna P, McCann HA, Sugrue DD. Emergency coronary angioplasty and stenting following acute myocardial infarction during pregnancy. *J Inv Card.* 1999;11:233–236.

Mahon NG, Maree A, McKenna P, McCann HA, Sugrue DD. Emergency coronary angioplasty and stenting following acute myocardial infarction during pregnancy. *J Inv Card.* 1999;11:233–236.

Mousa HA, McKinley CA, Thong J. Acute postpartum myocardial infarction after ergometrine administration in a woman with familial hypercholesterolemia. *BJOG.* 2000;107:939–940.

Movsesiam MA, Wray RB. Postpartum myocardial infarction. *Br Heart J.* 1989;62:154–156.

Ottman EH, Gall SA. Myocardial infarction in the third trimester of pregnancy secondary to an aortic valve thrombus. *Obstet Gynecol.* 1993;81:804–805.

Poh CL, Lee CH. Acute myocardial infarction in pregnant women. *Ann Acad Med Singap.* 2010;39:247–253.

Reizig K, Diar N, Walcker JL. [Myocardial infarction, pregnancy and anesthesia]. *Ann Fr Anesth Reanim.* 2000;19:544–548.

Roth A, Elkayam U. Acute myocardial infarction associated with pregnancy. *Ann Intern Med.* 1996;125:751–762.

Ruch A, Duhring JL. Postpartum myocardial infarction in a patient receiving bromocriptine. *Obstet Gynecol.* 1989;74:448–449.

Schumacher B, Belfort MA, Card RJ. Successful treatment of acute myocardial infarction during pregnancy with tissue plasminogen activator. *Am J Obstet Gynecol.* 1997;176:716–719.

Schumacher B, Belfort MA, Card RJ. Successful treatment of acute myocardial infarction during pregnancy with tissue plasminogen activator. *Am J Obstet Gynecol.* 1997;176:716–719.

Sebastian C, Scherlag M, Kugelmass A. Schechte19, Foading Deffo B. Myocardial infarction and pregnancy. *Acta Cardiol.* 2007;62:303–308.

Sebastian C, Scherlag M, Kugelmass A, Schechter E. Primary stent implantation for acute myocardial infarction during pregnancy: use of abciximab, ticlopidine, and aspirin. *Cathet Cardiovasc Diagn.* 1998;45:275–279.

Sutaria N, O'Toole L, Northridge D. Postpartum acute MI following routine ergometrine administration treated successfully by primary PTCA. *Heart.* 2000;83:97–98.

Tsui BC, Stewart B, Fitzmaurice A, Williams R. Cardiac arrest and myocardial infarction induced by postpartum intravenous ergonovine administration. *Anesthesiology.* 2001;94:363.

Mustard Repair

Clarkson PM, Wilson NJ, Neutze JM, North RA, Calder AL, Barratt-Boyes BG. Outcome of pregnancy after the Mustard operation for transposition of the great arteries with intact ventricular septum. *J Am Coll Cardiol.* 1994;24:190–193.

Guédès A, Mercier LA, Leduc L, Bérubé L, Marcotte F, Dore A. Impact of pregnancy on the systemic right ventricle after a Mustard operation for transposition of the great arteries. *J Am Coll Cardiol.* 1994;44:433–437.

Lynch-Salamon DI, Maze SS, Combs CA. Pregnancy after Mustard repair for transposition of the great arteries. *Obstet Gynecol.* 1993;82(4 Pt 2 suppl):676–679.

Pericardial Disease

Adam FU, Avcı B, Koc M. Purulent pericarditis and pericardiac tamponade in a pregnant hemodialysis patient. *Hemodial Int.* 2016;20(1):E5–E8.

Brucato A, Imazio M, Curri S, Palmieri G, Trinchero R. Medical treatment of pericarditis during pregnancy. *Int J Cardiol.* 2010;144:413–414.

Diav-Citirn O, Shechtman S, Schwartz V, et al. Pregnancy outcome after in utero exposure to colchicine. *Am J Obstet Gynecol.* 2010;203(2):144e1–144e6.

Imazio M, Brucato A, Rampello S, et al. Management of pericardial diseases during pregnancy. *J Cardiovasc Med.* 2010;11(8):557–562.

Krausz Y, Naparstek E, Eliakim M. Idiopathic pericarditis and pregnancy. *Aust N Z J Obstet Gynaecol.* 1978;18(1):86–89.

Rabinovitch O, Zemer D, Kukia E, Sohar E, Mashiach S. Colchicine treatment in conception and pregnancy: two hundred thirty-one pregnancies in patients with familial Mediterranean fever. *Am J Reprod Immunol.* 1992;28:245–346.

Richardson PM, Le Roux BT, Rogers NM, Gotsman MS. Pericardiectomy in pregnancy. *Thorax.* 1970;25:627.

Ristić AD, Seferović PM, Ljubić A, et al. Pericardial disease in pregnancy. *Herz.* 2003;28(3):209–215.

Watson PT, Havelda CJ, Sorosky J, Kochenour NK, Sohi GS, Gray Jr. L. Irradiation-induced constrictive pericarditis requiring pericardiectomy during pregnancy. *J Reprod Med.* 1980;24(3):127–130.

Peripartum Cardiomyopathy

Abboud J, Murad Y, Chen-Scarabelli C, Saravolatz L, Scarabelli TM. Peripartum cardiomyopathy: a comprehensive review. Int J Cardiol. 2007;118(3):295–303.

Albanesi Filho PM, et al. Natural course of subsequent pregnancy after peripartum cardiomyopathy. Arq Bras Cardiol. 1999;73:47–57.

Amos AM, Jaber WA, Russell SD. Improved outcomes in peripartum cardiomyopathy with contemporary. Am Heart J. 2006;152:509–513.

Amos AM, Jaber WA, Russell SD. Improved outcomes in peripartum cardiomyopathy with contemporary. Am Heart J. 2006;152:509–513.

Ansari AA, Fett JD, Carraway RE, et al. Autoimmune mechanisms as the basis for human peripartum cardiomyopathy. Clin Rev Allergy Immunol. 2002;23(3):301–324.

Arany Z, Elkayam U. Peripartum cardiomyopathy. Circulation. 2016;133:1397–1409.

Arora NP, Mohamad T, Mahajan N, et al. Cardiac magnetic resonance imaging in peripartum cardiomyopathy. Am J Me Sci. 2014;347:112–117.

Bajou K, Herkenne S, Thijssen VL, et al. PAI-1 mediates the antiangiogenic and profibrinolytic effects of 16K prolactin. Nat Med. 2014;20:741–747.

Baruteau AE, Leurent G, Martins RP, et al. Peripartum cardiomyopathy in the era of cardiac magnetic resonance imaging: first results and perspectives. Int J Cardiol. 2010;144(1):143–145.

Baughman KL. Risks of repeat pregnancy after peripartum cardiomyopathy: double jeopardy. J Card Fail. 2001;7:36–37.

Bello N, Rendon IS, Arany Z. The relationship between pre-eclampsia and peripartum cardiomyopathy: a systematic review and meta-analysis. J Am Coll Cardiol. 2013;62:1715–1723.

Biteker M, Duran NE, Kaya H, et al. Effect of levosimendan and predictors of recovery in patients with peripartum cardiomyopathy, a randomized clinical trial. Clin Res Cardiol. 2011;100:571–577.

Biteker M, Ilhan E, Biteker G, Duman D, Bozkurt B. Delayed recovery in peripartum cardiomyopathy: an indication for long-term follow-up and sustained therapy. Eur J Heart Fail. 2012;14:895–901.

Blauwet LA, Libhaber E, Forster O, et al. Predictors of outcome in 176 South African patients with peripartum cardiomyopathy. Heart. 2013;99:308–313.

Bouabdallaoui N, Mastroianni C, Revelli L, Demondion P, Lebreton G. Predelivery extracorporeal membrane oxygenation in a life-threatening peripartum cardiomyopathy: save both mother and child. Am J Emerg Med. 2015;33(11):1713 e1-2.

Bozkurt B, Villaneuva FS, Holubkov R, et al. Intravenous immune globulin in the therapy of peripartum cardiomyopathy. J Am Coll Cardiol. 1999;34:177–180.

Brar SS, Khan SS, Sandhu GK, et al. Incidence, mortality, and racial differences in peripartum cardiomyopathy. Am J Cardiol. 2007;100:302–304.

Brar SS, Khan SS, Sandhu GK, et al. Incidence, mortality, and racial differences in peripartum cardiomyopathy. Am J Cardiol. 2007;100(2):302–304.

Chapa JB, et al. Prognostic value of echocardiography in peripartum cardiomyopathy. Obstet Gynecol. 2005;105 (6):1303–1308.

Chapa JB, Heiberger HB, Weinert L, Decara J, Lang RM, Hibbard JU. Prognostic value of echocardiography in peripartum cardiomyopathy. Obstet Gynecol. 2005;105: 1303–1308.

Damp J, Givertz MM, Semigran M, et al. Relaxin-2 and soluble Flt1 levels in peripartum cardiomyopathy: results of the multicenter IPAC study. J Am Coll Cardiol Heart Fail. 2016;4(5):380–388.

de Souza JL, et al. Left ventricular function after a new pregnancy in patients with peripartum cardiomyopathy. J Card Fail. 2001;7:30–35.

DeBenedetti Zunino ME, Schuger C, Lahiri M. High rate of ventricular arrhythmias in women with peripartum cardiomyopathy and implanted cardioverter defibrillators. J Am Coll Cardiol. 2014;63(suppl 12):A313.

Desplantie O, Tremblay-Gravel M, Avram R, et al. The medical treatment of new-onset peripartum cardiomyopathy: a systematic review of prospective studies. Can J Cardiol. 2015;31:1421–1426.

Duncker D, Haghikia A, Konig T, et al. Risk for ventricular fibrillation in peripartum cardiomyopathy with severely reduced left ventricular function-value of the wearable cardioverter/defibrillator. Eur J Heart Fail. 2014;16(12): 1331–1336.

Duncker D, Haghikia A, König T, et al. Risk for ventricular fibrillation in peripartum cardiomyopathy with severely reduced left ventricular function: value of the wearable cardioverter/defibrillator. Eur J Heart Fail. 2014;16:1331–1336.

Egan DJ, Bisanzo MC, Hutson HR. Emergency department evaluation and management of peripartum cardiomyopathy. J Emerg Med. 2009;36(2):141–147.

Elkayam U. Clinical characteristics of peripartum cardiomyopathy in the United States: diagnosis, prognosis, and management. J Am Coll Cardiol. 2011;58:659–670.

Elkayam U. Pregnant again peripartum cardiomyopathy: be not be: Eur Heart J. 2002;23:753–756.

Elkayam U. Risk of subsequent pregnancy in women with a history of peripartum cardiomyopathy. J Am Coll Cardiol. 2014;64:1629–1636.

Elkayam U, Akhter MW, Singh H, et al. Pregnancy associated cardiomyopathy: clinical characteristics and a comparison between early and late presentation. Circulation. 2005;111:2050–2055.

Elkayam U, Akhter MW, Singh H, et al. Pregnancy-associated cardiomyopathy: clinical characteristics and a comparison between early and late presentation. Circulation. 2005;111(16):2050–2055.

Elkayam U, Akhter MW, Singh H, et al. Pregnancy-associated cardiomyopathy: clinical characteristics and a comparison between early and late presentation. Circulation. 2005;111:2050–2055.

Elkayam U, Tummala PP, Rao K, et al. Maternal and fetal outcomes of subsequent pregnancies in women with peripartum cardiomyopathy. N Engl J Med. 2001;344(21): 1567–1571.

Fett J, Ansari AA, Sundstrom JB, Combs GF. Peripartum cardiomyopathy: a selenium disconnection and an autoimmune connection. Int J Cardiol. 2002;86(2):311–316.

Fett JD, Christie LG, Carraway RD, Murphy JG. Five-year prospective study of the incidence and prognosis of peripartum cardiomyopathy at a single institution. Mayo Clin Proc. 2005;80:1602–1606.

Fett JD, Christie LG, Carraway RD, Murphy JG. Five-year prospective study of the incidence and prognosis of peripartum cardiomyopathy at a single institution. Mayo Clin Proc. 2005;80(12):1602–1606.

Fett JD, Shah TP, McNamara DM. Why do some recovered peripartum cardiomyopathy mothers experience heart failure with a subsequent pregnancy? Curr Treat Options Cardiovasc Med. 2015;17:354.

Gentry MB, Dias JK, Luis A, Patel R, Thornton J, Reed GL. African American women have a higher risk for developing peripartum cardiomyopathy. J Am Coll Cardiol. 2010;55:654–659.

Gevaert S, Van Belleghem Y, Bouchez S, et al. Acute and critically ill peripartum cardiomyopathy and "bridge to" therapeutic options: a single center experience with intra-aortic balloon pump, extra corporeal membrane oxygenation and continuous-flow left ventricular assist devices. Crit Care. 2011;15:R93.

Goland S, Bitar F, Modi K, et al. Evaluation of the clinical relevance of baseline left ventricular ejection fraction as a predictor of recovery or persistence of severe dysfunction in women in the United States with peripartum cardiomyopathy. J Card Fail. 2011;17:426–430.

Goland S, Bitar F, Modi K, et al. Evaluation of the clinical relevance of baseline left ventricular ejection fraction as a predictor of recovery or persistence of severe dysfunction in women in the United States with peripartum cardiomyopathy. J Card Fail. 2011;17:426–430.

Goland S, Modi K, Bitar F, et al. Clinical profile and predictors of complications in peripartum cardiomyopathy. J Card Fail. 2009;15:645–650.

Goland S, Modi K, Hatamizadeh P, Elkayam U. Differences in clinical profile of African-American women with peripartum cardiomyopathy in the United States. J Card Fail. 2013;19(4):214–218.

Gunderson EP, Croen LA, Chiang V, Yoshida CK, Walton D, Go AS. Epidemiology of peripartum cardiomyopathy: incidence, predictors, and outcomes. Obstet Gynecol. 2011;118:583–591.

Haghikia A, Podewski E, Libhaber E, et al. Phenotyping and outcome on contemporary management in a German cohort of patients with peripartum cardiomyopathy. Basic Res Cardiol. 2013;108:366.

Harper MA, Meyer RE, Berg CJ. Peripartum cardiomyopathy: population-based birth prevalence and 7-year mortality. Obstet Gynecol. 2012;120:1013–1019.

Hasan JA, Qureshi A, Ramejo BB, Kamran A. Peripartum cardiomyopathy characteristics and outcome in a tertiary care hospital. J Pak Med Assoc. 2010;60:377–380.

Hasan JA, Ramejo BB, Qureshi A, Kamran A. Peripartum cardiomyopathy characteristics and outcome in a tertiary care hospital. J Pak Med Assoc. 2010;64(5):377–380.

Herman DS, Lam L, Taylor MR, et al. Truncations of titin causing dilated cardiomyopathy. N Engl J Med. 2012;366:619–628.

Hilfiker-Kleiner D, Kaminski K, Podewski E, et al. A cathepsin D-cleaved 16 kDa form of prolactin mediates postpartum cardiomyopathy. Cell. 2007;128:589–600.

Hilfiker-Kleiner D, Kaminski K, Podewski E, et al. A cathepsin D-cleaved 16 kDa form of prolactin mediates postpartum cardiomyopathy. Cell. 2007;128(3):589–600.

Hilfiker-Kleiner D, Kaminski K, Podewski E, et al. A cathepsin D-cleaved 16 kDa form of prolactin mediates postpartum cardiomyopathy. Cell. 2007;128:589–600.

Hilfiker-Kleiner D, Sliwa K, Drexler H. Peripartum cardiomyopathy: recent insights in its pathophysiology. Trends Cardiovasc Med. 2008;18(5):173–179.

Horne BD, Rasmusson KD, Alharethi R, et al. Genome-wide significance and replication of the chromosome 12p11.22 locus near the PTHLH gene for peripartum cardiomyopathy. Circ Cardiovasc Genet. 2011;4:359–366.

Hu CL, Li YB, Zou YG, et al. Troponin T measurement can predict persistent left ventricular dysfunction in peripartum cardiomyopathy. Heart. 2007;93:488–490.

Hu CL, Li YB, Zou YG, et al. Troponin T measurement can predict persistent left ventricular dysfunction in peripartum cardiomyopathy. Heart. 2007;93(4):488–490.

Isezuo SA, Abubakar SA. Epidemiologic profile of peripartum cardiomyopathy in a tertiary care hospital. Ethn Dis. 2007;17:228–233.

Jahns BG, Stein W, Hilfiker-Kleiner D, Pieske B, Emons G. Peripartum cardiomyopathy—a new treatment option by inhibition of prolactin secretion. Am J Obstet Gynecol. 2008;199(4):e5–e6.

James P. A review of peripartum cardiomyopathy. Int J Clin Pract. 2004;58(4):363–365.

Kao DP, Hsich E, Lindenfeld J. Characteristics, adverse events, and racial differences among delivering mothers with peripartum cardiomyopathy. J Am Coll Cardiol Heart Fail. 2013;1:409–416.

Karaye KM, Lindmark K, Henein MY. Left ventricular structure and function among sisters of peripartum cardiomyopathy patients. Int J Cardiol. 2015;182:34–35.

Kim DY, Islam S, Mondal NT, Mussell F, Rauchholz M. Biventricular thrombi associated with peripartum cardiomyopathy. J Health Popul Nutr. 2011;29:178–180.

Kolte D, Khera S, Aronow WS, et al. Temporal trends in incidence and outcomes of peripartum cardiomyopathy in the United States: a nationwide population-based study. J Am Heart Assoc. 2014;3:e001056.

Laghari AH, Khan AH, Kazmi KA. Peripartum cardiomyopathy: ten year experience at a tertiary care hospital in Pakistan. BMC Res Notes. 2013;6:495.

Łasińska-Kowaraa M, Lango R, Kowalik M, Jarmoszewicz K. Accelerated heart function recovery after therapeutic plasma exchange in patient treated with biventricular mechanical circulatory support for severe peripartum cardiomyopathy. Eur J Cardiothorac Surg. 2014;46:1035–1036.

Lata I, Gupta R, Sahu S, Singh H. Emergency management of decompensated peripartum cardiomyopathy. J Emerg Trauma Shock. 2009;2(2):124–128.

Loyaga-Rendon RY, Pamboukian SV, Tallaj JA, et al. Outcomes of patients with peripartum cardiomyopathy who received mechanical circulatory support: data from the Interagency Registry for Mechanically Assisted Circulatory Support. Circ Heart Fail. 2014;7:300–309.

Marmursztejn J, Vignaux O, Goffinet F, Cabanes L, Duboc D. Delayed-enhanced cardiac magnetic resonance imaging features in peripartum cardiomyopathy. Int J Cardiol. 2009;137(3):e63–e64.

Massad LS, Reiss CK, Mutch DG, Haskel EJ. Familial peripartum cardiomyopathy after molar pregnancy. Obstet Gynecol. 1993;81(pt 2):886–888.

McNamara DM, Elkayam U, Alharethi R, et al. Clinical outcomes for peripartum cardiomyopathy in North America: results of the IPAC Study (Investigations of Pregnancy-Associated Cardiomyopathy). J Am Coll Cardiol. 2015;66:905–914.

McNamara DM, Holubkov R, Starling RC, et al. Controlled trial of intravenous immune globulin in recent-onset dilated cardiomyopathy. Circulation. 2001;103:2254–2259.

Mielniczuk LM, Williams K, Davis DR, et al. Frequency of peripartum cardiomyopathy. Am J Cardiol. 2006;97: 1765–1768.

Mielniczuk LM, Williams K, Davis DR, et al. Frequency of peripartum cardiomyopathy. Am J Cardiol. 2006;97(12): 1765–1768.

Moioli M, Valenzano Menada M, Bentivoglio G, Ferrero S. Peripartum cardiomyopathy. Arch Gynecol Obstet. 2010;281(2):183–188.

Morales A, Painter T, Li R, et al. Rare variant mutations in pregnancy-associated or peripartum cardiomyopathy. Circulation. 2010;121:2176–2182.

Morales A, Painter T, Li R, Siegfried JD, Li D, Norton N, et al. Rare variant mutations in pregnancy-associated or peripartum cardiomyopathy. Circulation. 2010;121(20): 2176–2182.

Murali S, Baldisseri MR. Peripartum cardiomyopathy. Crit Care Med. 2005;33:S340–S346.

Ntusi NB, Chin A. Characterisation of peripartum cardiomyopathy by cardiac magnetic resonance imaging. Eur Radiol. 2009;19(6):1324–1325.

Ntusi NB, Mayosi BM. Aetiology and risk factors of peripartum cardiomyopathy: a systematic review. Int J Cardiol. 2009;131:168–179.

Ntusi NB, Mayosi BM. Aetiology and risk factors of peripartum cardiomyopathy: a systematic review. Int J Cardiol. 2009;131(2):168–179.

Pandit V, Shetty S, Kumar A, Sagir A. Incidence and outcome of peripartum cardiomyopathy from a tertiary hospital in South India. Trop Doct. 2009;39:168–169.

Park SH, Chin JY, Choi MS, Choi JH, Choi YJ, Jung KT. Extracorporeal membrane oxygenation saved a mother and her son from fulminant peripartum cardiomyopathy. J Obstet Gynaecol Res. 2014;40:1940–1943.

Patten IS, Rana S, Shahul S, et al. Cardiac angiogenic imbalance leads to peripartum cardiomyopathy. Nature. 2012;485:333–338.

Pearl W. Familial occurrence of peripartum cardiomyopathy. Am Heart J. 1995;129:421–422.

Pierce JA, Price BO, Joyce JW. Familial occurrence of postpartal heart failure. Arch Intern Med. 1963;111:651–655.

Pillarisetti J, Kondur A, Alani A, et al. Peripartum cardiomyopathy: predictors of recovery and current state of implantable cardioverter-defibrillator use. J Am Coll Cardiol. 2014;63(pt A):2831–2839.

Pyatt JR, Dubey G. Peripartum cardiomyopathy: current understanding, comprehensive management review and new developments. Postgrad Med J. 2011;87(1023): 34–39.

Ramaraj R, Sorrell VL. Peripartum cardiomyopathy: causes, diagnosis, and treatment. Cleve Clin J Med. 2009;76(5): 289–296.

Rasmusson K, Brunisholz K, Budge D, et al. Peripartum cardiomyopathy: post-transplant outcomes from the United Network for Organ Sharing Database. J Heart Lung Transpl. 2012;31:180–186.

Rasmusson K, et al. Update on heart failure management. Current understanding of peripartum cardiomyopathy. Prog Cardiovasc Nurs. 2007;22(4):214–216.

Renz DM, Röttgen R, Habedank D, et al. New insights into peripartum cardiomyopathy using cardiac magnetic resonance imaging. Rofo. 2011;183:834–841.

Ro A, Frishman W. Peripartum cardiomyopathy. Cardiol Rev. 2006;14(1):35–42.

Roberts AM, Ware JS, Herman DS, et al. Integrated allelic, transcriptional, and phenomic dissection of the cardiac effects of titin truncations in health and disease. Sci Transl Med. 2015;7:270ra6.

Ruys TP, Roos-Hesselink JW, Hall R, et al. Heart failure in pregnant women with cardiac disease: data from the ROPAC. Heart. 2014;100:231–238.

Safirstein JG, Ro AS, Grandhi S, Wang L, Fett JD, Staniloae C. Predictors of left ventricular recovery in a cohort of peripartum cardiomyopathy patients recruited via the internet. Int J Cardiol. 2012;154:27–31.

Saltzberg MT, Szymkiewicz S, Bianco NR. Characteristics and outcomes of peripartum versus nonperipartum cardiomyopathy in women using a wearable cardiac defibrillator. J Card Fail. 2012;18:21–27.

Shimamoto T, Marui A, Oda M, et al. A case of peripartum cardiomyopathy with recurrent left ventricular apical thrombus. Circ J. 2008;72:853–854.

Sliwa K, Blauwet L, Tibazarwa K, et al. Evaluation of bromocriptine in the treatment of acute severe peripartum cardiomyopathy: a proof-of-concept pilot study. Circulation. 2010;121:1465–1473.

Sliwa K, Fett J, Elkayam U. Peripartum cardiomyopathy. Lancet. 2006;368(9536):687–693.

Sliwa K, Hilfiker-Kleiner D, Mebazaa A, et al. EURObservational Research Programme: a worldwide registry on peripartum cardiomyopathy (PPCM) in conjunction with the Heart Failure Association of the European Society of Cardiology Working Group on PPCM. Eur J Heart Fail. 2014;16:583–591.

Sliwa K, Hilfiker-Kleiner D, Petrie MC, et al. Current state of knowledge on aetiology, diagnosis, management, and therapy of peripartum cardiomyopathy: a position statement from the Heart Failure Association of the European Society of Cardiology Working Group on Peripartum Cardiomyopathy. Eur J Heart Fail. 2010;12(8): 767–778.

Sliwa K, Skudicky D, Candy G, Bergemann A, Hopley M, Sareli P. The addition of pentoxifylline to conventional therapy improves outcome in patients with peripartum cardiomyopathy. Eur J Heart Fail. 2002;4:305–309.

Sliwa K, Tibazarwa K, Hilfiker-Kleiner D. Management of peripartum cardiomyopathy. Curr Heart Fail Rep. 2008;5 (5):238–244.

Tidswell M. Peripartum cardiomyopathy. Crit Care Clin. 2004;20:777–788.

van Spaendonck-Zwarts KY, Posafalvi A, van den Berg MP, et al. Titin gene mutations are common in families with both peripartum cardiomyopathy and dilated cardiomyopathy. Eur Heart J. 2014;35:2165–2173.

van Spaendonck-Zwarts KY, van Tintelen JP, van Veldhuisen DJ, et al. Peripartum cardiomyopathy as a part of familial dilated cardiomyopathy. Circulation. 2010;121: 2169–2175.

Van Spaendonck-Zwarts KY, van Tintelen JP, van Veldhuisen DJ, et al. Peripartum cardiomyopathy as a part of familial dilated cardiomyopathy. Circulation. 2010;121 (20):2169–2175.

Vinay P, Sirish S, Ashwini K, Afrin S. Incidence and outcome of peripartum cardiomyopathy from a tertiary hospital in South India. Trop Doct. 2009;39:168–169.

Ware JS, Li J, Mazaika E, et al. Shared genetic predisposition in peripartum and dilated cardiomyopathies. N Engl J Med. 2016;374:233–241.

Zehir R, Karabay CY, Kocabay G, Kalayci A, Akgun T, Kirma C. An unusual presentation of peripartum cardiomyopathy: recurrent transient ischemic attacks. Rev Port Cardiol. 2014;33:561.e1–561.e3.

Zolt A, Elkayam E. Peripartum cardiomyopathy. Circulation. 2016;133:1397–1404.

Patent Ductus Arteriosus

Akintunde AA, Opadjio OG. Case report of a 26 year old primigravida with patent ductus arteriosus (PDA) in heart failure. Afr Health Sci. 2011;11(1):138–140.

Postural Orthostatic Tachycardia Syndrome

Blitshteyn S, Poya H, Bett GC. Pregnancy in postural tachycardia syndrome: clinical course and maternal and fetal outcomes. J Matern Fetal Neonatal Med. 2011;25(9): 1631–1634.

Glatter KA, Tuteja D, Chiamvimonvat N, Hamdan M, Park JK. Pregnancy in postural orthostatic tachycardia syndrome. Pacing Clin Electrophysiol. 2005;28(6):591–593.

Kanjwal K, Karabin B, Kanjwal Y, Grubb BP. Outcomes of pregnancy in patients with preexisting postural tachycardia syndrome. Pacing Clin Electrophysiol. 2009;32(8): 1000–1003.

Kimpinski K, Iodice V, Sandroni P, Low PA, et al. Effect of pregnancy on postural tachycardia syndrome. Mayo Clin Proc. 2010;85(7):639–644.

Lide B, Haeri S. A case report and review of postural orthostatic tachycardia syndrome in pregnancy. AJP Rep. 2015;5 (1):e33–e36.

Poless CA, Harms RW, Watson WJ. Postural tachycardia syndrome complicating pregnancy. J Matern Fetal Neonatal Med. 2010;23(8):850–853.

Pseudoxanthoma Elasticum

Bercovitch L, Leroux T, Terry S, Weinstock MA. Pregnancy and obstetrical outcomes in pseudoxanthoma elasticum. Br J Dermatol. 2004;151:1011–1018.

Pericardial Disease

Ristić AD, Seferović PM, Ljubić A, et al. Pericardial disease during pregnancy. Herz. 2003;28:209–215.

Spodick DH. Pericardial disorders during pregnancy. In: Spodick DH, ed. The Pericardium: A Comprehensive Text book. : Dekker; 1997:89–92.

Polyartcritis Nodosa

Malillos Pérez M, Ortega Carnicer O, Gutiérrez Millet V, Pazmiño Narváez L. Infarto agudo de miocardio posparto asociado a panarteritis nodosa [Postpartum acute myocardial infarction associated with panarteritis nodosa (author's transl)] Med Clin (Barc). 78198232–34.

Pulmonary Atresia

Averbuch M, Bojko A, Levo Y. Cardiac tamponade in the early post partum period as the presenting and predominant manifestation of systemic lupus. J Rheumatol. 1986: 13444–13445.

Connoly HM, Warnes CA. Outcome of pregnancy in patients with complex pulmonary atresia. Am J Cardiol. 1997;79: 519–521.

Drenthen W, Pieper PG, Zoon N, et al. Pregnancy after biventricular repair for pulmonary atresia with ventricular septal defect. Am J Cardiol. 2006;98:16–29.

Neumayer U, Somerville J. Outcome of pregnancies in patients with complex pulmonary atresia. Heart. 1997;78(1): 16–21.

Stangl V, Bamberg C, Schröder T, et al. Pregnancy outcome in patients with complex pulmonary atresia: case report and review of the literature. Eur J Heart Fail. 2010;12:202–207.

Pulmonary Hypertension

Avdalovic M, Sandrock C, Hoso A, Allen R, Albertson TE. Epoprostenol in pregnant patients with secondary pulmonary hypertension: two case reports and a review of the literature. Treat Respir Med. 2004;3(1):29–34.

Badalian SS, Silverman RK, Aubry RH, Longo J. Twin pregnancy in a woman on long term epoprostenol therapy for primary pulmonary hypertension. *J Reprod Med.* 2000;45(2):149–1152.

Bassily-Marcus AM, Yuan C, Oropello J, Manasia A, Kohli-Seth R, Benjamin E. Pulmonary hypertension in pregnancy: critical care management. *Pulm Med.* 2012;2012: 709407.

Bédard E, Dimopoulos K, Gatzoulis MA. Has there been any progress made on pregnancy outcomes among women with pulmonary hypertension? *Eur Heart J.* 2009;30: 256–265.

Bédard E, Dimopoulos K, Gatzoulis MA. Has there been any progress made on pregnancy outcomes among women with pulmonary arterial hypertension? *Eur Heart J.* 2009;30:256–265.

Bildrici I, Shumway JB. Intravenous and inhaled epoprostenol for primary pulmonary hypertension during pregnancy. *Am J Obstet Gynecol.* 2004;103(5 Pt 2):1102–1105.

Bonnin M, Mercier FJ, Sitbon O, et al. Severe pulmonary hypertension during pregnancy: mode of delivery and anesthetic management of 15 consecutive cases. *Anesthesiology.* 2005;102:1133–1137.

Decoene C, Bourzoufi K, Moreau D, Narducci F, Crepin F, Krivosic-Horber R. Use of inhaled nitric oxide for emergency cesarean section in a woman with unexpected primary pulmonary hypertension. *Can J Anaesth.* 2001;48:584–587.

Duarte AG, Thomas S, Safdar Z, et al. Management of pulmonary arterial hypertension during pregnancy: a retrospective, multicenter experience. *Chest.* 2013;143: 1330–1336.

Easterling TR, Ralph DD, Schmucker BC. Pulmonary hypertension in pregnancy: treatment with pulmonary vasodilators. *Obstet Gynecol.* 1999;93:494–498.

Hsu CH, Gomberg-Maitland M, Glassner C, Chen JH. The management of pregnancy and pregnancy-related medical conditions in pulmonary arterial hypertension patients. *Int J Clin Pract Suppl.* 2011;65(172):6–14.

Huang S, DeSantis ER. Treatment of pulmonary arterial hypertension in pregnancy. *Am J Health Syst Pharm.* 2007;64(18):1922–1926.

Huang S., Treatment of pulmonary arterial hypertension in pregnancy. 2007 Sep 15; doi: 10.2146/ajhp060391. PMID: 17823103.

Jaïs X, Olsson KM, Barbera JA, et al. Pregnancy outcomes in pulmonary arterial hypertension in the modern management era. *Eur Respir J.* 2012;40:881–885.

Katsuragi S, Yamanaka K, Neki R, et al. Maternal outcome in pregnancy complicated with pulmonary arterial hypertension. *Circ J.* 2012;76:2249–2254.

Kiely DG, Condliffe R, Webster V, et al. Improved survival in pregnancy using a multiprofessional approach. *BJOG.* 2010;117:565–574.

Ladouceur M, Benoit L, Radojevic J, et al. Pregnancy outcomes in patients with pulmonary arterial hypertension associated with congenital heart disease. *Heart.* 2017;103 :287–292.

Lam GK, Stafford RE, Thorp J, Moise Jr KJ, Cairns BA. Inhaled nitric oxide for primary pulmonary hypertension in pregnancy. *Obstet Gynecol.* 2001;98:895–898.

Madden BP. Pulmonary hypertension and pregnancy. *Int J Obstet Anesth.* 2009;18:156–164.

Monnery L, Nanson J, Charlton G. Primary pulmonary hypertension in pregnancy: a role for novel vasodilators. *Br J Anaesth.* 2001;87:295–298.

Nootens M, Rich S. Successful management of labour and delivery in primary pulmonary hypertension. *Am J Cardiol.* 1993;71:1124–1125.

Olsson KM, Channick R. Pregnancy in pulmonary arterial hypertension. *Eur Resp Rev.* 2016;25(142):431–437.

Pieper PG, Hoendermis ES. Pregnancy in women with pulmonary hypertension. *Neth Heart J.* 2011;19(12): 504–508.

Stewart R, Tuazon D, Olson G, Duarte AG. Pregnancy and primary pulmonary hypertension: successful outcome with epoprostenol therapy. *Chest.* 2001;119:973–975.

Stewart R, Tuazon D, Olson G, Duarte AG. Pregnancy and primary pulmonary hypertension: successful outcome with epoprostenol therapy. *Chest.* 2001;119:973–975.

Terek D, Kayikcioglu M, Kultursay H, et al. Pulmonary arterial hypertension and pregnancy. *J Res Med Sci.* 2013;18: 73–76.

Torres PJ, Gratacós E, Magriñá J, Martínez-Crespo JM, Cardrach V. Primary pulmonary hypertension and pre-eclampsia: a successful pregnancy. *Br J Obstet Gynaecol.* 1994;101:163–165.

Warnes CA. Pregnancy and pulmonary hypertension. *Int J Cardiol.* 2004;97:11–13.

Weiss BM, Zemp L, Seifert B, Hess OM. Outcome of pulmonary vascular disease in pregnancy; a systematic review from 1978 through 1996. *J Am Coll Cardiol.* 1998;31: 1650–1657.

Pulmonary Valve Regurgitation

Stout K, Otto CM. Pregnancy in women with valvular heart disease. *Heart.* 2007;93(5):552–558.

Pulmonic Stenosis

Drenthen W, Pieper PG, Roos-Hesselink JW, et al. Non-cardiac complications during pregnancy in women with isolated pulmonary valvar stenosis. *Heart.* 2006;92(12): 1838–1843.

Hameed AB, Goodwin TM, Elkayam U. Effect of pulmonary stenosis on pregnancy outcomes—a case control study. *Am Heart J.* 2007;154(5):852–854.

Pulmonary Vascular Disease

Weiss BM, Zemp L, Seifert B, Hess OM. Outcome of pulmonary vascular disease in pregnancy: a systematic overview from 1978 through 1996. *J Am Coll Cardiol.* 1998;31:1650–1657.

Single Ventricle

Stiller RJ, Vintzileos AM, Nochimson DJ, et al. Single ventricle in pregnancy: case report and review of the literature. *Obstet Gynecol.* 1984;64(3 suppl):18S–20S.

Sumner D, Melville C, Smith CD, Hunt T, Kenney A. Successful pregnancy in a patient with a single ventricle. *Eur J Obstet Gynecol.* 1992;44(3):239–240.

Rheumatic Heart Disease

Johnson MJ. Obstetric complications and rheumatic disease. *Rheum Dis Clin North Am.* 1997;23:169–182.

Sawhney H, Aggarwal N, Suri V, Vasishta K, Sharma Y, Grover A. Maternal and perinatal outcome in rheumatic heart disease. *Int J Gynecol Obstet.* 2003;80:9–14.

Right Ventricular Dysplasia

Lui CY, Marcus FI, Sobonya RE. Arrhythmogenic right ventricular dysplasia masquerading as peripartum cardiomyopathy with atrial flutter, advanced atrioventricular block and embolic stroke. *Cardiology.* 2002;97:49–50.

Systemic Lupus Erythematosus

Aggarwal N, Raveendran A, Suri V, Chopra S, Sikka P, Sharma A. Pregnancy outcome in systemic lupus erythematosus: Asia's largest single centre study. *Arch Gynecol Obstet.* 2011;284(2):281–285.

Al Arfaj AS, Khalil N. Pregnancy outcome in 396 pregnancies in patients with SLE in Saudi Arabia. *Lupus.* 2010;19:1665–1673.

Brucato A, Frassi M, Franceschini F, et al. Risk of congenital complete heart block in newborns of mothers with anti-Ro/SSA antibodies detected by counterimmunoelectrophoresis: a prospective study of 100 women. *Arthritis Rheum.* 2001;44:832–1835.

Buyon JP, Kim MY, Copel JA, Friedman DM. Anti-Rho/SSA antibodies and congenital heart block: necessary but not sufficient. *Arthritis Rheum.* 2001;44:1723–1727.

Buyon JP, Kim MY, Guerra MM, et al. Predictors of pregnancy outcomes in patients with lupus: a cohort study. *Ann Intern Med.* 2015;163(3):153–163.

Buyon JP, Rupel A, Clancy RM. Neonatal lupus syndrome. *Lupus.* 2004;13:705–712.

Cavallasca JA, Laborde HA, Ruda-Vega H, Nasswetter GG. Maternal and fetal outcomes of 72 pregnancies in Argentine patients with systemic lupus erythematosus (SLE). *Clin Rheumatol.* 2008;27:41–46.

Chen S, Sun X, Wu B, Lian X. Pregnancy in Women with systemic lupus erythematosus: a retrospective study of 83 pregnancies at a single centre. *Int J Envion Res Public Health.* 2015;12:9876–9888.

és-Hernández J, Ordi-Ros J, Paredes F, Casellas M, Castillo F, Vilardell-Tarres M. Clinical predictors of fetal and maternal outcome in systemic lupus erythematosus: a prospective study of 103 pregnancies. *Rheumatol (Oxf).* 2002;41(6):643–650.

Georgiou PE, Politi EN, Katsimbri P, Sakka V, Drosos AA. Outcome of lupus pregnancy: a controlled study. *Rheumatol (Oxf).* 2000;39(9):1014–10019.

Hughes G. The eradication of congenital heart block. *Lupus.* 2004;43(suppl):S5–S12.

Lateef A, Petri M. Managing lupus patients during pregnancy. *Best Pract Res Clin Rheumatol.* 2013;27(3):435–447.

McMillan E, Martin WL, Waugh J, et al. Management of pregnancy in women with pulmonary hypertension secondary to SLE and anti-phospholipid syndrome. *Lupus.* 2002;11:392–398.

Petri M, Howard D, Repke J. Frequency of lupus flare in pregnancy. The Hopkins Lupus Pregnancy Center experience. *Arthritis Rheum.* 1991;34:679–682.

Ruiz-Irastorza G, et al. Increased rate of lupus flare during pregnancy and the puerperium: a prospective study of 78 pregnancies. *Br J Rheumatol.* 1996;35:133–138.

Ruiz-Irastorza G, Khaashta MA. Evaluation of systemic lupus erythematosus activity during pregnancy. *Lupus.* 2004;13:679–682.

Ruiz-Irastorza G, Khaashta MA. Management of thrombosis in antiphospholipid syndrome and systemic lupus in pregnancy. *Ann NY Acad Sci.* 2005;1051:606–612.

Ruiz-Irastorza G, Khamashta MA, Nelson-Piercy C, Hughes GR. Lupus pregnancy: is heparin a risk factor for osteoporosis? *Lupus.* 2001;10:597–600.

Saaleb S, Copel J, Friedman D, Buyon JP. Comparison of treatment with fluorinated glucocorticoids to the natural history of autoantibody-associated congenital heart block. *Arthritis Rheum.* 1999;42:2335–2345.

Smyth A, Oliveira GH, Lahr BD, Bailey KR, Norby SM, Garovic VD. A systematic review and meta-analysis of pregnancy outcomes in patients with systemic lupus erythematosus and lupus nephritis. *Clin J Am Soc Nephrol.* 2010;5(11):2060–2068.

Soubassi L, Haidopoulos D, Sindos M, et al. Pregnancy outcome in women with pre-existing lupus nephritis. *J Obstet Gynaecol.* 2004;24(6):630–634.

Stojan G, Baer AN. Flares of systemic lupus erythematosus during pregnancy and the puerperium: prevention, diagnosis and management. *Expert Rev Clin Immunol.* 2012;8(5):439–453.

Wang PH, Teng SW, Lee FK. Disease activity of pregnant women with systemic lupus erythematosus. *J Chin Med Assoc.* 2015;78:193–194.

Zen M, Ghirardello A, Iaccarino L, et al. Hormones, immune response, and pregnancy in healthy women and SLE patients. *Swiss Med Wkly*. 2010;140(13-14):187–201.

Zhao CM, Zhao J, Huang Y, et al. New-onset systemic lupus erythematosus during pregnancy. *Clin Rheumatol*. 2013;32:815–822.

Still's Disease

Parry G, Goudevenos J, Williams DO. Coronary thrombosis postpartum in a young woman with Still's disease. *Clin Cardiol*. 1992;15:305307.

Syncope

Chatur S, Islam S, Moore LE, et al. Incidence of syncope during pregnancy: temporal trends and outcomes. *J Am Heart Assoc*. 2019;8(10):8 e011608.

Systemic Sclerosis

Steen VD. Scleroderma and pregnancy. *Rheum Dis Clin North Am*. 1997;23:133–147.

Steen VD, Conte C, Day N, Ramsey-Goldman R, Medsger Jr. TA. Pregnancy in women with systemic sclerosis. *Arthritis Rheum*. 1989;32:151–157.

Steen VD, et al. Prospective pregnancy study in women with systemic sclerosis. *Arthritis Rheum*. 1996;39:S151.

Takayasu Arteritis

Sharma BK, Jain S, Vasishta K. Outcome of pregnancy in Takayasu arteritis. *Int J Cardiol*. 2000;75(suppl 1):S159–S162.

Takotsubo Cardiomyopathy

Brezina P, Isler CM. Takotsubo cardiomyopathy in pregnancy. *Obstet Gynecol*. 2008;112(2 Pt 2):450–452.

Citro R, Giudice R, Mirra M, et al. Is Tako-tsubo syndrome in the postpartum period a clinical entity different from peripartum cardiomyopathy? *J Cardiovasc Med*. 2013;14: 568–575.

Citro R, Pascotto M, Provenza G, Gregorio G, Bossone E. Transient left ventricular ballooning (tako-tsubo cardiomyopathy) soon after intravenous ergonovine injection following caesarean delivery. *Int J Cardiol*. 2010;138(2): e31–e34.

Minatoguchi M, Itakura A, Takagi E, Nishibayashi M, Kikuchi M, Ishihara O. Takotsubo cardiomyopathy after cesarean: a case report and published work review of pregnancy . *J Obstet Gynaecol Res*. 2014;40(6):1534–1539.

Tetralogy of Fallot

Balci A, Drenthen W, Mulder BJ, et al. Pregnancy in women with corrected tetralogy of Fallot: occurrence and predictors of adverse events. *Am Heart J*. 2011;16(2):307–313.

Meijer JM, Pieper PG, Drenthen W, et al. Pregnancy, fertility, and recurrence risk in corrected tetralogy of Fallot. *Heart*. 1995;91:713–714.

Veldtman G, et al. Outcomes of pregnancy in women with tetralogy of Fallot. *J Am Coll Cardiol*. 2004;44910:174–180.

Transposition of the Great Vessels

Connolly HM, Grogan M, Warnes CA. Pregnancy among women with congenitally corrected transposition of the great arteries. *J Am Col Cardiol*. 1999;33(6):1962–1965.

Greutmann M, Von Klemperer K, Brooks R, et al. Pregnancy outcome in women with congenital heart disease and residual haemodynamic lesion of the right ventricular outflow tract. *Eur Heart J*. 2010;31(14):1764–1770.

Therrin J, Barnes I, Somerville J. Outcome of pregnancy in patients with congenitally corrected transposition of the great arteries. *Am J Cardiol*. 1999;84(7):820–824.

Tobler D, Fernandes SM, Wald RM, et al. Pregnancy outcomes in women with transposition of the great arteries and arterial switch operation. *Am J Cardiol*. 2010;106(3): 417–420.

Tricuspid Atresia

Bitsch M, et al. Tricuspid atresia and pregnancy. *Eur J Obstet Gynecol Reprod Biol*. 1989;31(3):277–282.

Carmona F, Martínez S, Periz A, Cararach V. Pregnancy after surgical correction of tricuspid atresia. *Acta Obstet Gynecol Scand*. 1993;72:498–499.

Collins MJ, et al. Tricuspid atresia and pregnancy. *Obstet Gynecol*. 1977;50(suppl 1):72S–73S.

Hess DB, Hess LW, Heath BJ, et al. Pregnancy after Fontan repair of tricuspid atresia. *South Med J*. 1991;84(4):532–534.

Tricuspid Stenosis

Silwa k, Johnson MR, Zilla P, Roos-Hesselink JW. Management of valvular disease in pregnancy. *Eur Heart J*. 2015;36(8):1078–1089.

Tricuspid Regurgitation

Limacher MC, Ware JA, O'Meara ME, Fernandez GC, Young JB. Tricuspid regurgitation during pregnancy: two-dimensional and pulsed Doppler echocardiographic observations. *Am J Cardiol*. 1985;55(8):1059–1062.

Soh MC, Sankaran S, Chung NY, et al. Mildly raised tricuspid regurgitant velocity 2.5-3.0 m/s in pregnant women with sickle cell disease is not associated with poor obstetric outcome—an observational study. *Obstet Med*. 2016;9(4): 160–163.

Valvular Heart Disease

Hameed A, Karaalp IS, Tummala PP, et al. The effect of valvular heart disease on maternal and fetal outcome during pregnancy. *J Am Coll Cardiol*. 2001;37:893–899.

Leśniak-Sobelga A, Tracz W, KostKiewicz M, Podolec P, Pasowicz M. Clinical and echocardiographic assessment of pregnant women with valvular heart disease—maternal and fetal outcome. *Int J Cardiol*. 2004;94:15–23.

Malhorta M, Sharma JB, Tripathii R, Arora P, Arora R. Maternal and fetal outcome in valvular heart disease. *Int J Gynecol Obstet.* 2004;84:11–16.

Reimold SC, Rutherford MB. Valvular heart disease in pregnancy. *N Engl J Med.* 2003;349:52–59.

Vasovagal Syncope

Burke D, Wildsmith JA. Severe vasovagal attack during regional anesthesia for cesarean section. *Br J Anaesth.* 2000;84(1):118–120.

Goncé-Mellgren A, Tamayo-Rojas O, Sánchez-Martinez M, Salvia-Roigés D, Ramírez-Ruz J, Cararach-Ramoneda V. Encefalopatía neonatal grave, secundaria a episodio vasovagal prolongado en una gestante de 31 semanas [Severe neonatal encephalopathy, secondary to a prolonged vasovagal episode in a woman 31 weeks pregnant]. *Rev Neurol.* 2002;34(9):833–835.

Huang MH, Roeske WR, Hu H, Indik JH, Marcus FI. Postural position and neurocardiogenic syncope in late pregnancy. *Am J Cardiol.* 2003;92(10):1252–1253.

Jang YE, Do SH, Song IA. Vasovagal cardiac arrest during spinal anesthesia for Cesarean section—a case report. *Korean J Anesthesiol.* 2013;64(1):77–81.

Jarvi K, Osborn N, Wall N. An obstetric patient with neurocardiogenic syncope. *Int J Obstet Anesth.* 2009;18(4):396–399.

Meek T. Severe vasovagal attack during regional anesthesia for cesarean section. *Br J Anaesth.* 2000;84(6):825.

Occhetta E, Bortnik M, Audoglio R, Vassanelli C. INVASY Study Investigators. Closed loop stimulation in prevention of vasovagal syncope. Inotropy controlled pacing in vasovagal syncope (INVASY): a multicentre randomized, single blind, controlled study. *Europace.* 2004;6(6):538–547.

Peterson AL, Isler WC. Applied tension treatment of vasovagal syncope during pregnancy. *Mil Med.* 2004;169(9):751–753.

Saqr LK. Neurocardiogenic syncope in the obstetric patient. *Anaesthesia.* 2007;62(1):79–84.

Tsai PS, Chen CP, Tsai MS. Perioperative vasovagal syncope with focus on obstetric anesthesia. *Taiwan J Obstet Gynecol.* 2006;45(3):208–214.

Watkins EJ, Dresner M, Calow CE. Severe vasovagal attack during regional anesthesia for cesarean section. *Br J Anaesth.* 2000;84(1):118–120.

Weksler N, Rozenstweig V, Shapira AR. Severe vasovagal attack: an unusual cause of abruptio placentae. *Arch Gynecol Obstet.* 2004;270(4):299–301.

Ventricular Septal Defects

Carson M. Hypertension and pregnancy. *Medscape.* May 3 2016 updated.

Roos-Hesselink JW, Duvekot JJ, Thorne SA. Pregnancy in high risk cardiac conditions. *Heart.* 2009;95:680–686.

Siu SC, Sermer M, Colman JM, et al. Prospective multicenter study of pregnancy outcomes in women with heart disease. *Circulation.* 2001;104:515–521.

8

Peripartum Cardiomyopathy

John H. Wilson, MD, FACC, FHRS

Peripartum cardiomyopathy (PPCM), a disorder specific to pregnancy, is one of the most feared complications for pregnant women and their medical care teams. It carries such a heightened risk for recurrence and subsequent morbidity and mortality that it warrants counseling against future conception. However, relatively little is understood about its underlying pathophysiology, risk factors, and early warning signs. This chapter explores the incidence and risk factors, diagnosis, proposed etiologies and pathophysiology, treatment, and prognosis of PPCM.

INCIDENCE AND RISK FACTORS

Owing to the tremendous overlap with other diseases and given that PPCM is a diagnosis of exclusion, its true incidence is unknown. In addition, the highly variable clinical presentation makes it difficult to determine an accurate incidence estimate in resource-poor countries. The World Health Organization (WHO) estimates that between 18 and 333 cases of PPCM occur for every 100,000 live births. The wide variation reflects regional differences, with rates as high as 1 in 50 live births within certain African countries and Haiti. Within the United States, the incidence ranges between 1 in 2066 to 1 in 4025 live births. Racial differences also can account for the relatively wide range of incidence estimates. A US study by Harper and colleagues demonstrated a significantly higher incidence in Black women versus Hispanic and White women. The incidence of PPCM was 9.2 cases per 10, 000 live births among Black women versus 2.34 per 10, 000 live births among White women and 0.32 per 10, 000 live births among Hispanic women. These differences appear to correlate with and can be partly explained by examining the identified risk factors for PPCM (Table 8.1).

DIAGNOSIS

Historically, the diagnostic criteria for PPCM have included the development of heart failure in the last month of pregnancy or within the first 6 months of the postpartum period, the absence of preexisting heart disease, and echocardiograph findings of left ventricular (LV) systolic failure (Box 8.1). Most cases occur within the first 3 months postpartum, with far fewer cases occurring during late pregnancy or between 3 and 6 months postpartum. Symptoms include dyspnea, peripheral edema, fatigue, orthopnea, paroxysmal nocturnal dyspnea, palpitations, chest pain, decreased exercise tolerance, anorexia, persistent cough, and abdominal discomfort. Signs on the physical examination include pulmonary rales, a loud second heart sound (S2), a third heart sound (S3) or gallop, mitral murmur, tricuspid murmur, lateral and downward displacement of the cardiac point of maximal impulse, jugular venous distension, hepatojugular reflux, hepatomegaly, peripheral edema, and ascites. These symptoms and signs overlap with several other disease processes, so it is essential to rule out other causes of heart failure in establishing the diagnosis of peripartum cardiomyopathy.

TABLE 8.1 Risk Factors for Peripartum Cardiomyopathy by Evidence Association

Demonstrated	Proposed	Emerging
Multifetal gestation (twins)	Smoking	Preeclampsia
High gravidity and parity	Chronic hypertension	Genetics
Extremes of reproductive age	Malnutrition	Obesity
Prolonged tocolysis	Cocaine abuse	
	African ancestry	
	Socioeconomic status	

BOX 8.1 Diagnostic Criteria of Peripartum Cardiomyopathy

- Development of systolic heart failure in last month of pregnancy or first 6 months of the postpartum period
- Absence of preexisting heart disease
- Echocardiograph findings of LV systolic heart failure
  - LV end-diastolic dimension >2.7 cm/m²
  - M-mode fractional shortening <30%
  - LV ejection fraction < 5%

LV, Left ventricular.

Often, a brain natriuretic peptide serum level is elevated markedly above the already heightened value seen in pregnancy; values greater than 120 pg/mL are incongruent with the normal physiologic changes of pregnancy and suggest a disease process. The electrocardiogram (ECG) may be useful in ruling out other causes of cardiac disease. ECG findings in patients with PPCM are somewhat nonspecific and include sinus tachycardia, nonspecific ST- and T-wave changes, Q waves in the anterior precordium, and mildly prolonged PR and QRS intervals. Rarer findings include atrial fibrillation, left bundle branch block, and left atrial enlargement. Chest radiographs and echocardiography likely will identify enlargement of the cardiac silhouette, left atrial and LV enlargement, pulmonary congestion, and possibly pulmonary edema. If LV function is markedly reduced (left ventricular ejection fraction [LVEF] <35%), a thrombus near the apex of the left ventricle may be witnessed.

Because we are able to estimate right ventricular systolic pressures with echocardiography, right heart catheterization is seldom necessary.

In establishing the diagnosis of PPCM, the major disease entity to rule out is hypertensive heart failure of pregnancy. Although both can be seen in the setting of hypertensive disorders of pregnancy, such as preeclampsia, the latter tends to demonstrate evidence of LV hypertrophy and diastolic dysfunction rather than the dilated and relatively thin-walled, poorly contractile left ventricle of PPCM. Additional differential diagnostic considerations include underlying acquired or congenital valvular heart disease that was unmasked by the burdens of pregnancy (e.g., mitral or aortic stenosis), preexisting cardiomyopathies (idiopathic dilated cardiomyopathy, familial dilated cardiomyopathy, HIV/AIDS cardiomyopathy), preexisting undetected congenital heart disease (e.g., ventricular septal defects), myocardial infarction, and pulmonary embolism.

PROPOSED ETIOLOGIES AND PATHOPHYSIOLOGY

Many research teams have investigated potential etiologies in the development of PPCM, and it is likely that the pathophysiology involves elements of several processes. The immune system likely plays a role through various inflammatory pathways, potentially in response to the pregnancy itself, the hemodynamic stresses of pregnancy, or subacute infection. The resultant inflammation may then lead to weakening of the cardiac myocytes with increased myocyte apoptosis. In the presence of an abnormal and potentially detrimental hormonal milieu within the maternal vasculature that increases systemic vascular resistance, myocyte apoptosis places more of a burden on the already weakened myocardium. Increased adrenergic tone throughout the cardiovascular system can be witnessed, supporting this theory.

One of the leading pathophysiologic theories behind the mechanism whereby PPCM develops focuses on the role of prolactin and potential genetic predispositions. Prolactin is produced and secreted by the anterior pituitary gland as a 23-kD protein. Most of the normal biologic functions attributable to the prolactin hormone are initiated by this 23-kDa form. An enzyme known as cathepsin D, along with various matrix metalloproteinases (MMPs), can cleave the 23-kDa prolactin molecule into a 16-kDa biologically active fragment (alternatively referred to as vasoinhibin). This smaller form (16kDa) of prolactin acts on the endothelium of the circulatory system, causing vasoconstriction, apoptosis, inflammation, and capillary destruction. Additionally, the 16-kDa prolactin molecule causes diminished cardiomyocyte metabolism, diminished contractility, and chamber dilation within the heart. Individuals lacking normal alleles of the cardiac tissue-specific signal transduction, an activator of transcription gene (STAT3), demonstrate a buildup of oxidative free radicals within the mitochondria of the cardiomyocytes. These oxidative free radicals promote release of MMPs and activation of the cathepsin D enzyme, leading to increased cleavage of the normal 23-kDa prolactin molecule and potentially the development of PPCM.

However, not all individuals with STAT3 mutations develop PPCM, suggesting a potential two-hit hypothesis. Researchers suggest that individuals lacking normal STAT3 function or other genetic variants (e.g., the *TTN* gene, which encodes for a sarcomere protein, titin) are genetically predisposed to PPCM, but the full development of the disease requires additional late-gestational or postpartum hormonal changes or vasotoxic effects. Emerging evidence suggests that several proangiogenic factors (vascular endothelial growth factor and placenta-like growth factor), and antiangiogenic factors (e.g., soluble FMS-like tyrosine kinase inhibitor 1, 16-kDa prolactin, placenta-derived soluble endoglin, and leptin) may play a role. The proangiogenic factors recruit and enhance the mobilization of circulating endothelial progenitor cells, which play a critical role in endothelial homeostasis and repair. The antiangiogenic factors neutralize the proangiogenic factors, and their serum concentrations have been demonstrated to be elevated in women with preeclampsia, PPCM, vasculitides, and atherosclerosis. Thus, women who develop PPCM may be predisposed to the disease by genetic abnormalities that prime the heart and vascular endothelium for a devastating hit when they subsequently experience an insult during the second wave of placentation; the result is upregulated placental production of antiangiogenic factors overwhelming the endothelium and leading to the downstream cascade of clinical signs and symptoms of PPCM.

TREATMENT

Standard heart failure regimens are the cornerstone of therapy for women with PPCM, in both the antepartum and postpartum periods. The focuses of this therapy are to minimize the afterload, improve contractility, and reduce preload at a time when the hormonal and circulatory changes attributable to pregnancy are increasing preload and afterload. A woman who presents in cardiogenic shock requires a multidisciplinary team focused on returning stable maternal cardiovascular function before efforts are made to deliver the fetus. Attempting to deliver the fetus when an unstable woman is in cardiogenic shock might cause her status to deteriorate and ultimately lead to her death. However, certain medications should be avoided while the woman is still pregnant. Table 8.2 lists the types of medications that make up the complete standard approach to patients with PPCM depending on whether they are still pregnant or are postpartum. Nearly all patients are prescribed

TABLE 8.2 Medications to Treat Patients With Peripartum Cardiomyopathy		
Type of Medication	**Options During Pregnancy**	**Options After Pregnancy**
Vasodilators	Hydralazine	ACE inhibitors
	Nitrates	ARBs
Diuretics	Hydrochlorothiazide	Hydrochlorothiazide
	Furosemide	Furosemide
Beta blockers	Carvedilol	Carvedilol
	Metoprolol	Atenolol and metoprolol
Anticoagulants	IV UFH	LWMH
	LMWH	Warfarin
Other	Digitalis	Digitalis
		Spironolactone

IACE, Angiotensin-converting enzyme; *ARB*, angiotensin receptor blocker; *IV, intravenous*; *LMWH*, Low-molecular-weight heparin; *UFH*, unfractionated heparin.

some form of vasodilator, diuretic, and beta blocker, but additional agents, such as antiarrhythmics, anticoagulants, and inotropic agents, can be added as the clinical circumstances demand. In pregnancy, angiotensin-converting enzyme inhibitors and receptor blockers should be avoided, and although some clinicians would recommend against spironolactone use, it is likely safe in late gestation. Therapeutic-dose anticoagulation medications should be initiated in the presence of a LV thrombus or atrial fibrillation, and they also should be considered for a LVEF below 35%. In pregnancy, intravenous unfractionated heparin should be initiated first, given the potential need for imminent delivery, whereas in the postpartum period, low-molecular-weight heparin can be initiated (1 mg/kg twice daily) to bridge to warfarin. For women who fail to respond to these measures, consider delivering the fetus first followed by mechanical support with a ventricular-assist device, which is generally continued until native heart function improves or a cardiac transplant is performed.

When a pregnant woman with PPCM is in stable condition, delivery should be entertained in the early term period (37–38 weeks). Cesarean delivery should be reserved for obstetric indications. An operative vaginal delivery should be considered, which will shorten the second stage of labor. Importantly, such women should undergo epidural analgesia early in the course of labor to minimize pain, anxiety, and the resultant catecholamine surge, which might overburden a sick myocardium. Given the potential link with prolactin, some have advocated against breastfeeding in women with PPCM, and this may be a reasonable recommendation for women with severely reduced systolic function or who are recalcitrant to therapies.

Like all patients with significant LV dysfunction, women with PPCM are at risk for serious ventricular arrythmias. Because women with PPCM are young and have dependents, they would seem to be an ideal target population for the defibrillator vest. A recent multicenter study seems to confirm this concept. Researchers identified a group of 49 patients from 16 German centers. All had newly diagnosed PPCM and an ejection fraction less than 35%. All were given a cardioverter defibrillator vest. In this group, five patients had ventricular fibrillation, and two had sustained ventricular tachycardia over a period of 3 to 6 months. All received appropriate shocks, and none died. Not all studies have found such dramatic results, but this is the largest study to date, and

it suggests that this therapy is appropriate. Patients who do not recover LV function and persist with an EF below 35% should receive an implantable defibrillator.

Bromocriptine, a medication that inhibits pituitary prolactin secretion, has been suggested as a possible treatment for patients with PPCM. Preliminary studies have demonstrated a possible benefit from bromocriptine; however, the data are insufficient to recommend widespread use in those with PPCM. Bromocriptine inhibits lactation, eliminating the possibility of breastfeeding. Additionally, it has been linked to an increased risk of thromboembolic complications; therefore, anticoagulation is recommended if bromocriptine is used for treatment of patients with PPCM.

PROGNOSIS

Compared with other forms of heart failure, PPCM has a relatively good prognosis. Older studies suggested that 50% of women recover normal heart function, 25% experience no recovery but remain stable, and 25% progress to severe failure. New literature highlights the benefits of modern therapies with improved rates of complete recovery (return of LV function to an LVEF >50%). However, certain factors are associated with lowered rates of complete recovery, including LVEF less than 30%, fractional shortening less than 20%, LV end-diastolic dimension greater than 6 cm, and elevated cardiac troponin T. Among those patients with a complete recovery of LVEF to above 50%, 20% may experience a significant decline in their LV function (20% drop in LVEF or more) during a subsequent pregnancy. Women with persistent LV dysfunction are at substantial risk for worsening LV dysfunction in subsequent pregnancies (~40%) and death (nearly 20%). As such, these women fall into the WHO class IV strata of cardiac disease in pregnancy, wherein subsequent pregnancies are not advised; moreover, if a woman does become pregnant inadvertently, termination should be offered.

BIBLIOGRAPHY

Bello N, Rendon IS, Arany Z. The relationship between pre-eclampsia and peripartum cardiomyopathy: a systematic review and meta-analysis. *J Am Coll Cardiol.* 2013;62:1715.

Blauwet LA, Cooper LT. Diagnosis and management of peripartum cardiomyopathy. *Heart.* 2011;97:1970.

Duncker D, Westenfeld R, Konrad T, et al. Risk for life-threatening arrhythmia in newly diagnosed peripartum cardiomyopathy with low ejection fraction: a German multi-centre analysis. *Clin Res Cardiol.* 2017;106(8):582–589.

Eklayam U, Akhter MW, Singh H, et al. Pregnancy-associated cardiomyopathy: clinical characteristics and a comparison between early and late presentation. *Circulation.* 2005;111:2050.

Hilfiker-Kleiner D, Kaminski K, Podewski E, et al. A cathepsin D-cleaved 16 kDa form of prolactin mediates postpartum cardiomyopathy. *Cell.* 2007;128:589.

Mandal D, Mandal S, Mukherjee D, et al. Pregnancy and subsequent pregnancy outcomes in peripartum cardiomyopathy. *J Obstetric Gynaecol Res.* 2011;37:222.

Patten IS, Rana S, Arany Z, et al. Cardiac angiogenic imbalance leads to peripartum cardiomyopathy. *Nature.* 2012;485:333.

Pearson GD, Veille JC, Rahimtoola S, et al. Peripartum cardiomyopathy: National Heart, Lung, and Blood Institute and Office of Rare Diseases (National Institutes of Health) workshop recommendations and review. *JAMA.* 2000;283:1183.

Podewski EK, Hilfiker-Kleiner D, Hilfiker A, et al. Alterations in Janus kinase (JAK)-signal transducers and activators of transcription (STAT) signaling in patients with end-stage dilated cardiomyopathy. *Circulation.* 2003;107:798.

Silwa K, Blauwet L, Tibazarwa K, et al. Evaluation of bromocriptine in the treatment of acute severe peripartum cardiomyopathy a proof of-of-concept pilot study. *Circulation.* 2010;121(13):1465–1473.

Sliwa K, Fett J, Elkayam U. Peripartum cardiomyopathy. *Lancet.* 2006;368:687.

9

Endocarditis in Pregnancy

John H. Wilson, MD, FACC, FHRS

Endocarditis usually occurs on previously damaged heart valves or is associated with shunt lesions or baffles. When seen on previously normal valves, endocarditis is most often on the right-sided valves and is associated with intravenous (IV) drug abuse. This chapter discusses the incidence and risk factors, diagnosis, and treatment of endocarditis in pregnancy.

INCIDENCE AND RISK FACTORS

Although endocarditis is rare in pregnancy (incidence of 0.03–0.14 per 1000 live births), it may be fatal. Pregnant women are at higher risk of endocarditis than their nonpregnant counterparts because pregnancy is an immunocompromised state, and certain infections, particularly urinary tract infections, are more common during pregnancy. Streptococcal infections are the most common cause of endocarditis.

The reported incidence of bacteremia with vaginal delivery is 0% to 5%. With cesarean section, it has been reported as high as 14%.

DIAGNOSIS

The diagnostic criteria for endocarditis are the same as in nonpregnant women. Most commonly used are the Duke criteria, outlined next.

Major Criteria

Two or more positive blood cultures with a typical organism and no primary source
Echocardiographic criteria of endocarditis

Minor Criteria

Predisposing cardiac condition or IV drug use
Fever greater than 38°C

Vascular features (emboli or mycotic aneurysms)
Immunologic features (Osler's nodes or glomerulonephritis)
Positive blood cultures not meeting major criteria
Definite endocarditis is diagnosed if:
Two major criteria are met or
One major criterion and three or more minor criteria are met or
Five minor criteria are met.
    Possible endocarditis is diagnosed if:
One major criterion and one minor criterion are met or
Three or four minor criteria are met.

TREATMENT

As with diagnosis, blood cultures are the key to the appropriate treatment of patients with endocarditis. Three to six sets should be obtained at separate sites and times, preferably before starting antibiotics. Antibiotic therapy is determined by the organism present and its antibiotic sensitivity. In a pregnant woman, treatment should always be done in consultation with an infectious disease specialist.

Certain antibiotics are known to produce adverse effects in the fetus if given during pregnancy. Aminoglycosides may cause ototoxicity, but they can be used if levels are monitored. Chloramphenicol can cause gray baby syndrome. Sulfonamides can cause neonatal jaundice if given after 34 weeks of gestation. Tetracyclines slow bone growth and can cause enamel hypoplasia. If used in the first trimester, trimethoprim has been associated with neural tube defects.

Antibiotic prophylaxis is generally not recommended for obstetric procedures, including vaginal delivery and cesarean section.

BIBLIOGRAPHY

Aoyagi S, Akasu K, Amako M, Yoshikawa K, Hori H. Infective endocarditis during pregnancy: report of a case. *Ann Thorac Cardiovasc Surg.* 2005;11:51–54.

Baker TH, Hubbell R. Reappraisal of asymptomatic puerperal bacteremia. *Am J Obstet Gynecol.* 1967;97:575–576.

Campuzano K, Roque H, Bolnick A, et al. Bacterial endocarditis complicating pregnancy: case report and systematic review of the literature. *Arch Gynecol Obstet.* 2003;268: 251–255.

Campuzano K, Roqué H, Bolnick A, Leo MV, Campbell WA. Bacterial endocarditis complicating pregnancy: a case report and systematic review of the literature. *Arch Gynecol Obstet.* 2003;268:251–255.

Connolly C, O'Donoghue K, Doran H, McCarthy FP. Infective endocarditis in pregnancy: case report and review of the literature. *Obstet Med.* 2015;8(2):102–104.

Datta S, Wykes C. Is labour safe in infective endocarditis patients with septic lung embolism? *J Obstet Gynecol.* 2007;27:858–859.

Marcoux J, Rosin M, Mycyk T. CPB-assisted aortic valve replacement in a pregnant 27-year old with endocarditis. *Perfusion.* 2009;24:361–364.

Montoya ME, Karnath BM, Ahmad M. Endocarditis during pregnancy. *South Med J.* 2003;96:1156–1157.

Ou TY, Chen RF, Hsu CS, et al. Pulmonary valve endocarditis in a pregnant woman with a ventricular septal defect. *J Microbiol Immunol Infect.* 2009;42:92–95.

Quiñones JN, Campbell F, Coassolo KM, Pytlewski G, Maran P. Tricuspid valve endocarditis during the second trimester of pregnancy. *Obstet Med.* 2010;3:78–80.

Shimada K, Nakazawa S, Ishikawa N, Haga M, Takahashi Y, Kanazawa H. Successful surgical treatment for infective endocarditis during pregnancy. *Gen Thorac Cardiovasc Surg.* 2007;55:428–430.

Vizzardi E, De Cicco G, Zanini G, et al. Infectious endocarditis during pregnancy, problems in the decision-making process: a case report. *Cases J.* 2009;2:6537–6546.

Yuan S. Infective endocarditis during pregnancy. *J Coll Phys Pakistan.* 2014;25(2):134–139.

10

Arrhythmias During Pregnancy

John H. Wilson, MD, FACC, FHRS

Arrhythmias of any type may occur during pregnancy. Patients who have a condition that predisposes them to develop arrhythmias may have their initial episodes during pregnancy, and patients who already have arrhythmias may have them continue during pregnancy. Some patients with supraventricular tachycardias (SVTs) have a reduction in the frequency of episodes while pregnant, and others have an increase. This chapter first provides an overview of arrhythmias in pregnancy and the drugs used to treat them and then discusses specific types of arrhythmias.

OVERVIEW: ARRHYTHMIAS

There are three physiologic mechanisms of arrhythmia: automaticity, reentry, and triggered activity. The physiologic changes of pregnancy enhance the probability of firing of an automatic focus and predispose to reentry. Increased catecholamine levels promote automaticity and shorten the refractory period of myocardial tissues, which also predisposes to reentry. By increasing the length of reentrant circuits, cardiac dilation predisposes to reentry as well.

The mainstays of modern diagnostic and therapeutic management of arrhythmias—electrophysiologic evaluation and ablation—could be performed during pregnancy, but they are rarely warranted because most arrhythmias can be diagnosed noninvasively and treated medically until after delivery.

In assessing a patient with arrhythmias, it is important to evaluate for causative factors, including structural heart disease, which usually can be diagnosed with an echocardiogram; electrolyte abnormalities; and hyperthyroidism. In pregnant patients, pulmonary emboli also should be considered. Channelopathies (a group of congenital disorders of the ion channels that predispose

patients to arrhythmias) may first present during pregnancy. Most often, they can be diagnosed with a 12-lead electrocardiogram (ECG).

For the most part, arrhythmias during pregnancy are treated in the same way as in nonpregnant patients. Digoxin; beta blockers; and antiarrhythmic drugs, such as flecainide, propafenone, and amiodarone, can be used with reasonable safety.

Antiarrhythmic drugs may sometimes have to be administered to a pregnant woman to treat fetal tachycardia. Sotalol, flecainide, and amiodarone may be used for this purpose. Amiodarone is usually reserved for resistant cases because of the potential for fetal thyrotoxicity.

SPECIFIC ARRHYTHMIAS: DIAGNOSIS AND MANAGEMENT

Specific arrhythmias include atrial fibrillation, atrial flutter, bradycardia, channelopathies, palpitations, premature contractions, tachycardia, SVT, VT, and Wolff-Parkinson-White (WPW) syndrome.

Atrial Fibrillation

Atrial fibrillation is rare in pregnancy, and typically it is associated with a causative factor, such as hyperthyroidism or structural heart disease. Unless associated with mitral stenosis, it is usually well tolerated. Atrial fibrillation in pregnant women is treated in a manner very similar to that in nonpregnant patients. Rate control, if necessary, can be achieved with intravenous (IV) verapamil. Verapamil is preferable to diltiazem because it has a good safety profile in pregnancy. There are limited data on diltiazem and reports of embryopathy in animal studies. For chronic rate control, oral verapamil or beta blockers can be used (avoid using atenolol in the first trimester). Digoxin is safe to use but not very effective; generally, it is used only as a second- or third-line drug in patients with left ventricular dysfunction. Anticoagulation with heparin is mandatory to prevent embolic events. Cardioversion should be undertaken as soon as practical. Propofol can be used safely for anesthesia during cardioversion. If long-term antiarrhythmic therapy is needed to maintain sinus rhythm, flecainide, sotalol, or amiodarone can be used. There is considerable experience using these drugs to treat fetal tachycardia, and they seem well tolerated by both the mother and baby. Amiodarone has the potential for fetal thyrotoxicity.

The difficult part of managing pregnant patients with either atrial fibrillation or atrial flutter is anticoagulation. Warfarin is generally contraindicated during pregnancy, particularly during weeks 6 to 12, because of embryopathy. The newer anticoagulants, non–vitamin K antagonist oral anticoagulants (NOACs), are probably contraindicated because they are small molecules that can cross the placenta. There have been accidental exposures of pregnant women to NOACs, but the data are very limited. At present, the best option is to use IV heparin or therapeutic doses of enoxaparin.

CHADS$_2$-VASc is a measure that helps predict the likelihood that a patient will have a stroke; the letters or contributing factors in the acronym stand for **c**ongestive heart failure, **h**igh blood pressure, **a**ge, **d**iabetes, and **s**troke (double weight). Women with normal hearts and low CHADS$_2$-VASc scores may not require anticoagulation throughout pregnancy, but they should receive it for a least 1 month after cardioversion because all guidelines (American Heart Association [AHA], American College of Cardiology [ACC], and Heart Rhythm Society [HRS]) recommend postcardioversion anticoagulation for all patients with atrial fibrillation with a duration of 48 hours or more. The AHA/ACC/HRS guidelines suggest the same anticoagulation regimen for patients with atrial flutter as for those with atrial fibrillation.

Atrial Flutter

Atrial flutter is rare in pregnancy and is usually associated with congenital heart disease. Atrial flutter in pregnant women is treated in a manner very similar to that in nonpregnant patients. Rate control, if necessary, can be achieved with IV verapamil. Verapamil is preferable to diltiazem because it has a good safety profile in pregnancy, but there are limited data on diltiazem, and there are reports of embryopathy in animal studies. For chronic

rate control, oral verapamil or beta blockers can be used (again, avoid using atenolol in the first trimester). Digoxin is safe to use but not very effective; generally, it is used only as a second- or third-line drug in patients with left ventricular dysfunction. Anticoagulation with heparin is mandatory to prevent embolic events. Cardioversion should be undertaken as soon as practical. Propofol can be used safely for anesthesia during cardioversion. If long-term antiarrhythmic therapy is needed to maintain sinus rhythm, flecainide, sotalol, or amiodarone can be used. There is considerable experience using these drugs to treat fetal tachycardia, and they seem well tolerated by both the mother and baby. Amiodarone has the potential for injury to the fetal thyroid gland.

Bradycardia

Bradycardia during pregnancy is rare. There are benign cases that are attributed to the supine hypotension syndrome of pregnancy, which is caused by uterine compression of the vena cava restricting blood return to the right atrium. In general, there is no effective medical treatment for bradycardia, so in severe cases, a pacemaker is implanted. Both temporary and permanent pacemakers can be used if necessary. Minimal exposure of the fetus to radiation should be a priority. Women with congenital third-degree atrioventricular (AV) block generally tolerate pregnancy well.

Channelopathies

Women with channelopathies who became pregnant have a variable risk depending on the specific syndrome they have. Patients with Brugada syndrome have little, if any, additional risk of arrhythmias while pregnant. Patients with long QT syndrome type 2 (LQT2) seem to be at increased risk in the postpartum period. Patients with either of these syndromes should avoid drugs known to precipitate arrhythmias. Patients with LQTS should continue their previously prescribed antiarrhythmic medications throughout pregnancy. Nadolol, a common medication used for LQTS, is safe to take while pregnant. Patients with LQTS should avoid all drugs that prolong the QT interval. Ondansetron, a common antiemetic used in pregnancy, may do this and should be avoided.

Palpitations

Palpitations are simply an awareness of the heartbeat. Patients complaining of palpitations may have a normal rhythm, single ectopic beats, or more sustained arrhythmias. The key to making a correct diagnosis is to record an ECG tracing during the episode. This can be done with a 12-lead ECG, a Holter monitor, or more sustained types of monitoring, such as a wearable event recorder. A number of cell phone apps can record, with good fidelity, single- or multilead ECGs. A cell phone recording is often the most practical option, although methods of transmission, storage, and appropriate confidentiality have not been standardized. Occasionally, patients with cardiac rhythm management devices, such as pacemakers, defibrillators, or implantable loop recorders, may be encountered, and these devices usually will have recorded ECGs of all arrhythmia the patient may have had.

Complaints of palpitations are common during pregnancy. Investigation will document ectopic beats, or nonsustained arrhythmias, in about half of patients complaining of palpitations. Sustained tachycardias are documented about 0.2% to 0.3% of the time.

Premature Contractions

Premature atrial contractions (PACs) are known to increase during pregnancy and may be a factor in increasing the incidence of SVT because most episodes of SVT are initiated by PACs. In and of themselves, PACs require no treatment.

Premature ventricular contractions also increase during pregnancy. Like PACs, they require no treatment.

Tachycardia

Sinus tachycardia is common during pregnancy, and although it may cause symptoms, it requires no treatment. The average patient has a heart rate increase of 10 beats/min during pregnancy. Sinus tachycardia with heart rates over 100 beats/min is common. If symptoms are disabling, consider treatment with a beta blocker. Atenolol should not be used during the first trimester because it has been associated with fetal growth restriction.

Supraventricular Tachycardia

Supraventricular tachycardia may have been present before pregnancy, and it is hard to predict whether the frequency of episodes will change during pregnancy. Some women seem to have more frequent episodes, likely because of the known increase in PAC frequency during pregnancy. As noted earlier, PACs often initiate sustained SVT episodes. Other women seem to have

a reduction in the frequency of SVT episodes, but the reason is unknown. The most common types of SVT encountered in pregnant patients include AV node reentry and AV reentry caused by accessory AV connections. Adenosine can be used safely for acute termination of SVT during pregnancy. Long-term treatment with beta blockers or verapamil can be recommended safely. Again, atenolol should not be used in the first trimester.

Ventricular Tachycardia

Ventricular tachycardia (VT) is usually divided into two groups, idiopathic and VT caused by structural heart disease. Idiopathic VT is relatively benign and has a prognosis similar to that of SVT. Sustained ventricular tachycardia associated with structural heart disease is potentially lethal and most often requires an implantable cardioverter-defibrillator (ICD) to protect the life of the patient.

When a patient presents with wide-complex tachycardia, the cause may not be immediately identifiable. If the patient is hemodynamically compromised, immediate cardioversion is necessary and can be accomplished safely in pregnant women, with propofol used for anesthesia. When the patient is hemodynamically stable, the cause of the wide complex tachycardia can be identified.

There are three possibilities for wide-complex tachycardia: aberrant conduction of an SVT, preexcited tachycardia, and ventricular tachycardia. One can usually make the correct diagnosis with the patient history and ECGs during the tachycardia and after resolution. Patients with VT most often have a history of structural heart disease. The exception is those presenting with idiopathic VT. Aberrant conduction exhibits either a typical right bundle or a typical left bundle branch block pattern on the ECG during tachycardia. VT, or a preexcited tachycardia, does not fall into either of these patterns. Patients with preexcitation show this on their posttachycardia ECGs.

If VT is identified and structural heart disease is known to be present, serious consideration should be given to using an ICD. Life vests may be considered as a temporary alternative, although their efficacy during pregnancy has not been established. To prevent recurrences, amiodarone can be used either intravenously or orally. If structural heart disease is not known to be present, an echocardiogram should be performed to look for it.

Idiopathic VT may respond to beta blockers, verapamil, or antiarrhythmic drugs. Flecainide, sotalol, and amiodarone can be used safely during pregnancy, although amiodarone may adversely affect the fetal thyroid gland.

Wolff-Parkinson-White Syndrome

Wolff-Parkinson-White syndrome is diagnosed by the presence of tachycardia in a patient with preexcitation on their ECG. The preexcitation seen on the ECG in sinus rhythm is a manifestation of conduction over an AV accessory connection. Patients with WPW syndrome are susceptible to AV reentrant arrhythmias involving conduction over the accessory connection in one direction and conduction through the AV node, His bundle, and bundle branches in the other. If the antegrade conduction is through the AV node, a narrow QRS complex will be seen during tachycardia, and the tachycardia is called *orthodromic reciprocating tachycardia*. If the antegrade limb of the tachycardia is via the accessory connection, a wide QRS complex will be seen during the tachycardia, and the tachycardia is called *antidromic reciprocating tachycardia*. Patients with WPW syndrome are susceptible to atrial fibrillation, which may be life threatening, because of the possibility of very rapid AV conduction over the accessory connection, which may then lead to ventricular fibrillation.

Patients with hypertrophic cardiomyopathy and Ebstein's anomaly have an increased incidence of WPW syndrome.

Patients with asymptomatic preexcitation may or may not develop tachycardia during pregnancy. No therapy is warranted, but it is prudent (on the part of both patients and care givers) to be aware of the possibility of tachycardia.

Treat AV reentrant tachycardias with beta blockers or adenosine. Digoxin should be avoided because it may accelerate conduction over an accessory connection. For atrial fibrillation, consider cardioversion or treatment with IV amiodarone. Definitive treatment with ablation should be deferred until after delivery.

BIBLIOGRAPHY

Ferrero S, Colombo BM, Ragni N. Maternal arrhythmias during pregnancy. *Arch Gynecol Obstet.* 2004;269:244–253.
Gowada RM, et al. Cardiac arrhythmias in pregnancy: clinical and therapeutic considerations. *Int J Cardiol.* 2003;88:19–133.
Joglar JA, Page RL. Management of arrhythmia syndromes during pregnancy. *Curr Opin Cardiol.* 2014;29:36–44.
Knots RJ, Garan H. Cardiac arrhythmias in pregnancy. *Semin Perinatol.* 2014;38:285–288.
Mendelson CL. Disorders of the heartbeat in pregnancy. *Am J Obstet Gynaecol.* 1956;72:1268.
Page RI. Treatment of arrhythmias in pregnancy. *Am Heart J.* 1995;130:871–876.
Perez-Silva Merino JI. Tachyarrhythmias in pregnancy. *EJ Cardiol Pract.* 2011;9:31.
Shotan A, Ostrzega E, Mehra A. Incidence of arrhythmias in normal pregnancy and relation to palpitations, dizziness, and syncope. *Am J Cardiol.* 1997;79:1061–1064.
Silversides CK, Harris L, Haberer K, Sermer M, Colman JM, Siu SC. Recurrence rates of Arrhythmias during pregnancy in women with previous tachyarrhythmia and impact on fetal and neonatal outcomes. *Am J Cardiol.* 2006;97:1206–1212.
Tan HL, Lie KI. Treatment of tachyarrhythmias during pregnancy and lactation. *Eur Heart J.* 2001;22(6). 4558-4464.

Antiarrhythmic Drugs
Bryerly WG, Hartmann A, Foster DE, Tannenbaum AK. Verapamil in the treatment of maternal paroxysmal supraventricular tachycardia. *Ann Emerg Med.* 1991;20 552-544.
Chow T, Galvin J, McGovern B. Antiarrhythmic drug therapy in pregnancy and lactation. *Am J Cardiol.* 1998;82:581–621.
Rotmensch HH, Elkayam U, Frishman W. Antiarrhythmic drug therapy during pregnancy. *Ann Intern Med.* 1983;98:487–497.
Widerhorn J, Bhandrari AK, Bughi S. Fetal and neonatal adverse effects profile of amiodarone treatment during pregnancy. *Am Heart J.* 1991;122:1162–1166.

Atrial Fibrillation
Dicarlo-Meacham LTA, Dahlke J. Atrial fibrillation in pregnancy. *Obstet Gynecol.* 2011;117(2):489–492.
Lee MS, Chen W, Zhang Z, et al. Atrial fibrillation and atrial flutter in pregnant women—a population based study. *J Am Heart Assoc.* 2016;5:e003182.

Atrial Flutter
Lee MS, Chen W, Zhang Z, et al. Atrial fibrillation and atrial flutter in pregnant women—a population based study. *J Am Heart Assoc.* 2016:e003182.

Cardioversion
Barnes EJ, Eben F, Patterson D. Direct current cardioversion during pregnancy should be performed with facilities available for fetal monitoring and emergency caesarean section. *Br J Obstet Gynaecol.* 2002;109(12):1406–1407.

Finlay AY, Edmunds V. DC cardioversion in pregnancy. *Br J Clin Pract*. 1979;33:88–94.

Klepper I. Cardioversion in late pregnancy. *Anaesthesia*. 1981;36:611–616.

Long QT Syndromes

Rasaba EJ, Zareba W, Moss AJ, et al. Influence of pregnancy on the risk for cardiac events in patients with hereditary long Qt syndrome LQTS investigators. *Circulation*. 1998;97:451–456.

Palpitations

Adamson DL, Nelson-Piercy C. Managing palpitations and arrhythmias during pregnancy. *Heart*. 2007;93(12): 1630–1636.

Supraventricular Tachycardia

Dunn JS, Brost BC. Fetal bradycardia after IV adenosine for maternal PSVT. *Am J Emerg Med*. 2000;18:234–235.

Elkayam U, Goodwin TM. Adenosine therapy for supraventricular tachycardia during pregnancy. *Am J Cardiol*. 1995;75:521–523.

Harrison JK, Greenfield RA, Wharton JM. Acute termination of supraventricular tachycardia by adenosine during pregnancy. *Am Heart J*. 1992;5:1386–1388.

Klein V, Repke JT. Supraventricular tachycardia in pregnancy: cardioversion with verapamil. *Obstet Gynecol*. 1984;63: 165–185.

Lee SH, Chen SA, Wu TJ, et al. Effects of pregnancy on first onset and symptoms of paroxysmal supraventricular tachycardia. *Am J Cardiol*. 1993;76:675–678.

Mason BA, et al. Adenosine in the treatment of maternal paroxysmal supraventricular tachycardia. *Am J Cardiol*. 1995;76:675–678.

Robins K, Lyons G. Supraventricular tachycardia in pregnancy. *Br J Anaesth*. 2004;92(1):140–143.

Tawam M, Levine J, Mendelson M, Goldberger J, Dyer A, Kadish A. Effect of pregnancy on paroxysmal supraventricular tachycardia. *Am J Cardiol*. 1993;72:838–840.

VanZijl DHS, Dyer A, Scott Millar RN, James MFM. Supraventricular tachycardia during spinal anaesthesia for caesarean section. *Int J Obstet Anesth*. 2001;10:202–205.

Ventricular Tachycardia

Kotchetkov R, Patel A, Salehian O. Ventricular tachycardia in pregnant patients. *Clin Med Insights Cardiol*. 2010;4: 39–44.

Nakagawa M, Katou S, Ichinose M, et al. Characteristics of new-onset ventricular arrhythmias in pregnancy. *J Electrocardiol*. 2004;37:47–53.

Ventricular Fibrillation

Columbo J, Lawal AH, Bhandari A, Hawkins JL, Atlee JL. Case 1: a patient with severe peripartum cardiomyopathy and persistent ventricular fibrillation supported by a biventricular assist device. *J Cardiothorac Vasc Anesth*. 2002;16:107–113.

Wolf Parkinson White Syndrome

Ahmad A, et al. Wolff-Parkinson syndrome in pregnancy: risks and management dilemmas—a review of literature. *Eur Clin Obstet Gynaecol*. 2008;3(3):123–126.

Gleicher N, Mellor J, Sandler RZ, Sullum S. Wolf-Parkinson-White syndrome in pregnancy. *Obstet Gynaecol*. 1981;58: 748–751.

Widerhorn J, Widerhorn ALM, Rahimtoola SH, Elkayam U. WPW syndrome in pregnancy: increased incidence of supraventricular arrhythmias. *Am Heart J*. 1992;123: 796–798.

11

Fetal Tachycardia

Timothy K. Knilans, MD

Fetal tachycardia complicates about 0.5% of pregnancies and is a significant contributor to fetal mortality and morbidity. Defined as a fetal heart rate over 180 beats/min, it may be caused by various forms of supraventricular tachycardia (SVT) or ventricular tachycardia (VT). One serious consequence of untreated fetal tachycardia may be nonimmune hydrops fetalis.

DIAGNOSIS

Fetal tachycardia is often initially diagnosed by auscultation or Doppler evaluation, which can indicate a rapid ventricular rate but does not elucidate the mechanism of the tachycardia. Fetal electrocardiography (ECG) can be performed with specialized equipment by attaching electrodes to the maternal abdomen; it is limited in later pregnancy by electrical insulation of the fetus because of the development the vernix caseosa, a cheeselike coating made of shed skin cells and sebaceous secretions. Fetal magnetocardiography, measurement of the magnetic field created by cardiac electrical activity, can provide a tracing similar to the ECG, but few centers have the necessary specialized equipment.

Fetal echocardiography is the most commonly used method to determine the mechanism of fetal tachycardia. This is done by using M-mode imaging with the sector oriented through the fetal atrium and ventricle to assess mechanical contraction of both chambers and their relative timing. Doppler interrogation directed at ventricular inflow and simultaneous recording of inferior vena cava and aortic flow also can be used to identify occurrence and timing of atrial and ventricular contraction. Using these techniques, fetal tachycardia can be subdivided into rhythms with a one-to-one atrioventricular (AV) relationship or those with atrial rates faster or slower than the ventricular rate.

Fetal tachycardia with one-to-one AV relationship is most commonly supraventricular in mechanism, but VT with retrograde conduction to the atrium is not excluded. AV reentrant tachycardia using an accessory AV connection is the most common form of SVT with a one-to-one AV relationship in the fetus with SVT. Junctional tachycardia and AV nodal reentrant tachycardia account for a much smaller proportion of cases. The specific timing of the atrial and ventricular activity can be helpful in differentiating these mechanisms with AV reentry having short ventricular-to-atrial (VA) intervals and atrial tachycardia and the permanent form of junctional reciprocating tachycardia (AV reentry with slowly conducting accessory pathway) having longer VA intervals. AV nodal reentry and junctional tachycardia with one-to-one VA conduction, which are rare in fetuses, have simultaneous atrial and ventricular activation. Careful assessment of paroxysmal (sudden in onset) fetal tachycardia to ascertain the specifics of initiation and termination can be helpful in diagnosis. Repeated termination of tachycardia with the last event being an atrial contraction suggests an AV nodal–dependent mechanism or ventricular origin.

Fetal SVT is associated with cardiac structural abnormalities in only about 2% of cases, and Ebstein's anomaly of the tricuspid valve is the most frequently associated abnormality. Sometimes frequent premature atrial contractions (PACs) are detected. In and of themselves, they are not harmful and require no therapy. However, the rare fetus with frequent PACs detected may go on to develop tachycardia. This is likely caused by the origin of PACs being single accessory pathway echo beats to the atrium.

Fetal tachycardia with atrial rates exceeding the ventricular rate is atrial in origin. Atrial flutter is the most frequently seen of these and the second most common cause of fetal tachycardia, comprising between 21% and 50% of cases. The atrial rate is typically between 350 and 500/min, and often there are two or three atrial contractions for every ventricular contraction.

Atrial tachycardia is less commonly seen and typically presents with a slower atrial rate than atrial flutter and may at times have one-to-one conduction. Coexistence of atrial flutter and AV reentrant tachycardia in the same fetus is common and may be related to prolonged AV reentry resulting in atrial dilation and subsequent atrial flutter.

Ventricular tachycardia is rare as a cause of fetal tachycardia. It is usually paroxysmal. Cases of polymorphic VT related to congenital long QT syndromes have been reported and should be strongly suspected if there is family history of the disease.

TREATMENT

In most cases, it is best to treat fetal tachycardia because of the risk of fetal tachycardia-induced cardiomyopathy, congestive heart failure, and hydrops fetalis. In cases when the tachycardia burden is low and there is no indication of hydrops, it may be reasonable not to initiate therapy, but careful monitoring is indicated with or without treatment. Both the tachycardia burden and the heart rate have been shown to be predictors of fetal hydrops; the type of tachycardia and the gestational age at onset are also predictive. Even so, the ability to identify which babies will get into trouble is limited. Therapy is usually with antiarrhythmic drugs given to the mother. Previously, digoxin has been the first-line therapy because of its limited side effects and risk to the mother, but recent experience suggests that flecainide is superior in efficacy, especially for the most common form of fetal tachycardia (AV reentry). Sotalol appears to be more effective for atrial flutter, but often only ventricular rate control can be achieved with this rhythm. If these drugs fail, amiodarone can be quite effective.

Digoxin reportedly achieves fetal-to-maternal plasma concentration ratios that vary between 0.4 and 0.9. However, in case of fetal hydrops, this ratio is reduced, which may cause the treatment to fail. Conversion to sinus rhythm is reported in approximately 50% of cases of SVT and 45% of cases of atrial flutter. In tachycardia complicated by hydrops, conversion rates are lower, in the range of 15% to 25%. Maternal adverse effects are confined to nausea, vomiting, and headache, mostly related to overdosing. Cardiac adverse effects are ventricular extrasystoles and heart block. Digoxin seems to have a relatively low fetal mortality rate. Direct fetal administration has been reported, but it clearly carries its own risks.

Sotalol is a class III antiarrhythmic drug with beta-blocking properties. The transplacental transfer is excellent, with a fetal-to-maternal ratio of 1:1. The success rate of sotalol as a single agent in the treatment of patients with atrial flutter is approximately 65%, rising to 80% with the addition of digoxin. The success rate in fetal SVT is approximately 55% with sotalol as a single drug and 75% with the addition of digoxin. Maternal adverse effects are mostly related to its beta-blocking properties. Sotalol has been associated with intrauterine deaths, mainly in hydropic cases. Whether these intrauterine deaths are caused by proarrhythmia is unknown, as death from fetal hydrops is a well-known complication.

Flecainide, a class IC antiarrhythmic agent, is used mainly in cases of AV reentry. If used as a sole agent in cases of atrial flutter, it could lead to faster ventricular rates because it can slow the tachycardia and does not block the AV node. The transplacental transfer is good, with fetal-to-maternal ratios ranging from 0.5 to 0.97. Reported conversion rates for SVT range from 75% to 92%. The adverse effects of flecainide are dizziness, headache, visual disturbances, paresthesia, tremors, flushing, and nausea and vomiting. It has been associated with intrauterine deaths, some possibly from proarrhythmia.

Amiodarone is an antiarrhythmic agent with actions of all four antiarrhythmic drug classes. The transplacental transfer is relatively low, with fetal-to-maternal ratios of 0.2 to 0.4. In a large study by Strasburger et al. (2004), amiodarone was initiated in drug-refractory fetal tachycardia complicated by hydrops. They reported a high success rate of 93% in SVT, a lower conversion rate of 33% in atrial flutter, and no fetal deaths. Some infants treated with amiodarone may develop hypothyroidism.

In severely hydropic fetuses or those with therapy-resistant tachycardia, direct fetal therapy is sometimes initiated. Several modes of administration have been described, including intraumbilical, intraamniotic, intraperitoneal, intramuscular, and intracardiac. To minimize the number of invasive procedures, fetal intramuscular or intraperitoneal injections that provide a more sustained release are preferred. On occasion, early delivery is necessary, but complications and mortality in premature infants, especially those with hydrops fetalis, must be weighed against the risk of continuing the pregnancy.

BIBLIOGRAPHY

Allan LD, Anderson RH, Sullivan ID, et al. Evaluation of fetal arrhythmias by echocardiography. *Br Heart J*. 1983;50:240–245.

Allan LD, Chita SK, Sharland GK, et al. Flecainide in the treatment of fetal tachycardias. *Br Heart J*. 1991;65:46–48.

Allan LD. Cardiac ultrasound of the fetus. *Arch Dis Childhood*. 1984;59:603–604.

Alsaied T, Baskar S, Fares M, et al. First-line antiarrhythmic transplacental treatment for fetal tachyarrhythmia: a systematic review and meta-analysis. *J Am Heart Assoc*. 2017;6:e007164.

Azancot-Benisty a, Jacqz-Aigrain E, Guirgis NM, et al. Clinical and pharmacologic study of fetal supraventricular tachyarrhythmias. *J Pediatr*. 1992;121:608–613.

Barjot P, Hamel P, Calmelet P, et al. Flecainide against fetal supraventricular tachycardia complicated by hydrops fetalis. *Acta Obstet Gynecol Scand*. 1998;77:353–354.

Bergmans MGM, Jonker GJ, Kock HCL, et al. Fetal supraventricular tachycardia: review of the literature. *Obstet Gynecol Surv*. 1985;40:61–68.

Bourget P, Pons JC, Delouis C, et al. Flecainide distribution, transplacental passage, and accumulation in the amniotic fluid during the third trimester of pregnancy. *Ann Pharmacother*. 1994;28:1031–1034.

Chan V, Tse TF, Wong V. Transfer of digoxin across the placenta and into breast milk. *Br J Obstet Gynaecol*. 1978;85:605–609.

Copel JA, Friedman AH, Kleinman CS, et al. Management of fetal cardiac arrhythmias. *Fetal Diagn Ther*. 1997;24:201–211.

Cuneo BF, Ovadia M, Strasburger JF, et al. Prenatal diagnosis and in utero treatment of torsades de pointes associated with congenital long QT syndrome. *Am J Cardiol*. 2003;91:1395–1398.

Cuneo BF, Strasburger JF. Management strategy for fetal tachycardia. *Obstet Gynecol*. 2000;96:575–581.

Cuneo BF. Treatment of fetal tachycardia. *Heart Rhythm*. 2008;5(5):1216–1218.

Donn SM, Bowerman RA. Association of paroxysmal supraventricular tachycardia and periventricular leukomalacia. *Am J Perinatol*. 1993;10:212–214.

Ebenroth ES, Cordes TM, Darragh RK. Second-line treatment of fetal supraventricular tachycardia using flecainide acetate. *Pediatr Cardiol*. 2001;22:483–487.

Echt DS, Liebson PR, Mitchell LB, et al. Mortality and morbidity in patients receiving encainide, flecainide, or placebo, the cardiac arrhythmia suppression trial. *N Engl J Med*. 1991;324:781–788.

Ekiz A, Kaya B, Bornaun H, et al. Flecainide as first line treatment for fetal supraventricular tachycardia. *J Matern Fetal Neonatal Med*. 2018;31(4):407–412.

Fouron JC, Fournier A, Proulx F, et al. Management of fetal tachyarrhythmia based on superior vena cava/aorta Doppler flow recordings. *Heart*. 2003;89:1211–1216.

Fouron JC, Proulx F, Miro J, et al. Doppler and M-mode ultrasonography to time fetal atrial and ventricular contractions. *Obstet Gynecol*. 2000;96:732–736.

Frohn-Mulder IM, Stewart PA, Witsenburg M, et al. The efficacy of flecainide versus digoxin in the management of fetal supraventricular tachycardia. *Prenat Diagn*. 1995;15:1297–1302.

Gembruch U, Manz M, Bald R, et al. Repeated intravascular treatment with amiodarone in a fetus with refractory supraventricular tachycardia and hydrops fetalis. *Am Heart J*. 1989;118:1335–1338.

Gest AL, Hansen TN, Moise AA, et al. Atrial tachycardia causes hydrops in fetal lambs. *Am J Physiol*. 1990;258:H1159–H1163.

Grimm B, Haueisen J, Huotilainen M, et al. Recommended standards for fetal magnetocardiography. *Pacing Clin Electrophysiol*. 2003;26:2121–2126.

Gunteroth WG, Cyr DR, Shields LR, et al. Rate-based management of fetal supraventricular tachycardia. *J Ultrasound Med*. 1996;13:453–458.

Hallak M, Neerhof MG, Perry R, et al. Fetal supraventricular tachycardia and hydrops fetalis: combined intensive, direct, and transplacental therapy. *Obstet Gynecol*. 1991;78:523–525.

Hamada H, Horigome H, Asaka M, et al. Prenatal diagnosis of long QT syndrome using fetal magnetocardiography. *Prenat Diagn*. 1999;19:677–680.

Hansmann M, Gembruch U, Bald R, et al. Fetal tachyarrhythmias: transplacental and direct treatment of the fetus. A report of 60 cases. *Ultrasound Obstet Gynecol*. 1991;1:162–170.

Hijazi ZM, Rosenfeld LE, Copel JA, et al. Amiodarone therapy of intractable atrial flutter in a premature hydropic neonate. *Pediatr Cardiol*. 1992;13:227–229.

Hill GD, Kovach JR, Saudek DE, et al. Transplacental treatment of fetal tachycardia: a systematic review and meta-analysis. *Prenat Diagn*. 2017;37:1076–1083.

Hosono T, Chiba Y, Shinto M, et al. A fetal Wolff-Parkinson-White syndrome diagnosed prenatally by magnetocardiography. *Fetal Diagn Ther*. 2001;16:215–217.

Jaeggi E, Fouron JC, Drblik SP, et al. Fetal atrial flutter: diagnosis clinical features, treatment and outcome. *J Pediatr*. 1998;132:335–339.

Jaeggi E, Fouron JC, Fournier A, et al. Ventriculo-atrial time interval measured on M-mode echocardiography: a determining element in diagnosis, treatment and prognosis of fetal supraventricular tachycardia. *Heart.* 1998;79:582–587.

Jouannic JM, LeBidois J, Fermont L, et al. Prenatal ultrasound may predict fetal response to therapy in non-hydropic fetuses with supraventricular tachycardia. *Fetal Diagn Ther.* 2002;17:120–123.

Kleinman CS, Copel JA, Weinstein EM, et al. Treatment of fetal supraventricular tachyarrhythmias. *J Clin Ultrasound.* 1985;13:265–273.

Kleinman CS, Nehgme R, Copel JA, et al. Fetal cardiac arrhythmias: diagnosis and therapy. In: Creasy RK, Resnik R, eds. *Matern-Fetal Medicine.* : Saunders; 1998:301–318.

Kofinas AD, Simon NV, Sagel H, et al. Treatment of fetal supraventricular tachycardia with flecainide acetate after digoxin failure. *Am J Obstet Gynecol.* 1991;165:630–631.

Kohl T, Tercanli S, Kececioglu D, et al. Direct fetal administration of adenosine for the termination of incessant supraventricular tachycardia. *Obstet Gynecol.* 1995;85:873–874.

Krapp M, Baschat AA, Gembruch U, et al. Flecainide in the intrauterine treatment of fetal supraventricular tachycardia *Ultrasound Obstet Gynecol.* 2002;19:158–164.

Krapp M, Baschat AA, Gembruch U, et al. Flecainide in the intrauterine treatment of fetal supraventricular tachycardia. *Ultrasound Obstet Gynecol.* 2002;19:158–164.

Krapp M, Kohl T, Simpson JM, et al. Review of diagnosis, treatment, and outcome of fetal atrial flutter compared with supraventricular tachycardia. *Heart.* 2003;89 923-917.

Lisowski LA, Verheijen PM, Benatar AA, et al. Atrial flutter in the perinatal age group: diagnosis, management and outcome. *J Am Coll Cardiol.* 2000;35:771–777.

Mangione R, Guyon F, Vergnaud A, et al. Successful treatment of refractory supraventricular tachycardia by repeat intravascular injection of amiodarone with long term follow-up. *Prenat Diagn.* 2000;20:449–452.

Maxwell DJ, Crawford DC, Curry PVM, et al. Obstetric importance, diagnosis, and management of fetal tachycardias. *Br Med J.* 1988;297:107–110.

Menendez T, Achenbach S, Beinder E, et al. Fetal cardiac arrhythmias: diagnosis and therapy. *Am J Cardiol.* 2001;88:334–336.

Naheed ZJ, Strasburger JF, Deal BJ, et al. Fetal tachycardia: mechanisms and predictors of hydrops fetalis. *J Am Coll Cardiol.* 1996;27:1736–1740.

Nijhuis IJM, Hof J, ten, Mulder EJH, et al. Antenatal fetal heart rate monitoring; normograms and minimal duration of recordings. *Prenat Neonat Med.* 1998;3:314–322.

Oudijk MA, Michon MM, Kleinman CS, et al. Sotalol in the treatment of fetal dysrhythmias. *Circulation.* 2000;101:2721–2726.

Oudijk MA, Ruskamp JM, Ambachtsheer EB, et al. Drug treatment of fetal tachycardias. *Pediatr Drugs.* 2002;4:49–63.

Oudijk MA, Ruskamp JM, Ververs FF, et al. Treatment of fetal tachycardia with sotalol: transplacental pharmacokinetics and pharmacodynamics. *J Am Coll Cardiol.* 2003;42:765–770.

Oudijk MA, Stoutenbeek Ph, Sreeram N, et al. Persistent junctional reciprocating tachycardia in the fetus. *J Matern Fetal Neonatal Med.* 2003;13:191–196.

Oudijk MA. Fetal tachycardia, diagnosis and treatment and the fetal QT interval in hypoxia. 2003.

Oudjik MA, Visser GHA, Meijboom EJ. Fetal tachyarrhythmia—part I: diagnosis. *Indian Pacing Electrophysiol J.* 2004;4(3):104–113.

Oudjik MA, Visser GHA, Meijboom EJ. Fetal tachyarrhythmia—part II: treatment. *Indian Pacing Electrophysiol J.* 4(4):185–194.

Parilla BV, Strasburger JF, Socol ML. Fetal supraventricular tachycardia complicated by hydrops fetalis: a role for direct fetal intramuscular therapy. *Am J Perinatol.* 1996;13:483–486.

Quartero HWP, Stinstra JG, Golbach EGM, et al. Clinical implications of fetal magnetocardiography. *Ultrasound Obstet Gynecol.* 2002;20:142–153.

Rogers MC, Willerson JT, Goldblatt A, et al. Serum digoxin concentrations in the human fetus, neonate and infant. *N Engl J Med.* 1972;16 1010-10.

Schade RP, Stoutenbeek PH, de Vries LS, et al. Neurological morbidity after fetal supraventricular tachyarrhythmia. *Ultrasound Obstet Gynecol.* 1999;13:43–47.

Simpson JM, Sharland GK. Fetal tachycardias: management and outcome of 127 consecutive cases. *Heart.* 1998;79 576-561.

Simpson LL, Marx GR, D'Alton ME. Supraventricular tachycardia in the fetus: conservative management in the absence of hemodynamic compromise. *J Ultrasound Med.* 1997;16:459–464.

Sonesson SE, Winberg P, Lidegran M, et al. Foetal supraventricular tachycardia and cerebral complications. *Acta Paediatr.* 1996;85:1249–1252.

Strasburger JF, Cuneo BF, Michon MM, et al. Amiodarone therapy for drug-refractory fetal tachycardia. *Circulation.* 2004;109:375–379.

Strasburger JF. Fetal arrhythmias. *Prog Pediatr Cardiol.* 2000;11:1–17.

Strasburger JF. Radiofrequency catheter ablation of ventricular tachycardia in patients without structural heart disease. *Prog Pediatr Cardiol.* 2000;11:1–17.

Van Engelen AD, Weijtens O, Brenner JL, et al. Management, outcome and follow-up of fetal tachycardia. *J Am Coll Cardiol.* 1994;24:1371–1375.

Villazon E, Fouron JC, Fournier A, et al. Prenatal diagnosis of junctional ectopic tachycardia. *Pediatr Cardiol.* 2001;22:160–162.

Wacker-Gussmann A, Strasburger JF, Srinivassan S, et al. Fetal atrial flutter: electrophysiology and association with rhythms involving an accessory pathway. *J Am Heart Assoc.* 2016;5:e003673.

Wagner X, Jouglard J, Moulin M, et al. Coadministration of flecainide acetate and sotalol during pregnancy: lack of teratogenic effects, passage across the placenta, and excretion in human breast milk. *Am Heart J.* 1990;119: 700–702.

Wladimiroff JW, Stewart PA. Treatment of fetal cardiac arrhythmias. *Br J Hosp Med.* 1985;34:134–140.

Younis JS, Granat M. Insufficient transplacental digoxin transfer in severe hydrops fetalis. *Am J Obstet Gynecol.* 1987;157:1268–1269.

12

An Overview: Pharmacology During Pregnancy

John H. Wilson, MD, FACC, FHRS

Pregnancy affects almost every aspect of pharmacology, including volume of distribution, protein binding, absorption, and metabolism. Consequently, when giving drugs to pregnant patients, the maternal cardiac care team must consider these changes in the maternal handling of drugs as well as how the drug will affect the fetus—not only potential teratogenesis but also the pharmacologic effects on the baby.

VOLUME OF DISTRIBUTION

A major effect of pregnancy is on the volume of distribution of many drugs. Starting at 6 to 8 weeks' gestation, maternal blood volume surges by 40% to 50%, with a concomitant increase in total body water, significantly increasing the volume of distribution for hydrophilic drugs. Another effect of hemodilution is the reduced peak concentration of hydrophilic drugs.

PROTEIN BINDING

During pregnancy, there is a relatively greater increase in plasma than in the cellular and protein components of blood, which leads to hemodilutional anemia and a decrease in the concentration of albumin and other drug-binding proteins. Therefore, drugs that are protein bound display a higher free level.

Respiratory changes in pregnancy also can affect pharmacology. Pregnancy is associated with an increased tidal volume of 30% to 50%, which begins during the first trimester and is driven by progesterone. The increase in tidal volume leads to an elevation in PaO_2 and a drop in PCO_2. The drop in PCO_2 leads to a respiratory alkalosis, with an increase in blood pH to 7.40 to 7.45. This change in pH may alter the protein binding of drugs. During pregnancy, the upper respiratory mucosa develops edema and increased vascularity, which in theory could increase the absorption of inhaled medications.

Renal blood flow and glomerular filtration rate increase by about 50% as early as 14 weeks' gestation. As a result, serum creatinine falls to an average of 0.8 mg/dL, and renal clearance of drugs increases by 20% to 65%. This increase may be an important consideration for renally cleared drugs such as many antibiotics, digoxin, and atenolol.

ABSORPTION

In pregnancy, gastric emptying and bowel transit time are prolonged by 30% to 50%, altering the bioavailability of drugs by reducing maximum concentration and the time to maximum concentration. This is most significant for drugs in which a rapid onset of action is desired. In addition, drug absorption may be reduced by the nausea and vomiting often associated with early pregnancy. During pregnancy, gastric pH increases, potentially ionizing drugs that are acidic and reducing their absorption. The increase in gastric pH also may enhance chelation by iron or antacids of co-administered drugs.

Opioid use for pain relief, during delivery or postpartum, also may delay intestinal transit time and drug absorption.

METABOLISM

Drug metabolism is enhanced in pregnancy because of increased activity of the enzymes involved in both phase I metabolism (reduction, oxidation, and hydrolysis) and phase II metabolism (glucuronidation, acetylation, methylation, and sulfation). The activity of the cytochrome P450 system, a family of oxidative liver enzymes involved in the metabolism of many drugs, is enhanced, resulting in faster metabolism of many drugs. One example of a drug metabolized by this system is nifedipine, which is metabolized by CYP3A4.

EFFECTS ON THE FETUS

The risk of a drug causing a fetal malformation is greatest when the drug is given during organogenesis, which occurs between weeks 3 and 8 of gestation. Drugs given during the second and third trimesters may affect fetal growth and functional development, or they may have a direct tissue toxicity or simply pharmacologic effects. The degree to which a drug affects the fetus depends on its ability to cross the placenta, and this ability is based primarily on its size. On average, no more than 10% of a drug will cross the placenta.

General principles guiding drug administration during pregnancy are that if a drug can be avoided, it should be avoided. However, if withholding a drug will adversely affect the mother's health, then it (or a safer alternative, if available) should be given. Low doses should be initiated and titrated up as necessary. Established drugs with known safety profiles are preferred. Both the mother and the fetus should be monitored for potential adverse effects.

The Food and Drug Administration (FDA) has classified most drugs based on the risk posed to the fetus. The classes are as follows:

A: Controlled studies have failed to demonstrate a risk to the fetus.

B: Animal studies have not demonstrated a risk, or animal studies found a risk, but it was not confirmed in humans.

C: Animal studies have demonstrated a risk, or no data is available.

D: There is evidence of risk to the fetus in humans.

X: The risk to the fetus is great enough to outweigh any potential benefit. Should not be used.

N: The FDA has not classified the drug.

BIBLIOGRAPHY

Anderson GD. Pregnancy-induced changes in pharmacokinetics: a mechanistic-based approach. *Clin Pharmacokinet.* 2005;44(10):989–1008.

Bogen DL, Perel JM, Helsel JC, et al. Pharmacologic evidence to support clinical decision making for peripartum methadone treatment. *Psychopharmacology.* 2013;225 (2):441–451.

Chambers CD, Polifka JE, Friedman JM. Drug safety in pregnant women and their babies: ignorance not bliss. *Clin Pharmacol Ther.* 2008;83(1):181–183.

Cheung CK, Lao T, Swaminathan R. Urinary excretion of some proteins and enzymes during normal pregnancy. *Clin Chem.* 1989;35(9):1978–1980.

Davison JM, Dunlop W. Renal hemodynamics and tubular function normal human pregnancy. *Kidney Int.* 1980;18 (2):152–161.

Erman A, Neri A, Sharoni R, et al. Enhanced urinary albumin excretion after 35 weeks of gestation and during labour in normal pregnancy. *Scand J Clin Lab Invest.* 1992;52 (5):409–413.

Feghali M, Venkataramanan R, Caritis S. Pharmacokinetics of drugs in pregnancy. *Semin Perinatol.* 2016;39(7): 512–519.

Hebert MF, Easterling TR, Kirby B, et al. Effects of pregnancy on CYP3A and P-glycoprotein activities as measured by disposition of midazolam and digoxin: a University of Washington specialized center of research study. *Clin Pharmacol Ther.* 2008;84(2):248–253.

Luxford AM, Kellaway GS. Pharmacokinetics of digoxin in pregnancy. *Eur J Clin Pharmacol.* 1983;25(1):117–121.

Maged MC. Physiologic and pharmacokinetic changes in pregnancy. *Front Pharmacol.* 2014;5:65–83.

Mitchell AA, Gilboa SM, Werler MM, et al. Medication use during pregnancy, with particular focus on prescription drugs: 1976-2008. *Am J Obstet Gynecol.* 2011;205(1). 51. e51-51.e58.

Pirani BB, Campbell DM, MacGillivray I. Plasma volume in normal first pregnancy. *J Obstet Gynaecol Br Commonw.* 1973;80(10):884–887.

Qasqas SA, McPherson C, Frishman WH, Elkayam U. Cardiovascular pharmacotherapeutic considerations during pregnancy and lactation. *Cardiol Rev.* 2004;12(4):201–221.

Syme MR, Paxton JW, Keelan JA. Drug transfer and metabolism by the human placenta. *Clin Pharmacokinet.* 2004;43(8):487–514.

Thomas SH, Yates LM. Prescribing without evidence—pregnancy. *Br J Clin Pharmacol*. 2012;74(4):691–697.

Tracy TS, Venkataramanan R, Glover DD, Caritis SN. National Institute for Child Health and Human Development Network of Maternal-Fetal-Medicine Unit. Temporal changes in drug metabolism (CYP1A2, CYP2D6 and CYP3A Activity) during pregnancy. *Am J Obstet Gynecol*. 2005;192(2):633–639.

Tsutsumi K, Kotegawa T, Matsuki S, et al. The effect of pregnancy on cytochrome P4501A2, xanthine oxidase, and N-acetyltransferase activities in humans. *Clin Pharmacol Ther*. 2001;70(2):121–125.

13

The Use of Cardiac Drugs During Pregnancy

John H. Wilson, MD, FACC, FHRS

In Chapter 12, we presented an overview of pharmacology during pregnancy; in this chapter, we focus on drugs specifically used to treat cardiac conditions in expecting mothers. These conditions include acute coronary syndromes and postoperative care (after angioplasty, stenting, or coronary bypass surgery), angina, arrhythmias, heart failure, and hypertension. The chapter concludes with a list of drugs commonly used to treat cardiac disease with recommendations for their use in breastfeeding mothers.

Note: Some drugs that are commonly used to treat patients with heart conditions should not be used during pregnancy in general. These include atenolol, which has been associated with fetal growth restriction when given in the first trimester; propafenone; and diltiazem, which, although it has been used safely in pregnancy, has caused embryopathy in animal studies. In most instances, verapamil can be used in place of diltiazem. In addition, angiotensin-converting enzymes (ACE) inhibitors and angiotensin receptor blockers (ARBs), both of which are mainstays in the treatment of systolic left-sided heart failure in nonpregnant patients, have been associated with fetal hypoperfusion, dysgenesis, and renal failure. They may be used postpartum.

ACUTE CORONARY SYNDROMES AND POSTOPERATIVE CARE

Antiplatelet drugs are used to treat women with acute coronary syndromes and after angioplasty, stenting, or coronary bypass surgery. Often, aspirin is used throughout pregnancy to prevent preeclampsia, and it is generally considered safe during pregnancy. The safety of other antiplatelet drugs is not clearly established. A case of ticagrelor administration throughout pregnancy has been reported. The baby was small for gestational age, but the pregnancy was otherwise uneventful.

ANGINA

Drugs used to treat angina include nitroglycerin, isosorbide mononitrate, beta blockers, and verapamil.

Nitroglycerin SL (class B2) can be used safely, but it may lower maternal blood pressure. Isosorbide mononitrate is also generally safe to use in pregnancy (class B2), but it can lower maternal blood pressure in high doses. Beta blockers are effective in treating patients with angina and are generally safe; all are class C unless otherwise noted. There is considerable experience with metoprolol, propranolol, and labetalol. As already noted, atenolol (class D) should not be used in the first trimester because of concerns about fetal growth restriction. One may wish to use nadolol to treat channelopathies, but compared with other beta blockers, experience with this drug is limited. Verapamil (class C) can be used to treat patients with angina, and it also has been used extensively in pregnancy to treat patients with arrhythmias. It can be given both orally and intravenously. Amlodipine (class C) and nifedipine (class C) are other calcium channel blockers that may be used to treat patients with angina.

ARRHYTHMIAS

The pharmacological treatment of arrhythmias varies according to the specific condition: atrial fibrillation and atrial flutter, supraventricular tachycardia (SVT), and ventricular tachycardia (VT).

Atrial Fibrillation and Atrial Flutter

These arrhythmias usually require treatment with an atrioventricular (AV) nodal blocking agent to slow the rate. For acute situations, intravenous (IV) verapamil (class C) is the drug of choice. Long term, beta blockers such as metoprolol or oral verapamil (both class C) are best. Digoxin (class C) is not as effective and should be used only in rare situations when heart failure is present and beta blockers are ineffective or cannot be used. To prevent recurrences, an antiarrhythmic, such as flecainide (class C) or sotalol (class C), can be used; because both are proarrhythmic drugs, they should not be used in women with left ventricular dysfunction. In these cases, amiodarone (class D) is less likely to be proarrhythmic, but it should be used cautiously because of concerns for fetal thyroid dysfunction. Anticoagulation should be initiated. Acutely, IV heparin (class B) can be used; long term, low-molecular-weight heparin given subcutaneously (class B) is now the standard. In general, warfarin (class X) should not be used.

Supraventricular Tachycardia

For the acute treatment of patients with SVT, IV adenosine (class C) is quite effective; it is the most commonly used treatment in both pregnant women and the general population. If adenosine fails or arrhythmias recur, IV verapamil (class C) can be used.

For long-term prevention of SVT recurrences, AV nodal blocking agents are the drugs of choice. Digoxin (class C) has been used for many years and is effective. The dose generally should be increased during pregnancy because of increased renal clearance. Beta blockers also are effective. Metoprolol (class C) is widely used, but propranolol (class C) or labetalol (class C) can be used as well. As noted earlier, atenolol (class D) has been associated with fetal growth restriction when given in the first trimester. The calcium channel blocker verapamil (class C) is also effective.

In the rare cases when an antiarrhythmic drug is needed, flecainide (class C) or sotalol (class C) can be used. Amiodarone (class D) is used in pregnancy to treat fetal tachycardia, but it should be used only as a last resort because of concerns for fetal thyroid dysfunction.

Ventricular Tachycardia

Idiopathic VT can be treated with beta blockers (class C) or verapamil (class C). If these drugs are unsuccessful, antiarrhythmics such as flecainide (class C) or sotalol (class C) could be tried. Amiodarone (class D) may be considered. However, it may not be necessary to eliminate all nonsustained VT.

Ventricular tachycardia associated with LV dysfunction is usually quite intermittent, and if the patient has an implantable cardioverter-defibrillator, it may not need to be treated. If there are recurrent episodes of VT, amiodarone (class D) is the best option.

Adenosine (class C), which is given intravenously, transiently blocks conduction through the AV node. It can be used diagnostically if the diagnosis of a tachycardia is uncertain. If the patient is in atrial flutter with two-to-one conduction, adenosine may bring out the flutter waves and allow a correct diagnosis. It also may be used as a diagnostic tool in wide complex tachycardias. SVT with aberrancy will usually break. Idiopathic VT may convert to sinus rhythm. Usually, adenosine has no effect on VT associated with structural heart disease.

Quinidine (class C) is rarely used today, but it may be a good option in extremely rare cases, such as VT storm in Brugada syndrome.

Pronestyl (class C) is still available for IV use and occasionally may be helpful in pregnant patients.

In current practice, lidocaine (class C) is rarely used in treating patients with ventricular arrhythmias; the lidocaine-like drug tocainamide has been used to treat idiopathic VT of pregnancy, but it is no longer available.

HEART FAILURE

Heart failure can be classified as systolic or diastolic or as right or left sided, and the treatment varies for each.

Left-Sided Systolic Heart Failure

To treat left-sided systolic heart failure, diuretics are used to relieve pulmonary congestion and edema, and beta blockers are used to help prevent recurrences. In nonpregnant patients, carvedilol is the most commonly used drug, but there is little experience with it in pregnancy, so metoprolol is probably the best choice. Digitalis can be used to treat symptoms. As noted earlier, ACE inhibitors and ARBs, both of which are mainstays of therapy in nonpregnant patients, should not be used.

Right-Sided Diastolic Heart Failure

To treat right-sided diastolic heart failure, diuretics are used. Beta blockers and verapamil are sometimes used, but there is little evidence that they are effective. Similarly, there is no convincing evidence that digitalis is helpful. Long-acting nitrates such as isosorbide dinitrate are also sometimes helpful in relieving symptoms.

HYPERTENSION

There are many options for treating hypertension in pregnancy, including beta blockers, calcium channel blockers, and diuretics.

Numerous beta blockers are used to treat hypertension, including atenolol, bisoprolol, labetalol, metoprolol, nadolol, and propranolol. All are class C drugs unless otherwise noted. Atenolol (class D) should not be used in the first trimester because of concerns about fetal growth restriction. Bisoprolol is cardioselective. Labetalol also blocks alpha receptors and has been used extensively to treat hypertension in pregnancy. Nadolol is the drug of choice to treat long QT syndrome type II (LQTS2), but experience in pregnancy is limited.

Calcium channel blockers include amlodipine, nifedipine, and verapamil. All are class C drugs. Nifedipine may cause reflex tachycardia. Verapamil tends to slow the heart rate, and because it is a negative inotrope, it may cause heart failure (left ventricular dysfunction).

Diuretics also may be used to lower blood pressure in certain circumstances, particularly if edema is present or a vasodilator has been used and is ineffective or produces edema. Thiazides are class D drugs; loop diuretics are class C. Methyldopa, a class B drug, is considered a first-line drug for treating hypertension in pregnancy because of extensive experience and a good safety profile. Hydralazine is a class C drug and is considered a second-line antihypertensive in pregnancy. It can be given intravenously in hypertensive emergencies.

BREASTFEEDING

The following is a list of commonly used cardiac drugs and a recommendation about their use in breastfeeding mothers.

ACE inhibitors	yes
ARBs	no data
Adenosine	yes
Amiodarone	no
Amlodipine	no data
Aspirin	yes
Atenolol	yes
Bisoprolol	no data
Clonidine	yes
Clopidogrel	no data
Digoxin	yes
Diltiazem	yes, but freely diffusible into breast milk
Doxazocin	no
Flecainide	yes
Heparin	yes
Hydralazine	yes
Isosorbide mononitrate	no data
Lidocaine	yes
Loop diuretics	yes, but excreted in breast milk
Methyldopa	yes
Nifedipine	yes
Procainamide	yes
Propafenone	no
Propranolol	yes
Quinidine	yes
Sotalol	yes
Spironolactone	no
Thiazide diuretics	yes
Verapamil	yes, but excreted in breast milk
Warfarin	yes

BIBLIOGRAPHY

General
Frishman WH, Elkayam U, Aronow WS. Cardiovascular drugs in pregnancy. *Cardiol Clin.* 2012;30:463–491.
Qasqas SA, McPherson C, Frishman WH, Elkayam U. Cardiovascular pharmacotherapeutic considerations during pregnancy and lactation. *Cardiol Rev.* 2004;12(4):201–221.

Angiotensin-Converting Enzyme Inhibitors
Bateman BT, Patorno E, Desai RJ, et al. Angiotensin-converting enzyme inhibitors and the risk of congenital malformations. *Obstet Gynecol.* 2017;129(1):171–184.
Bullo M, Tschumi S, Bucher BS, Bianchetti MG, Simonetti GD. Pregnancy outcome following exposure to angiotensin-converting enzyme inhibitors or angiotensin receptor antagonists. *Hypertension.* 2012;60(2):444–450.
Burrows RF, Burrows EA. Assessing the teratogenic potential of angiotensin-converting enzyme inhibitors in pregnancy . *Aust NZJ Obstet Gynaecol.* 1998;38:306–311.
Cooper WO, et al. Major congenital malformations after first-trimester exposure to ACE inhibitors. *N Engl J Med.* 2006;354:2443–2451.
Lambot MA, Vermeylen D, Noel JC. Angiotensin-II-receptor inhibitors in pregnancy. *Lancet.* 2001;357:1619–1620.
Li DK, Yang C, Andrade S, Tavares V, Ferber JR. Maternal exposure to angiotensin-converting enzyme inhibitors in the first trimester and risk of malformations in offspring: a retrospective cohort study. *BMJ.* 2011;343:d5931.
Mitchell A. Fetal risk from ACE inhibitors in the first trimester. *BMJ.* 2011;343:d6667.
Walfisch A, Al-maawali A, Moretti ME, Nickel C, Koren G. Teratogenicity of angiotensin converting enzyme inhibitors or receptor blockers. *J Obstet Gynecol.* 2011;31(6):465–472.

Antiarrhythmics

Chow T, Galvin J, McGovern B. Antiarrhythmic drug therapy in pregnancy and lactation. *Am J Cardiol.* 1998;82:581–621.

Amiodarone

Magee BA, Downar E, Sermer M, Boulton BC, Allen LC, Koren G. Pregnancy outcome after gestational exposure to amiodarone in Canada. *Am J Obstet Gynecol.* 1995;172: 1307–1311.

Ovadia M, Brito M, Hoyer GL, Marcus FI. Human experience with amiodarone in the embryonic period. *Am J Cardiol.* 1994;73:316–317.

Antihypertensives

Abalos E, Duley L, Steyn D, Henderson-Smart D. Antihypertensive drug therapy for mild to moderate hypertension during pregnancy. *Cochrane Database Syst Rev.* 2007(2). CD002252.

Abalos E, Duley L, Steyn DW, Henderson-Smart DJ. Antihypertensive drug therapy for mild to moderate hypertension during pregnancy. *Cochrane Database Syst Rev.* 2001(1). CD002252.

Brown MA, Hague WM, Higgins J, et al. The detection, investigation and management of hypertension in pregnancy: full consensus statement. *Aust N Z J Obstet Gynaecol.* 2000;40:139–155.

Duley L, Henderson-Smart DJ, Meher S. Drugs for treatment of very high blood pressure during pregnancy. *Cochrane Database Syst Rev.* 2006;3 CD001449.

Magee LA. Drugs in pregnancy. Antihypertensives. *Best Pract Res Clin Obstet Gynaecol.* 2001;15:827–845.

Podymow T, August P. Update on the use of antihypertensive drugs in pregnancy. *Hypertension.* 2008;51:960–969.

Rosenthal T, Oparil S. The effect of antihypertensive drugs on the fetus. *J Hum Hypertens.* 2002;16:293–298.

Sibai BM. Antihypertensive drugs during pregnancy. *Semin Perinatol.* 2001;25:159–164.

Sibai BM. Chronic hypertension in pregnancy. *Obstet Gynecol.* 2002;100:369–377.

von Dadelszen P, Magee LA. Antihypertensive medications in management of gestational hypertension-preeclampsia. *Clin Obstet Gynecol.* 2005;48:441–459.

Waterman EJ, Magee LA, Lim KI, Skoll A, Rurak D, von Dadelszen P. Do commonly used oral antihypertensives alter fetal or neonatal heart rate characteristics? A systematic review. *Hypertens Pregnancy.* 2004;23:155–169.

Angiotensin Receptor Blockers

Saji H, Yamanaka M, Hagiwara A, Ijiri R. Losartan and fetal toxic effects. *Lancet.* 2001;357:363.

Antiplatelet Drugs

Kozer E, et al. Effects of aspirin consumption during pregnancy on pregnancy outcomes: meta analysis. *Birth Defects Res B Dev Reprod Toxicol.* 2003;68(1):70–84.

Verbruggen M, Mannaerts D, Muys J, Jacquemyn Y. Use of ticagrelor in human pregnancy, the first experience. *BMJ Case Rep.* 2015 2015:bcr2015212217.

Beta Blockers

Butters L, Kennedy S, Rubin PC. Atenolol in essential hypertension during pregnancy. *BMJ.* 1990;301:587–589.

Lip GY, Beevers M, Churchill D, Shaffer LM, Beevers DG. Effect of atenolol on birth weight. *Am J Cardiol.* 1997;79: 1436–1438.

Mabie WC, Gonzalez AR, Sibai BM, Amon E. A comparative trial of labetalol and hydralazine in the acute management of severe hypertension complicating pregnancy. *Obstet Gynecol.* 1987;70:328–333.

Magee LA, Duley L. Oral beta-blockers for mild to moderate hypertension during pregnancy. *Cochrane Database Syst Rev.* 2000(3). CD002863.

Magee LA, Elran E, Bull SB, Logan A, Koren G. Risks and benefits of beta-receptor blockers for pregnancy hypertension: overview of the randomized trials. *Eur J Obstet Gynecol Reprod Biol.* 2000;88:15–26.

Munshi UK, Deorari AK, Paul VK, Singh M. Effects of maternal labetalol on the newborn infant. *Indian Pediatr.* 1992;29:1507–1512.

Paran E, Holzberg G, Mazor M, Zmora E, Insler V. Beta-adrenergic blocking agents in the treatment of pregnancy-induced hypertension. *Int J Clin Pharmacol Ther.* 1995;33:119–123.

Pickles CJ, Broughton Pipkin F, Symonds EM. A randomized placebo controlled trial of labetalol in the treatment of mild to moderate pregnancy induced hypertension. *Br J Obstet Gynaecol.* 1992;162:960–966.

Pickles CJ, Symonds EM, Pipkin FB. The fetal outcome in a randomized double-blind controlled trial of labetalol versus placebo in pregnancy-induced hypertension. *Br J Obstet Gynaecol.* 1989;96:38–43.

Sibai BM, Gonzalez AR, Mabie WC, Moretti M. A comparison of labetalol plus hospitalization versus hospitalization alone in the management of preeclampsia remote from term. *Obstet Gynecol.* 1987;70:323–327.

Sibai BM, Mabie WC, Shamsa F, Villar MA, Anderson GD. A comparison of no medication versus methyldopa or labetalol in chronic hypertension during pregnancy. *Am J Obstet Gynecol.* 1990;162:960–966.

Calcium Channel Blockers

Bartels PA, Hanff LM, Mathot RA, Steeges EA, Vulto AG, Visser W. Nicardipine in pre-eclamptic patients: placental transfer and disposition in breast milk. *BJOG.* 2007;114:230–233.

Belfort MA, Anthony J, Buccimazza A, Davey DA. Hemodynamic changes associated with intravenous infusion of the calcium antagonist verapamil in the treatment of severe gestational proteinuric hypertension. *Obstet Gynecol.* 1990;75:970–974.

Brown MA, Buddle ML, Farrell T, Davis GK. Efficacy and safety of nifedipine tablets for the acute treatment of severe hypertension in pregnancy. *Am J Obstet Gynecol.* 2002;187:1046–1050.

Casele IIL, Windley KC, Prieto JA, Gratton R, Laifer SA. Felodipine use in pregnancy. *Report of three cases. J Reprod Med.* 1997;42:378–381.

Constantine G, Beevers DG, Reynolds AL, Luesley DM. Nifedipine as a second line antihypertensive in pregnancy. *Br J Obstet Gynaecol.* 1987;11:36–42.

Jannet D, Carbonne B, Sebban E, Milliez J. Nicardipine versus metoprolol in the treatment of hypertension during pregnancy: a randomized comparative trial. *Obstet Gynecol.* 1994;84:354–359.

Magee LA, Schick B, Donnenfeld AE, et al. The safety of calcium channel blockers in human pregnancy: a prospective, multicenter cohort study. *Am J Obstet Gynecol.* 1996;174:823–828.

Papatsonis DN, Lok CA, Bos JM, Geijn HP, Dekker GA. Calcium channel blockers in the management of preterm labor and hypertension in pregnancy. *Eur J Obstet Gynecol Reprod Biol.* 2001;97:122–140.

Wide-Swensson DH, Ingemarsson I, Lunell NO, et al. Calcium channel blockade (isradipine) in treatment of hypertension in pregnancy: a randomized placebo-controlled study. *Am J Obstet Gynecol.* 1995;173:872–878.

Clonidine

1. Horvath JS, Phippard A, Korda A, Henderson-Smart DJ, Child A, Tiller DJ. Clonidine hydrochloride—a safe and effective antihypertensive agent in pregnancy. *Obstet Gynecol.* 1985;66:634–638.
2. Huisjes HJ, Hadders-Algra M, Touwen BC. Is clonidine a behavioural teratogen in the human? *Early Hum Dev.* 1986;14:43–48.

Digitalis

1. Soyka LF. Digoxin: placental transfer, effects on the fetus, and therapeutic use in the newborn. *Clin Perinatol.* 1975;2(1):23–35.

Diuretics

1. Collins R, Yusuf S, Peto R. Overview of randomised trials of diuretics in pregnancy. In: Clin BMJ, editor. *Res.* 290;198517–23.
2. Groves TD, Corenblum B. Spironolactone therapy during human pregnancy. *Am J Obstet Gynecol.* 1995;172:1655–1656.

Hydralazine

1. Magee LA, Cham C, Waterman EJ, Ohlsson A, von Dadelszen P. Hydralazine for treatment of severe hypertension in pregnancy: meta-analysis. *BMJ.* 2003;327:955–960.
2. Paterson-Brown S, et al. Hydralazine boluses for the treatment of severe hypertension in pre-eclampsia. *Br J Obstet Gynaecol.* 1994:409–413.

Methyldopa

1. Montan S, Anandakumar C, Arulkumaran S, Ingemarsson I, Ratnam SS. Effects of methyldopa on uteroplacental and fetal hemodynamics in pregnancy-induced hypertension. *Am J Obstet Gynecol.* 1993;168:152–156.

Nitrates

1. Nevo O, Thaler I, Shik V, Vortman T, Soustiel JF. The effect of isosorbide dinitrate, a donor of nitric oxide, on maternal cerebral blood flow in gestational hypertension and preeclampsia. *Am J Obstet Gynecol.* 2003;188:1360–1365.

Breastfeeding

Atkinson H, Begg EJ. Concentrations of beta-blocking drugs in human milk. *J Pediatr.* 1990;116:156.

Atkinson HC, Begg EJ, Darlow BA. Drugs in human milk. *Clinical pharmacokinetic considerations. Clin Pharmacokinet.* 1988;14:217–240.

Beardmore KS, Morris JM, Gallery ED. Excretion of antihypertensive medication into human breast milk: a systematic review. *Hypertens Pregnancy.* 2002;21:85–95.

Breitzka RL, Sandritter TL, Hatzopoulos FK. Principles of drug transfer into breast milk and drug disposition in the nursing infant. *J Hum Lact.* 1997;13:155–158.

Ehrenkranz RA, Ackerman BA, Hulse JD. Nifedipine transfer into human milk. *J Pediatr.* 1989;114:478–480.

Makris A, Thornton C, Hennessy A. Postpartum hypertension and nonsteroidal analgesia. *Am J Obstet Gynecol.* 2004;190:577–578.

Shannon ME, Malecha SE, Cha AJ. Angiotensin converting enzyme inhibitors (ACEIs) and angiotensin II receptor blockers (ARBs) and lactation: an update. *J Hum Lact.* 2000;16:152–155.

White WB. Management of hypertension during lactation. *Hypertension.* 1984;6:297–300.

14

Anticoagulation During Pregnancy

John H. Wilson, MD, FACC, FHRS

Anticoagulation during pregnancy is required in patients with mechanical prosthetic valves and those with atrial fibrillation. It should be considered in patients with pulmonary hypertension. Patients who develop a left ventricular (LV) thrombus because of LV dysfunction also should receive anticoagulation; in those at risk because of severely reduced LV dysfunction (LV ejection factor <35%), it may be considered. Furthermore, anticoagulation may be required for patients who develop thromboembolic disease during pregnancy.

To mitigate the risk of pulmonary embolus, prophylactic anticoagulation is recommended for women at high risk of deep vein thrombosis (DVT) during pregnancy, including those with previous recurrent DVT, prior unprovoked or estrogen-related DVT, or prior DVT associated with a coagulopathy. These patients should receive low-molecular-weight heparin (LMWH) during pregnancy and for 6 weeks postpartum.

Warfarin, which has been the standard anticoagulant for mechanical valves and is often used in these and other conditions, is quite toxic to fetuses. It has been associated with embryopathy, intracranial hemorrhage, and miscarriage. Consequently, its use in pregnancy is discouraged, particularly during weeks 3 to 8 of gestation, when organogenesis is occurring. Occasionally, it may be needed in patients with highly thrombogenic mechanical valves in the mitral position.

The guidelines from various specialty societies for anticoagulation of pregnant women with mechanical prosthetic valves are listed in Table 14.1.

If warfarin is used during pregnancy, the international normalized ratio (INR) should be monitored and maintained at the same levels as for nonpregnant women: 2.0 to 3.0 for all patients except those with metallic prosthetic valves and 2.5 to 3.5 for patients with metallic valves.

Low-molecular-weight heparin has become the most widely used anticoagulant in pregnancy. It does not cross placentas and is therefore relatively safe for fetuses. It is administered subcutaneously and can cause injection-site irritation and allergic skin reactions. LMWH is effective in virtually all the conditions encountered in pregnancy that require anticoagulation. It is problematic in that the degree of anticoagulation cannot be readily measured, and there is no reversal agent. Heparin may cause osteoporosis in the mother, so it is prudent to check vitamin D and calcium levels and supplement as necessary.

Anticoagulation with LMWH is monitored by measuring factor Xa levels. Factor Xa peak levels should be measured at 4 hours after the dose. It is recommended that they be maintained at

- 0.8 to 1.0 IU/ML for aortic metal valves
- to 1.2 IU/ML for mitral metal valves
- 0.6 to 0.9 IU/ML for patients with venous thromboemboli

In high-risk women, trough levels should be measured also; they should be kept at 0.4 to 0.7 IU/ML.

Three different LMWHs are available: enoxaparin, dalteparin, and tinzaparin. The starting doses are

- Enoxaparin: 1 mg/kg twice a day antenatal; 1.5 mg/kg postnatal.
- Dalteparin: 100 units/kg antenatal; 200 units/kg postnatal
- Tinzaparin: 175 units every other day both antenatal and postnatal

Heparin-induced thrombocytopenia (HIT) is rare, but platelet counts should be checked periodically.

If patients with metallic valves are maintained on LMWH, low-dose aspirin (81 mg/day) should be added.

Unfractionated heparin (UFH) is cumbersome to use because it must be administered intravenously or, if given subcutaneously, three times a day. Its main advantages are that the anticoagulant effect can be directly measured with a partial thromboplastin time and that it can be quickly reversed with protamine. It carries a higher risk of HIT. During pregnancy, the subcutaneous

TABLE 14.1   Guidelines for Anticoagulation in Pregnant Women

Recommendation	ACC/AHA	ACCP	ESC
Oral anticoagulation	Can be used throughout pregnancy, with substitution of UFH or LMWH during 6–12 weeks if preferred by patient	Can be used throughout pregnancy in high-risk patients with substitution by LMWH or UHF close to term (48 hr antepartum)	If the warfarin dosage is <5 mg/day, oral anticoagulants throughout pregnancy are the safest option (<3% embryopathy)
Heparin derivatives	Monitored UHF or LMWH might be options throughout gestation or during weeks 6–12 of gestation; LMWH dose should be adjusted to give an anti-Xa activity 0.7–1.2 U/mL 4–6 hr after dose	LMWH should be given twice daily and adjusted to achieve peak inhibition of factor Xa 4 hours after dose	LMWH dose should be adjusted to give an anti-Xa activity of 0.8–1.2 U/mL 4–6 hr after dose
Aspirin	Low-dose aspirin in addition to anticoagulation in second and third trimesters	Low-dose aspirin in addition to anticoagulation in high-risk patients	Aspirin in addition to anticoagulation not recommended
Anticoagulation target	INR of 3 for all mechanical valves	INR of 2–3 for bileaflet aortic valves without high-risk features	No INR target given

ACC, American College of Cardiology; ACCP, American College of Chest Physicians; AHA, American Heart Association; ESC, European Society of Cardiology; LMWH, low-molecular-weight heparin; UFH, unfractionated heparin.

use of UFH has been associated with a 25% risk of prosthetic metal valve thrombosis.

If pregnancy is anticipated in a patient taking warfarin, the most commonly used strategy is to start LMWH and stop warfarin at 5 to 6 weeks' gestation. Another strategy may be to continue warfarin through most of pregnancy but switch to LMWH during weeks 3 to 8, when organogenesis is occurring.

Vaginal delivery is preferable to cesarean section in patients on anticoagulation. Peripartum, women on anticoagulation are at risk for bleeding related to both operative- and anesthetic-related conditions. Therefore, when contractions start, LMWH should be stopped. Hydration and compression stockings may be beneficial in reducing the risk of thrombosis.

If labor is prolonged for more than 24 hours after the last dose of LMWH, several options are available. A prophylactic dose of LMWH can be given every 24 hours. Doses of subcutaneous heparin can be given, typically 7500 units every 12 hours, or a continuous infusion of UFH can be started. IV heparin infusions should be stopped with the onset of the second stage of labor.

If it is necessary to induce labor, LMWH should be stopped 12 to 24 hours before induction, depending on parity and cervical Bishop score.

If a cesarean section is planned, LMWH should be held the morning before and restarted the evening after delivery (in the absence of bleeding complications).

If a patient is taking warfarin at time of delivery, it may be preferable to plan the delivery either by induction or by cesarean section to minimize the time off warfarin. There is a reported high risk of thrombosis if the patient is converted to either intravenous heparin or subcutaneous LMWH.

If labor is prolonged, a continuous infusion of UFH can be used at the time of delivery.

Postpartum, LMWH is usually restarted 6 to 12 hours after both vaginal delivery and cesarean section if there has been no bleeding. Typically, long-term warfarin is resumed on day 5 to 7 postpartum. If the patient has a metal valve, she is maintained on LMWH until the INR is 2.5 to 3.5.

Both warfarin and LMWH are safe to use during breastfeeding.

BIBLIOGRAPHY

Alshawbkeh L, Economy KE, Valente AM. Anticoagulation during pregnancy: evolving strategies. *JACC.* 2016;68: 804–1813.

Bates SM, et al. Use of antithrombotic agents during pregnancy: the seventh ACCP conference on antithrombotic and thrombolytic therapy. *Chest.* 2004;126(3 suppl): 627s–644s.

Castellano JM, et al. Guidleines for anticoagulation therapy in pregnant women with mechanical prosthetic vales. *Nat. Rev. Cardiol.* 2012;9:415–424.

Chan WC, et al. Anticoagulation of pregnant woen with mechanical valves: a systematic review of the literature. *Arch Intern Med.* 2000;160:191–196.

Chong MKB, et al. Follow up study of children whose mothers were treated with warfarin during pregnancy. *Br J Obstet Gynaecol.* 1984;91:1070–1073.

Gibson Paul S, Powrie R. Anticoagulants an pregnancy: When are they safe? *Cleve Clin J Med.* 2009;76:113–127.

Ginsberg JS, et al. Heparin therapy during pregnancy – risk to he fetus and the mother. *Arch Intern Med.* 1989;149: 2233–2236.

Ginsberg JS, Hirsh J. Anticoagulants during pregnancy. *Annu Rev Med.* 1989;40:79–86.

Jurcut R. How to anticoagulate the pregnant or lactating cardiac patient. *E journal of the ESC Council for Cardiology Practice.* 12;5.

Lee LH, et al. Low molecular weight heparin for thromboprophylaxis during pregnancy in 2 patients with mechanical mitral valve replacement. *Thromb Haemost.* 1996;6: 628–630.

Oakley CM. Anticoagulation in pregnancy. *Br Heart J.* 1995;74:107–111.

Oakley CM. Clinical and pregnancy perspectives: anticoagulation. *Eur Heart J.* 1995;16:1317–1319.

Oran B, et al. Low molecular weight heparin for the prophylaxis of thromboembolism in women with prosthetic mechanical heart valves during pregnancy. *Thromb Haemost.* 2004;92:747–751.

Rowan JA, et al. Enoxaparin treatment in women with mechanical heart valves during pregnancy. *Am J Obstet Gynecol.* 2001;185:633–637.

Salazar E, et al. The problem of crdiac valve prostheses: anticoagulants and pregnancy. *Circulation.* 1984;70: 169–177.

Sareli P, et al. Maternal and fetal sequelae of anticoagulation durin pregnancy in patients with mechanical heat valve prostheses. *J Am Coll Cardiol.* 1989;63:1462–1465.

Steinberg Maternal and fetal outcomes of anticoagulation in pregnant women with mechanical heart valves. *JACC.* 2017;69(22):2681–2691.

Vitale N, et al. Dose dependent fetal complications of warfarin in pregnant women with mechanical heart valves. *J Am Coll Cardiol.* 1995;33:1637–1641.

Whittfield LLR, et al. Effect of pregnancy on the relationship between concentration and anticoagulation action of heparin. *Clin Pharacol Ther.* 1983;34:23–28.

Wong V, et al. Fetal and neonatal outcome of exposure to anticoagulation during pregnancy. *Am J Med Genet.* 1993;45:17–21.

15

Cardiac Effects of Drugs Commonly Used in Obstetrics

John H. Wilson, MD, FACC, FHRS

The following drugs are commonly used in obstetrics and may affect the cardiovascular system. Depending on the effect and its degree, a drug may be contraindicated in women with specific cardiac conditions. Note: Drugs are listed alphabetically.

Atosiban, an oxytocin receptor analog, is used to inhibit labor. No serious cardiac side effects have been reported.

Carboprost (prostaglandin F2α) is a prostaglandin used for induction. It is contraindicated in patients with myocardial ischemia.

Dinoprostone (prostaglandin E) is a vaginally delivered prostaglandin that causes cervical thinning and dilation. No serious cardiac side effects have been reported.

Ergometrine is used to stimulate uterine contraction. It causes an increase in peripheral vascular resistance and can induce coronary artery spasm. It should be avoided in patients with preeclampsia or aortic root disorders.

Indomethacin is a nonsteroidal antiinflammatory drug (NSAIDs) that can be used to postpone delivery. It can cause fluid retention, and similar to all NSAIDs, it increases the risk of myocardial infarction. A number of serious fetal side effects have been reported, including constriction of ductus arteriosus, pulmonary hypertension (reversible), decreased renal function, oligohydramnios, intraventricular hemorrhage, hyperbilirubinemia, and necrotizing enterocolitis.

Misoprostol (a prostaglandin E1 analog) is used to dilate the cervix and induce labor. It is contraindicated in patients with myocardial ischemia.

Magnesium sulfate ($MgSO_4$) is used to treat patients with eclampsia. There are no known serious cardiac effects.

Nifedipine is a calcium channel blocker used to delay delivery. It relaxes smooth muscle and can cause hypotension. It may initiate a reflex tachycardia; therefore, it can exacerbate angina. Nifedipine is a negative inotrope and can worsen left ventricular dysfunction.

Oxytocin is often given after delivery to cause uterine contraction to limit bleeding. It can cause a decrease in blood pressure because of peripheral vasodilation. Oxytocin causes decreased cardiac contractility and bradycardia. It has an antidiuretic hormone–like effect and may cause fluid retention. It should be avoided in conditions in which vasodilation is poorly tolerated, such as pulmonary hypertension, aortic stenosis, and hypertrophic cardiomyopathy.

Sulindac is an NSAID that can be used to postpone delivery. It can cause fluid retention, and similar to all NSAIDs, it increases the risk of myocardial infarction. A number of serious fetal side effects have been reported, including constriction of ductus arteriosus, pulmonary hypertension (reversible), decreased renal function, oligohydramnios, intraventricular hemorrhage, hyperbilirubinemia, and necrotizing enterocolitis.

Terbutaline is a β_2 agonist that is used to inhibit preterm labor. It can cause arrhythmias, pulmonary edema, myocardial ischemia, hypertension, and sinus tachycardia. In animal studies, alterations in fetal brain development have been reported. No definite long-term adverse effects on human fetuses have been reported.

16

Cardiac Effects of Anesthetic Agents That May Be Used in Labor and Delivery

Kristin Horton, MD, and Andrea Girnius, MD

With the increasing number of women with cardiac disease presenting to labor and delivery, anesthesiologists must be equipped to manage their analgesia and anesthesia in the peripartum period. Therefore, it is important to consider the potential cardiovascular effects of the anesthetic agents encountered during the process of labor and delivery and how they may affect patients with cardiac disease. This chapter reviews the most common classes of anesthetics encountered during this time as well as important considerations regarding cardiac disease in pregnant women.

MEDICATIONS FOR NEURAXIAL ANESTHESIA

Local anesthetics are the predominate agents used for neuraxial analgesia and anesthesia in parturients. The most common agents in use are lidocaine, bupivacaine, ropivacaine, and 3-chloroprocaine. These agents exert their effects by binding to sodium channels, decreasing the influx of sodium and preventing action potential initiation. This leads to a decreased rate of depolarization of excitable membranes. Local anesthetics exhibit a "state-dependent blockade," preferentially binding to the activated form of sodium channels. As such, neurons with high-frequency firing rates, such as cardiac myocytes, will be more sensitive to blockade by local anesthetics. This property contributes to the use of

these medications in tachyarrhythmias as class I antiarrhythmics and explains the bradycardia occasionally encountered after administration. Of note, bupivacaine is known to bind more strongly to and dissociate more slowly from cardiac sodium channels, making cardiac resuscitation more difficult in bupivacaine-induced local anesthetic toxicity.

Other than their antiarrhythmic properties, the hemodynamic effects of local anesthetics are indirect and result from the blockade of sympathetic output to blood vessels. The magnitude of the effect varies with epidural versus intrathecal administration, with more significant hemodynamic effects occurring with the latter because of its more rapid onset. Neuraxial local anesthetics block sensory, motor, and sympathetic nerves. The sympathectomy induced by these agents leads to a significant decrease in systemic vascular resistance, resulting in a decrease in both preload and afterload. A subsequent decrease in cardiac output is seen from reduced preload. The end effects of these changes in parturients with cardiac disease will depend on the patient's specific cardiac physiology; however, they will be particularly problematic for patients with lesions that are preload dependent and those relying on optimal coronary perfusion.

During epidural placement, a test dose with lidocaine and epinephrine is given to assess for an inadvertent intrathecal or intravascular catheter placement. If the catheter is intravascular, the epinephrine commonly causes hypertension and tachycardia, which can have detrimental effects in patients with coronary artery disease or those prone to tachyarrhythmias.

MEDICATIONS FOR GENERAL ANESTHESIA

Benzodiazepines

Benzodiazepines, most commonly midazolam and diazepam, can be administered to the parturient for anxiolysis. They enhance binding of gamma-aminobutyric acid (GABA) to its receptor complex leading to increased central nervous system inhibitory effects. However, these agents are often avoided if possible in the labor and delivery setting because these drugs can cross the placenta and exert effects on the fetus.

If administered for anxiolysis, there are very few reported cardiovascular effects. Several studies have demonstrated a 15% to 19% reduction in mean arterial pressures (MAPs) after administration of midazolam. The heart rate was noted to mildly increase; however, there were no statistically significant changes in heart rate, cardiac output, or stroke volume.

Analgesics

Opiates are frequently used for pain control during labor and delivery via multiple routes of administration. They may be used as an adjunct to local anesthetic for an epidural infusion or spinal injection or used independently, either through intravenous administration or bolused through an epidural catheter. Meperidine is also occasionally used to treat postoperative shivering

As a class, these agents may decrease systemic vascular resistance through a reduction in circulating catecholamines and a resultant decrease in sympathetic tone. This can potentially cause hemodynamic changes including hypotension, bradycardia, and decreased cardiac output. Some opioids, including morphine and meperidine, can cause histamine release, which may further contribute to hypotension. Fentanyl and hydromorphone do not cause a histamine release and therefore cause less hypotension when administered. These drugs, however, do cause varying degrees of vasodilation leading to decreased cardiac output and hypotension. Meperidine, a synthetic opioid with additional anticholinergic properties, can cause tachycardia. In addition, it has also been reported to cause QT-c prolongation.

Induction Agents

Multiple agents are available for use in parturients for induction of general anesthesia.

Propofol is the most common intravenous agent used for induction of general anesthesia. It is thought to work via central $GABA_A$ receptors with some involvement of action on the sleep pathways in the hypothalamus. Propofol has multiple hemodynamic effects, of which the most commonly encountered is hypotension. Multiple studies have attempted to elucidate whether this is caused by a decrease in preload from a reduction in systemic vascular resistance, reduced afterload, decreased contractility from negative inotropic effects of the drug, or a combination of these effects. Heart rate is often minimally affected secondary to blunting of the sympathetic nervous system and the baroreceptor reflex.

Etomidate acts at the GABA receptor complex and is a good choice as an induction agent when strict hemodynamic stability is of particular clinical importance. Multiple studies have demonstrated minimal changes in hemodynamic parameters, including blood pressure, cardiac output, stroke volume, and systemic and pulmonary vascular resistance. There was noted a statistically significant decrease of up to 10% in heart rate. Although seen more often postoperatively than during induction, this agent can also lead to hypotension via adrenal suppression; this can be especially profound in the setting of septic shock. Etomidate has several side effects that preclude its more routine use, including burning on administration, severe postoperative nausea and vomiting, and the potential for adrenal suppression.

Ketamine is an N-methyl D-aspartate (NMDA) receptor antagonist that is well suited for use in cases of cardiac tamponade, significant hypovolemia, and shock. Hemodynamically, an increase in sympathetic outflow results in increased heart rate, myocardial oxygen consumption, systemic vascular resistance, and pulmonary artery pressures. As such, this agent could have detrimental effects in patients at risk for ischemia as well as those with right ventricular dysfunction. Although ketamine is known to have direct myocardial depressant effects, clinically this is often overshadowed by the effects of sympathetic stimulation. However, the cardiac depressant effects may be much more pronounced in catecholamine-depleted states.

Thiopental is a barbiturate whose use has waned in recent years because of lack of availability in the United

States. Barbiturates work via binding to the GABA receptor complex at a different site than benzodiazepines. Thiopental-induced hypotension, less common than propofol-induced hypotension, is a result of both peripheral vasodilation and histamine release. This can lead to a reflex tachycardia via the baroreceptor response and can precipitate ischemic events in those patients with significant coronary artery disease. In addition, thiopental also has negative inotropic effects derived from a decreased influx of calcium into the myocardial cells.

Volatile Anesthetics

After induction of general anesthesia, volatile anesthetic agents are commonly used to maintain an appropriate level of anesthesia. Inhalational agents in common clinical use in the United States are sevoflurane, desflurane, and isoflurane. Multiple clinical trials have demonstrated that all volatile agents can induce hypotension secondary to vasodilation and negative inotropy. This decrease in contractility can be beneficial in that it decreases myocardial oxygen demand, leading to lower risk of ischemia. However, reductions in cardiac output secondary to decreased preload can decrease uptake of these agents from the lungs, leading to increased alveolar concentrations and further reductions in cardiac output. This occurs more often with isoflurane and becomes clinically significant when inhalational agents are used to maintain general anesthesia in those patients with critically reduced ejection fractions. It has been noted that rapid increases in both isoflurane and desflurane beyond 1 minimum alveolar concentration (MAC) can actually lead to sympathetic stimulation and result in tachycardia and occasionally hypertension.

Inhalation of nitrous oxide is occasionally used during labor and delivery for analgesia. At subanesthetic doses (0.1–0.5 MAC), there are minimal changes in cardiac output, stroke volume, or heart rate. Higher doses, however, lead to sympathetic stimulation and can increase these factors. This is important to keep in mind when administering opioids concurrently because these agents can actually decrease sympathetic flow and can unmask cardiac depressant effects of nitrous oxide.

Muscle Relaxants

Succinylcholine is a depolarizing short-acting neuromuscular blocking agent with a dose-dependent cardiovascular effect. Single doses typically do not cause significant cardiovascular effects, but repeat dosing can stimulate sinus node muscarinic receptors, leading to bradycardia. Although this effect is much more common in children, it can be seen in adults as well. Succinylcholine can cause hyperkalemia, with an average increase in serum potassium level of approximately 0.5 mEq with an intubating dose of succinylcholine (1–1.5 mg/kg). However, this increase in potassium can be exaggerated to a lethal degree by precipitating cardiac arrhythmias in patients with burn or crush injuries or in disease processes leading to upregulation of extrajunctional acetylcholine receptors (prolonged bed rest, stroke, muscular sclerosis, spinal cord injuries with paralysis, etc.).

Vecuronium and rocuronium are both intermediate-acting nondepolarizing aminosteroid neuromuscular blocking agents. There have been no clinically significant cardiovascular effects discovered with use of vecuronium, although some studies have shown a statistically significant transient decrease in MAPs. Compared with vecuronium, rocuronium has been noted to have more vagolytic properties, which can lead to slightly higher rate of tachycardia and transient increase in MAPs. These changes are not considered to be clinically significant.

Pancuronium, a long-acting nondepolarizing aminosteroid neuromuscular blocking agent, is used less frequently than shorter acting and more reversible agents. In addition, it can cause tachycardia and arrhythmias stemming from sympathetic stimulation, vagolytic effects, and inhibition of catecholamine reuptake.

Cis-atracurium is a nondepolarizing benzylisoquinoline and is a stereoisomer of atracurium. Unlike atracurium, which can cause histamine release leading to hypotension, cis-atracurium has relatively few hemodynamic effects even in large doses.

Reversal Agents

Neostigmine is an acetylcholinesterase inhibitor and has been the mainstay for reversal of neuromuscular blocking agents. It causes an increase of acetylcholine at the neuromuscular junction and increases stimulation of both nicotinic and muscarinic receptors. Stimulation of the cholinergic muscarinic receptors of cardiac myocytes leads to increased parasympathetic output and a resulting bradycardia. It is commonly paired with an anticholinergic agent such a glycopyrrolate or atropine to attenuate the systemic cholinergic effects.

Atropine and glycopyrrolate are reversible, competitive antagonists of acetylcholine receptors. The decrease in parasympathetic input after administration of these medications leads to increases in heart rate, cardiac output, and contractility. Myocardial oxygen consumption increases with the increase in heart rate. These medications should be administered with caution in patients at risk for ischemic events or those with valvular disorders such as aortic stenosis in whom tachycardia could lead to decreases in cardiac output.

Although these medications have similar mechanisms of action, atropine is a tertiary amine and glycopyrrolate is a quaternary amine, the latter of which cannot cross the blood–brain barrier or the placenta. As such, atropine is the preferred anticholinergic agent to use in the parturient to offset the bradycardic effects of neostigmine in the fetus.

Sugammadex is a γ-cyclodextrin that is used for reversal of aminosteroid neuromuscular blocking agents, specifically rocuronium. At low doses, vecuronium and pancuronium can also be reversed. Sugammadex works by binding to the neuromuscular blockers without interfering with acetylcholine receptors or other neurotransmitters. There is no need to administer an anticholinergic or acetylcholinesterase inhibitor, thus avoiding the potential cardiovascular responses seen with those medications. As a single agent, there have been no significant cardiovascular derangements noted.

Antiemetics

Antiemetics are frequently used throughout the course of pregnancy and during the peripartum period. The most common agents used include ondansetron, promethazine, dexamethasone, and, occasionally, droperidol. Both ondansetron and droperidol have been shown to increase QT interval through unclear mechanisms and can lead to torsades de pointes in critically ill patients, those with congenital long QT syndrome, or those receiving other QT prolonging agents.

Although there have been some adverse effects associated with long-term use of glucocorticoids, associated adverse effects of single-dose dexamethasone have not conclusively been shown to have significant adverse cardiac effects.

Promethazine is known to cause sedation and has the potential to cause extrapyramidal effects. However, there are no significant cardiovascular affects associated with its use.

BIBLIOGRAPHY

Allolio B, Dörr H, Stuttmann R, Knorr D, Engelhardt D, Winkelmann W. Effect of a single bolus of etomidate upon eight major corticosteroid hormones and plasma ACTH. *Clin Endocrinol (Oxf)*. 1985;22(3):281–286.

Becker DE, Rosenberg M. Nitrous oxide and the inhalation anesthetics. *Anesth Prog*. 2008;55(4):121–131.

Caldwell JE, Miller RD. Clinical implications of sugammadex. *Anaesthesia*. 2009;64(suppl 1):66–72.

Cousins MJ, Carr DB, Horlocker TT, Bridenbaugh PO. *Neural Blockade in Clinical Anesthesia and Management of Pain*. 4th ed. Lippincott: Williams, &Wilkins; 2009.

Dahl V, Pendeville PE, Hollmann MW, Heier T, Abels EA, Blobner M. Safety and efficacy of sugammadex for the reversal of rocuronium-induced neuromuscular blockade in cardiac patients undergoing noncardiac surgery. *Eur J Anaesthesiol*. 2009;26(10):874–884.

Ebert TJ. Sympathetic and hemodynamic effects of moderate and deep sedation with propofol in humans. *Anesthesiology*. 2005;103(1):20–24.

Flacke JW, Flacke WE, Bloor BC, Van Etten AP, Kripke BJ. Histamine release by four narcotics: a double-blind study in humans. *Anesth Analg*. 1987;66(8):723–730.

Gooding JM, Corssen G. Effect of etomidate on the cardiovascular system. *Anesth Analg*. 1977;56(5):717–719.

Hug Jr CC, McLeskey CH, Nahrwold ML, et al. Hemodynamic effects of propofol: data from over 25,000 patients. *Anesth Analg*. 1993;77(4 suppl):S21–S29.

Hunter JM. New neuromuscular blocking drugs. *N Engl J Med*. 1995;332(25):1691–1699.

Keller GA, Ponte ML, Di Girolamo G. Other drugs acting on nervous system associated with QT-interval prolongation. *Curr Drug Saf*. 2010;5(1):105–111.

Keller GA, Villa Etchegoyen MC, Fernández N, et al. Meperidine-induced QTc-interval prolongation: prevalence, risk factors, and correlation to plasma drug and metabolite concentrations. *Int J Clin Pharmacol Ther*. 2017;55 (3):275–285.

Kirkbride DA, Parker JL, Williams GD, Buggy DJ. Induction of anesthesia in the elderly ambulatory patient: a double-blinded comparison of propofol and sevoflurane. *Anesth Analg*. 2001;93(5):1185–1187. table of contents.

Kizilay D, Dal D, Saracoglu KT, Eti Z, Gogus FY. Comparison of neostigmine and sugammadex for hemodynamic parameters in cardiac patients undergoing noncardiac surgery. *J Clin Anesth*. 2016;28:30–35.

Landoni G, Biondi-Zoccai GG, Zangrillo A, et al. Desflurane and sevoflurane in cardiac surgery: a meta-analysis of randomized clinical trials. *J Cardiothorac Vasc Anesth*. 2007;21(4):502–511.

Langesaeter E, Rosseland LA, Stubhaug A. Continuous invasive blood pressure and cardiac output monitoring during cesarean delivery: a randomized, double-blind comparison of low-dose versus high-dose spinal anesthesia with intravenous phenylephrine or placebo infusion. *Anesthesiology.* 2008;109(5):856–863.

Lawrence KR, Nasraway SA. Conduction disturbances associated with administration of butyrophenone antipsychotics in the critically ill: a review of the literature. *Pharmacotherapy.* 1997;17(3):531–537.

Lebowitz PW, Cote ME, Daniels AL, et al. Comparative cardiovascular effects of midazolam and thiopental in healthy patients. *Anesth Analg.* 1982;61(9):771–775.

Leykin Y, Pellis T, Vincenti E. Highlights in muscle relaxants. *Expert Rev Neurother.* 2006;6(12):1833–1843.

Mace SE. Challenges and advances in intubation: rapid sequence intubation. *Emerg Med Clin North Am.* 2008;26 (4):1043–6108. x.

Maneglia R, Cousin MT. A comparison between propofol and ketamine for anaesthesia in the elderly. Haemodynamic effects during induction and maintenance. *Anaesthesia.* 1988;43(suppl):109–111.

Muravchick S, Owens WD, Felts JA. Glycopyrrolate and cardiac dysrhythmias in geriatric patients after reversal of neuromuscular blockade. *Can Anaesth Soc J.* 1979;26 (1).22–25.

Naguib M. Sugammadex: another milestone in clinical neuromuscular pharmacology. *Anesth Analg.* 2007;104(3): 575–581.

Navari RM, Koeller JM. Electrocardiographic and cardiovascular effects of the 5-hydroxytryptamine3 receptor antagonists. *Ann Pharmacother.* 2003;37(9):1276–1286.

Nelson LE, Guo TZ, Lu J, Saper CB, Franks NP, Maze M. The sedative component of anesthesia is mediated by GABA(A) receptors in an endogenous sleep pathway. *Nat Neurosci.* 2002;5(10):979–984.

Riss J, Cloyd J, Gates J, Collins S. Benzodiazepines in epilepsy: pharmacology and pharmacokinetics. *Acta Neurol Scand.* 2008;118(2):69–86.

Rosow CE, Moss J, Philbin DM, Savarese JJ. Histamine release during morphine and fentanyl anesthesia. *Anesthesiology.* 1982;56(2):93–96.

Russo H, Bressolle F. Pharmacodynamics and pharmacokinetics of thiopental. *Clin Pharmacokinet.* 1998;35(2): 95–134.

Salmenperä M, Peltola K, Takkunen O, Heinonen J. Cardiovascular effects of pancuronium and vecuronium during high-dose fentanyl anesthesia. *Anesth Analg.* 1983;62(12): 1059–1064.

Schumacher MA, Basbaum AI, Way WL. Opioid analgesics and antagonists. In: Katzung MS, Trevor BG, Trevor AJ, eds. *Basic and Clinical Pharmacology.* : McGraw-Hill; 2012.

Sunzel M, Paalzow L, Berggren L, Eriksson I. Respiratory and cardiovascular effects in relation to plasma levels of midazolam and diazepam. *Br J Clin Pharmacol.* 1988;25 (5):561–569.

Swenson JD. BP. Opioids in cardiovascular anesthesia. *Semin Cardiothorac Vasc Anesth.* 1997;2:146–163.

Tsen LC. Anesthesia for cesarean delivery. In: Chestnut DH, Wong CA, Tsen LC, Kee WDN, Beilin Y, Mhyre J, eds. *Chestnut's Obstetric Anesthesia: Principles and Practice.* 5th ed. : Elsevier Saunders; 2014:545–603.

Tullock WC, Diana P, Cook DR, et al. Neuromuscular and cardiovascular effects of high-dose vecuronium. *Anesth Analg.* 1990;70(1):86–90.

Wang GK, Strichartz GR. State-dependent inhibition of sodium by local anesthetics: a 40 year evolution. *Biochem (Mosc) Suppl Ser A Membr Cell Biol.* 2012;6(2):120–127.

Weiskopf RB, Moore MA, Eger 2nd EI, et al. Rapid increase in desflurane concentration is associated with greater transient cardiovascular stimulation than with rapid increase in isoflurane concentration in humans. *Anesthesiology.* 1994;80(5):1035–1045.

Yang LP, Keam SJ. Sugammadex: a review of its use in anaesthetic practice. *Drugs.* 2009;69(7):919–942.

Zecharia AY, Nelson LE, Gent TC, et al. The involvement of hypothalamic sleep pathways in general anesthesia: testing the hypothesis using the GABAA receptor beta3N265M knock-in mouse. *J Neurosci.* 2009;29(7): 2177–2187.

17

Anesthesia for Cardiac Patients During Labor and Delivery

Jay Conhaim, MD, and Andrea Girnius, MD

Pregnant women with preexisting cardiac disease provide a unique challenge to anesthesiologists in the peripartum period. Pregnancy-related death has been increasing over the past three decades, and cardiovascular disease is the number one cause of pregnancy-related death in the United States. Caring for this challenging patient population depends on an understanding of the cardiovascular changes associated with pregnancy, effective communication between all members of the care team, adequate and accurate physiologic monitoring during labor and delivery, and an understanding of how peripartum anesthesia and analgesia may affect existing cardiac lesions. In formulating a plan of care, the anesthesiologist must consider the mode of delivery, the nature and severity of cardiac disease, the anticipated location of delivery and recovery, the anticipated physiologic consequences of each method of anesthesia, and the necessary monitors. This chapter reviews the main considerations for anesthetic care of patients with cardiac disease during labor and delivery.

CARDIAC CHANGES DURING LABOR AND DELIVERY

The cardiovascular changes associated with pregnancy, labor, and delivery are dramatic. Compared with the majority of pregnant women, those with heart disease may not tolerate these changes as well. During the course of pregnancy, cardiac output increases by 50% through increases in both heart rate and stroke volume. Increased plasma volume and stroke volume results in increased left ventricular (LV) end-diastolic dilation. Systemic vascular resistance (SVR) is decreased, and central filling pressures remain unchanged. These

physiologic changes are exacerbated during labor and immediately postpartum, with increases in cardiac output by an additional 50% to 100% during labor. This is largely caused by autotransfusion from uterine contractions. Labor pain complicates cardiovascular physiology further by elevating heart rate and mean arterial pressure (MAP). Immediately after delivery, autotransfusion from the involuting uterus rapidly increases circulatory volume by an additional 30%, further increasing preload and cardiac output. Collectively, these remarkable hemodynamic changes can strain a previously weakened cardiovascular system. With appropriate planning, pain control, and physiologic monitoring, the difficulty that these changes pose can be anticipated and mitigated.

THE BASICS OF NEURAXIAL ANESTHESIA AND ANALGESIA

Although women have various choices for labor analgesia, neuraxial analgesia is a common and effective method of labor pain relief, especially for those with cardiac disease. Neuraxial anesthesia and analgesia involve delivery of local anesthetics, analgesics, or both to the epidural or subarachnoid space. Typically, this is achieved in one of three ways: spinal (intrathecal) injection, epidural catheter placement, or combination spinal and epidural (CSE). Each technique works by blocking preganglionic afferent and efferent nerve fibers, including pain and temperature, motor, and sympathetic fibers. The blockade is typically achieved with a local anesthetic, such as bupivacaine or ropivacaine, which acts as a sodium channel blocker, and/or an opiate receptor agonist, such as fentanyl. Blockade of sensory fibers provides effective pain relief during labor, which mitigates the hypertension and tachycardia that can accompany uterine contractions. However, blockade of sympathetic fibers can cause hypotension and decreased venous return. These effects can be anticipated and treated by the anesthesiologist.

Certain women may not be eligible for neuraxial techniques. Contraindications to spinal or epidural placement include patient refusal, certain infections, bleeding disorders, active maternal use of anticoagulants, or certain spine disorders. The main risks to the patient include infection, bleeding, postdural puncture headache, and nonfunctional or one-sided epidural catheter resulting in ineffective analgesia.

ANALGESIA FOR VAGINAL DELIVERY

Pudendal and Paracervical Blocks

Infiltration of the pudendal or paracervical nerve bundles with local anesthetic can be used for pelvic floor or cervical analgesia, respectively. The benefit of these procedures is the absence of sympatholysis and hypotension that may occur with neuraxial analgesia. Blockade of L2 to L3 nerve fibers at the paracervical ganglion, if successful, can help reduce pain associated with cervical dilation in the first stage of labor. However, even if successful, a paracervical block does not affect pain associated with distension of the vagina, vulva, and perineum. A pudendal nerve block can provide pain relief to the aforementioned structures and may provide some relief during the second stage of labor. However, pudendal nerve blocks have not demonstrated reduction in pain associated with the first stage of labor and are not as effective as neuraxial analgesia at reducing labor pain. Although there are data that compare paracervical blockade and epidural analgesia with regard to maternal blood pressure, the 44 patients included were described as healthy, making the data difficult to generalize to patients with existing cardiac disease.

Patient-Controlled Analgesia

For parturients who cannot receive neuraxial or regional analgesia, intravenous (IV) patient-controlled analgesia (PCA) presents an alternative that may be effective for some women. Short-acting opioid analgesics, such as remifentanil and fentanyl, are typically used for labor analgesia. The available data show that pain relief from PCA is acceptable to many patients but inferior to epidural analgesia. It also has documented fetal effects

because these medications cross the placenta. In nulliparous patients without access to alternative pain control, 74% of those who used a fentanyl-containing PCA reported adequate pain relief in the first stage of labor compared with control participants without any form of analgesia. Apgar scores did not differ at time of delivery. However, for patients who used fentanyl PCA throughout both stages of labor, 44% of neonates had an Apgar score less than or equal to 6. This physiologic depression remained statistically significant at 5 minutes of life compared with the infants who had a 1-minute Apgar score greater than or equal to 7. An isolated study that compared remifentanil with fentanyl PCA use demonstrated that the only difference in pain control efficacy exists during the first hour of use, when remifentanil was more successful. Compared with epidural analgesia, patient satisfaction with a remifentanil PCA was comparable, although pain relief was inferior. Compared with epidural analgesia, women using remifentanil PCA required more oxygen supplementation and experienced lower rates of hypotension. Most studies that evaluate PCA use in parturients exclude high risk deliveries or women with significant comorbidities. Given the paucity of data in women with cardiac disease, use of opioid PCA for labor analgesia needs to carefully weigh the risks of hypoxia against the risk of blood pressure and heart rate lability if other forms of analgesia are contraindicated or refused.

Nitrous Oxide

Nitrous oxide is an inhaled hypnotic agent commonly used in labor and delivery units throughout the world. Ease of administration and rapid onset of effect make nitrous oxide an appealing option. Although it does not achieve analgesic equivalency with epidural analgesia, it does provide greater overall satisfaction with the birthing experience compared with other forms of analgesia. The cardiovascular effects of inhalational nitrous oxide are secondary to an associated catecholamine release that can result in mild elevations in heart rate and blood pressure. These effects are exacerbated during uterine contractions, resulting in measurable increases in heart rate, stroke volume, MAP, and cardiac output. Nitrous oxide depresses myocardial contractility in vitro and has the potential to unmask existing myocardial depression in vivo. There are no studies that have evaluated the use of nitrous oxide for labor and delivery in women with known cardiovascular disease;

however, a large randomized trial in general surgery patients showed no increase in major cardiovascular events at 1 year in patients with preexisting cardiac disease undergoing general anesthesia with nitrous oxide. Because of its noted vasodilatory effects on the pulmonary vasculature, nitrous oxide should not be used in patients with elevated pulmonary artery pressures and intracardiac shunts to avoid ventilation/perfusion mismatch and pulmonary to systemic flow ratio (Qp:Qs) imbalance, respectively. Patients receiving nitrous oxide are also at increased risk of nausea and vomiting. The use of nitrous oxide for parturients with cardiovascular disease should be considered on a case-by-case basis in consultation with the entire care team.

Neuraxial Analgesia

Epidural analgesia a very common analgesic administered by anesthesiologists during childbirth. For labor and anticipated vaginal delivery, local anesthetic is administered through a catheter into the epidural space, just superficial to the dura mater. This results in a blockade of sensory, motor, and sympathetic nerve fibers. Adequate analgesia for the first stage of labor (cervical dilation) requires blocking nociceptive afferents to the level of T10. For the second stage of labor, the blockade must include S2 to S4 fibers. Therefore, to obtain coverage of these dermatomes, labor epidurals are placed in the lumbar region (L3–L4 or L4–L5 is most common). After placement of an epidural catheter, a test dose of lidocaine with epinephrine is typically used to evaluate for intravascular or intrathecal placement of the catheter. This practice should be carefully considered in patients with a high potential for arrhythmia, and a plain 2% lidocaine or fentanyl test dose can be used instead. A mixture of local anesthetic (bupivacaine or ropivacaine) with or without fentanyl (1–2 mcg/mL) is the most commonly used agent. To cover the appropriate dermatomes and provide satisfactory analgesia, additional local anesthetic can be bolused through the catheter, and the rate of infusion can be titrated as necessary.

Inhibition of ascending pain neurotransmission mitigates catecholamine-induced fluctuations in heart rate and blood pressure seen with uterine contractions. However, the sympathetic blockade can cause vasodilation, leading to decreased preload and hypotension, a common complication of epidural analgesia. This can be mitigated by a slow, controlled rate of local anesthetic administration through the catheter, lessening the acuity of the sympathectomy and allowing the body time to compensate for the changes occurring. Prophylactic crystalloid boluses, left lateral tilt, and vasopressors are also commonly used to prevent and treat hypotension after epidural analgesia. Prophylactic crystalloid boluses are not always effective in preventing hypotension, likely because of redistribution into the extracellular space. Cautious use of crystalloid prehydration should be used in patients with known heart failure.

Overall, women with preexisting cardiac disease can benefit greatly from the analgesia provided by an epidural. A large descriptive study found that patients with heart disease successfully received epidurals at the same rate as healthy pregnant women. Prevention of hypertension and tachycardia with uterine contractions can reduce the stress on the heart during labor, and the vasodilation and reduction in preload can help accommodate the increased circulating volume associated with labor and delivery. Before an epidural catheter is placed, adequate hemodynamic monitoring is required. This varies depending on the severity of the lesion. Pulse oximetry and noninvasive blood pressure monitoring during placement and maintenance of the epidural are indicated for all women undergoing epidural placement. For women with severe cardiac lesions, intraarterial blood pressure monitoring may be indicated before placement of an epidural. For most women with cardiac disease, titrating epidural infusions slowly helps prevent the development of poor venous return and hypotension. If hypotension does develop, preload and afterload support can be provided by the anesthesiologist. Phenylephrine and ephedrine are currently the vasopressors of choice for mitigation of neuraxial-induced hypotension. Phenylephrine is favored because it has been shown to depress fetal pH less than ephedrine; however, the two agents have shown no difference in Apgar scores. Appropriate vasoactive agents also depend on the type of cardiac disease, further stressing the importance of communication and planning before labor and delivery.

ANESTHESIA FOR CESAREAN SECTION

Neuraxial Anesthesia

Neuraxial anesthesia is currently the preferred method of providing anesthesia for cesarean section. Between 1981 and 2001, the use of spinal and epidural anesthesia for both elective and urgent cesarean section increased.

This was partly caused by improvements in technique and quality of neuraxial blockade as well as increased understanding of the risks of general anesthesia in parturients.

Several techniques can be used to provide anesthesia for cesarean section, including spinal, epidural, CSE, and general anesthesia. The technique selected depends on the patient's comorbidities as well as the circumstances surrounding the cesarean section. For single-shot spinal anesthesia, local anesthetic is injected directly into the intrathecal space, but epidural anesthesia uses a catheter in the epidural space just outside the dura mater. CSE involves an intrathecal injection followed by an epidural catheter placement, which can provide more flexibility in dosing. In all cases, the goal is blockade of preganglionic spinal cord fibers to provide adequate surgical sensory blockade. Sensory block to the level of the T4 dermatome is required for cesarean section. In addition to sensory blockade, motor and sympathetic fibers are blocked by the local anesthetic. The sympathetic blockade is the cause of the hemodynamic effects observed after neuraxial anesthesia.

The hemodynamic effects of spinal and epidural anesthesia can be quite profound, and they may be more poorly tolerated in a parturient with preexisting heart disease. The nature and severity of hemodynamic change depend on the level of blockade and the speed with which it is achieved. Sympathetic blockade inhibits sympathetic outflow to vascular smooth muscle, causing vasodilation. This results in decreased SVR, preload, and circulating catecholamines, leading to significant hypotension. Bradycardia also can be seen with spinal anesthesia, although this is less common. The sympathetic blockade can extend up to six levels beyond the sensory blockade, although it is not always complete.

When single-shot spinal anesthesia is used, these hemodynamic changes occur in the space of a few minutes. However, when epidural anesthesia is used, the spread of local anesthetic can be controlled, resulting in slower onset of blockade. This gives the body's compensatory mechanisms time to adjust to the changes. Less hypotension is seen with epidural anesthesia for cesarean section. For this reason, epidural or CSE with opioid only or low-dose intrathecal local anesthetic injection is usually preferred for parturients with cardiac disease. As with neuraxial analgesia for vaginal deliveries, prehydration with crystalloids and boluses of phenylephrine can be used to mitigate downtrending arterial blood pressure

measurements. Having a prepared phenylephrine infusion ready can allow for gradual titration to maintain relative normotension for each individual patient.

General Anesthesia

General anesthesia is not a preferred method of anesthesia for cesarean section. It involves greater risk to the mother and fetus. The incidence of failed intubation is reported to be about 1 in 300 for pregnant women compared with about 1 in 2000 in the setting of elective surgery. Pregnant women are at higher risk for pulmonary aspiration of gastric contents. In addition, volatile general anesthetic agents are uterine relaxants and may contribute to increased intraoperative bleeding after delivery of the infant. Finally, anesthetic agents cross the placenta, leading to increased drug exposure of the fetus and neonate. However, in certain situations, general anesthesia is the most appropriate anesthetic choice. These situations include patient refusal of neuraxial anesthesia, the presence of contraindications to neuraxial anesthesia (e.g., anticoagulation), or the need for emergent surgery. A study of anesthesia in women with heart disease found that women with complex congenital heart disease and premature delivery were more likely to receive general anesthesia.

Rapid-sequence induction is typically indicated for pregnant women undergoing general anesthesia for cesarean section given their increased risk of aspiration. However, if high-risk cardiovascular lesions will not tolerate a rapid induction, the risks and benefits of rapid-sequence induction (aspiration risk vs potential hemodynamic instability) should be weighed. Choice of induction agents should tailored to each patient. Propofol, if delivered rapidly or in large quantities, decreases SVR, preload, and blood pressure. Etomidate does not depress myocardial contractility or vascular smooth muscle tone; however, it does not effectively suppress the sympathetic response to laryngeal stimulation, which can lead to increases in heart rate and blood pressure with laryngoscopy unless an adjunct agent is used. Ketamine is typically associated with development of hypertension and increased heart rate caused by sympathetic stimulation. IV opiates are not typically given before delivery for neonatal considerations, but they should be considered for women who cannot tolerate mild to moderate increases in blood pressure or cardiac output, to depress sympathetic stimulation during laryngoscopy despite the risk of neonatal depression.

If opioids are used during induction of anesthesia, the neonatal resuscitation team should be alerted before delivery. Muscle relaxation is typically achieved with the depolarizing paralytic succinylcholine if hyperkalemia is not a concern or there is no underlying maternal myopathy. Succinylcholine is preferred given its short onset and duration of action compared with intermediate-acting nondepolarizing paralytics such as rocuronium or vecuronium. After intubation, inhaled volatile anesthetics such as sevoflurane or desflurane are used for maintenance of anesthesia. Nitrous oxide can be used as a supplement; however, the use of nitrous oxide as an inhaled anesthetic should be avoided in patients with intracardiac shunts or noted pulmonary hypertension.

Anesthetic Considerations for Specific Conditions

The general hemodynamic goals for parturients with heart disease during labor and delivery include maintenance of adequate cardiac output, avoidance of wide blood pressure swings while maintaining adequate perfusion pressure, avoidance of fluid overload, and avoidance of tachycardia and bradycardia. Although slowly titrated epidural analgesia is appropriate for almost all of these patients, each individual cardiac condition has its own considerations that must be accounted for when devising an anesthetic plan.

Atrial Septal Defects

Patients with atrial septal defects and left-to-right shunting may benefit from an epidural placed early in the course of labor and delivery. This may reduce the degree of left-to-right shunting by lowering systemic blood pressure. Filters should be placed on IV tubing to reduce the risk of paradoxical air embolism.

Cyanotic Congenital Heart Disease and Eisenmenger Syndrome

Patients with intracardiac shunts and Eisenmenger syndrome can be very difficult to manage in the peripartum period. The maternal mortality rate is approximately 24% to 50%. The prevention of right-to-left intracardiac shunting and maintenance of right ventricular function are the primary management targets. Reduction of the pulmonary vascular resistance and maintenance of adequate SVR helps prevent right-to-left shunting.

Neuraxial analgesia and anesthesia have been used for epidural analgesia for laboring patients and cesarean section. The use of general anesthesia has been successfully reported in patients with Eisenmenger syndrome; however, its use in patients with cyanotic congenital heart disease or Eisenmenger syndrome has shown a trend toward increased mortality rates. If general anesthesia cannot be avoided, maintenance of SVR is critical. Avoidance of hypoxia and hypercarbia helps prevent increases in pulmonary vascular resistance, as does minimizing positive end-expiratory pressure and peak inspiratory pressures.

Aortic and Mitral Regurgitation

Regurgitant lesions are generally well tolerated in pregnancy. Goals of management include preservation of forward flow into the systemic vasculature and avoidance of retrograde flow into the pulmonary vasculature through SVR modulation. Elevated SVR can increase the regurgitant fraction. To avoid pain-related increases in SVR, neuraxial analgesia should be used early in labor. Successful use of epidural analgesia and general anesthesia for cesarean section has been reported. Forward flow can be maintained with mild tachycardia and goal heart rates of 80 to 100 beats/min. Moderate to severe aortic and mitral regurgitation may be associated with left atrial dilation and atrial fibrillation. If this is the case, sinus rhythm should be maintained. If sinus rhythm cannot be maintained, rapid ventricular rates should be avoided if possible. Controlled afterload reduction also enables forward flow, preventing the development of pulmonary congestion. Bradycardia allows for retrograde flow in these lesions and should therefore be avoided.

Mitral Stenosis

Pulmonary edema is the main cardiac risk in patients with mitral stenosis. Careful attention to fluid balance is critical, and diuretics can be used if needed for fluid overload. Beta blockers can be used to elicit bradycardia, which allows for increased diastolic filling time. Tachycardia, including tachyarrhythmias, are quite detrimental and should be avoided. Maintenance of sinus rhythm is ideal. Reductions in LV preload caused by hypovolemia or hypotension can have disastrous effects in this patient population.

Neuraxial analgesia for vaginal delivery should be slowly titrated to avoid a sudden loss of preload to the heart. Early initiation of epidural analgesia can prevent tachycardia or hypertension secondary to labor pains.

Neuraxial analgesia can be successfully used for cesarean section but should be titrated slowly to achieve the desired level of sensory blockade. General anesthesia can also be used if necessary, although the uterine relaxation effects of volatile anesthetics may increase blood loss, which is poorly tolerated in these patients. The use of methergine and oxytocin elevate SVR, and oxytocin may cause a reflex tachycardia, so their use should be carefully considered.

Aortic Stenosis

In patients with severe aortic stenosis, it is critical to avoid hypotension, which can lead to impaired coronary artery perfusion. This can lead to impaired LV function, further impairment of coronary perfusion, and rapid hemodynamic deterioration. Blood loss should be minimized, and volume replacement may be critical. Tachycardia should be avoided because these patients are likely to have diastolic dysfunction and need longer diastolic filling time. Both regional and general anesthesia have been used with success, although single-shot spinal anesthesia is typically avoided because the rapid sympathectomy is more likely to cause hypotension. Phenylephrine can be used safely to maintain afterload.

Prosthetic Heart Valves

Properly functioning bioprosthetic valves create few issues in pregnancy. The complications created by mechanical valves result from the need for anticoagulation. Patients with mechanical heart valves are commonly anticoagulated with warfarin, which is associated with significant fetal anomalies and is usually avoided in pregnancy. Its use, however, has been reported in patients with mechanical prosthetic valves because it provides superior anticoagulation. Low-molecular-weight heparin is often used during pregnancy, but unfractionated heparin is preferred during labor and delivery because it has a shorter half-life and can be more easily monitored and reversed. If regional anesthesia is to be used, heparin must be interrupted to avoid the risk of spinal hematoma. It may be restarted after an appropriate interval after regional anesthesia has been established. Heparin is typically discontinued before the second stage of labor; prolonged labor should be avoided so that it can be restarted as soon as possible. Labor augmentation with oxytocin may be used.

Endocarditis prophylaxis may be considered.

Hypertrophic Cardiomyopathy

Women with hypertrophic cardiomyopathy usually tolerate pregnancy well. The increased blood volume tends to reduce obstruction. If patients have severe diastolic dysfunction, fluid overload may cause pulmonary edema. Beta blockers may be used during pregnancy if indicated. Some of these patients may have implantable cardioverter-defibrillators for primary or secondary prevention. The devices should be interrogated before delivery to ensure that they are working properly. Fluid overload may also occur after delivery of the infant, when uterine involution results in a large-volume autotransfusion. The safe use of neuraxial anesthesia for both vaginal delivery and cesarean section is reported in patients with hypertrophic cardiomyopathy.

Adequate fluid replacement is mandatory to maintain filling pressures in the left ventricle and thereby avoid obstruction. Tachycardia is generally harmful. Anything that reduces afterload or increases myocardial contractility can worsen obstruction. Oxytocin and methergine are generally well tolerated.

Dilated Cardiomyopathy

Epidural anesthesia reduces afterload and may be helpful in promoting forward flow; its safe use is described in the literature. General anesthesia can also be used if necessary for cesarean section. Hydralazine, nitrates, and beta blockers are commonly used during pregnancy. Angiotensin-converting enzyme inhibitors are contraindicated because of a risk of birth defects.

Ischemic Heart Disease

Management goals include maintenance of myocardial perfusion by avoiding hypotension and tachycardia. Epidural analgesia may be useful in blunting the sympathetic pain response during labor. Local anesthetic should be dosed cautiously to avoid hypotension. Sedation should be administered cautiously to avoid hypotension and hypoventilation. Nitroglycerin causes uterine relaxation.

BIBLIOGRAPHY

2015 ESC Guidelines fothe management of infective endocarditis. *EuHeart J.* 2015;36(44):3036-3037.

Alshawabkeh L, Economy KE, Valente AM. Anticoagulation during pregnancy: evolving strategies with a focus on mechanical valves. *J Am Coll Cardiol.* 2016;68(16):1804–1813.

Ashikhmina E, Farbe MK, Mizuguchi KA. Parturients with hypertrophic cardiomyopathy: case series and review of pregnancy outcomes and anesthetic management of laboand delivery. *Int J Obstet Anesth.* 2015;24(4):344–355.

Bates SM, Middeldorp S, Rodge M, James AH, Gree I. Guidance fothe treatment and prevention of obstetric-associated venous thromboembolism. *J Thromb Thrombolysis.* 2016;41(1):92–128.

Bucklin BA, Hawkins JL, Anderson JR, Ullrich FA. Obstetric anesthesia workforce survey: twenty-yeaupdate. *Anesthesiology.* 2005;103(3):645–653.

Cappiello E. Complications and side effects of central neuraxial techniques. In: Wong CA, ed. *Spinal and Epidural Anesthesia.* : McGraw-Hill; 2007:151–182.

Chestnut DH. Alternative regional analgesic techniques folaboand vaginal delivery. In: Chestnut DH, Wong CA, Tsen LC, Kee WDN, Beilin Y, Mhyre J, eds. *Chestnut's Obstetric Anesthesia: Principles and Practice.* 5th edition : ElsevieSaunders; 2014:518–529.

Cook TM, MacDougall-Davis SR. Complications and failure of airway management. *BJ Anaesth.* 2012;109(suppl 1): i68–i85.

Creanga AA, Syverson C, Seed K, Callaghan WM. Pregnancy-related mortality in the United States, 2011-2013. *Obstet Gynecol.* 2017;130(2):366–373.

Douma MR, Verwey RA, Kam-Endtz CE, van deLinden PD, Stienstra R. Obstetric analgesia: a comparison of patient-controlled meperidine, remifentanil, and fentanyl in labour. *BJ Anaesth.* 2010;104(2):209–215.

European Society of Gynecology (ESG), Association foEuropean Paediatric Cardiology (AEPC), German Society foGendeMedicine (DGesGM) ESC Guidelines on the management of cardiovasculadiseases during pregnancy: the Task Force on the Management of Cardiovascula-Diseases during Pregnancy of the European Society of Cardiology (ESC). *EuHeart J.* 2011;32(24):3147–3197.

Fang G, Tian YK, Mei W. Anaesthesia management of caesarean section in two patients with Eisenmenger's syndrome. *Anesthesiol Res Pract.* 2011;2011:972671.

Freeman LM, Bloemenkamp KW, Franssen MT, et al. Patient controlled analgesia with remifentanil versus epidural analgesia in labour: randomised multicentre equivalence trial. *BMJ.* 2015;350:h846.

Fujita M, Satsumae T, Tanaka M. [General anesthesia using remifentanil focesarean section in a parturient with Marfan syndrome associated with heart failure due to severe mitral regurgitation]. *Masui.* 2016;65(5):530–534.

Gaise R. Physiologic changes of pregnancy. In: Chestnut DH, Wong CA, Tsen LC, Kee WDN, Beilin Y, Mhyre J, eds. *Chestnut's Obstetric Anesthesia: Principles and Practice.* 5th edition : ElsevieSaunders; 2014:15–38.

Gleiche N, Midwall J, Hochberge D, Jaffin H. Eisenmenger's syndrome and pregnancy. *Obstet Gynecol Surv.* 1979;34 (10):721–741.

Goldszmidt E, Macarthu A, Silversides C, Colman J, Serme M, Siu S. Anesthetic management of a consecutive cohort of women with heart disease folaboand delivery. *Int J Obstet Anesth.* 2010;19(3):266–272.

Gooding JM, Corssen G. Effect of etomidate on the cardiovasculasystem. *Anesth Analg.* 1977;56(5):717–719.

Horlocke TT, Wedel DJ, Rowlingson JC, et al. Regional anesthesia in the patient receiving antithrombotic othrombolytic therapy: American Society of Regional Anesthesia and Pain Medicine Evidence-Based Guidelines (Third Edition). *Reg Anesth Pain Med.* 2010;35(1):64–101.

Hug Jr CC, McLeskey CH, Nahrwold ML, et al. Hemodynamic effects of propofol: data from ove25,000 patients. *Anesth Analg.* 1993;77(4 suppl):S21–S29.

Hung L, Rahimtoola SH. Prosthetic heart valves and pregnancy. *Circulation.* 2003;107(9):1240–1246.

Ioscovich AM, Goldszmidt E, Fadeev AV, Grisaru-Granovsky S, Halpern SH. Peripartum anesthetic management of patients with aortic valve stenosis: a retrospective study and literature review. *Int J Obstet Anesth.* 2009;18(4): 379–386.

Ituk US, Habib AS, Polin CM, Allen TK. Anesthetic management and outcomes of parturients with dilated cardiomyopathy in an academic centre. *Can J Anaesth.* 2015;62 (3):278–288.

Kinsella SM, Winton AL, Mushambi MC, et al. Failed tracheal intubation during obstetric general anaesthesia: a literature review. *Int J Obstet Anesth.* 2015;24(4):356–374.

Leong EW, Sivanesaratnam V, Oh LL, Chan YK. Epidural analgesia in primigravidae in spontaneous labouat term: a prospective study. *J Obstet Gynaecol Res.* 2000;26(4): 271–275.

Leslie K, Myles PS, Kasza J, et al. Nitrous oxide and serious long-term morbidity and mortality in the Evaluation of Nitrous Oxide in the Gas Mixture foAnaesthesia (ENIGMA)-II trial. *Anesthesiology.* 2015;123(6):1267–1280.

Maneglia R, Cousin MT. A comparison between propofol and ketamine foanaesthesia in the elderly. Haemodynamic effects during induction and maintenance. . *Anaesthesia.* 1988;43(suppl):109–111.

Manninen T, Aantaa R, Salonen M, Pirhonen J, Palo P. A comparison of the hemodynamic effects of paracervical block and epidural anesthesia folaboanalgesia. *Acta Anaesthesiol Scand.* 2000;44(4):441–445.

Martin JT, Tautz TJ, Antognini JF. Safety of regional anesthesia in Eisenmenger's syndrome. *Reg Anesth Pain Med.* 2002;27(5):509–513.

Miyakoshi K, Tanaka M, Morisaki H, et al. Perinatal outcomes: intravenous patient-controlled fentanyl versus no analgesia in labor. *J Obstet Gynaecol Res.* 2013;39(4):783–789.

Morgan PJ, Halpern SH, Tarshis J. The effects of an increase of central blood volume before spinal anesthesia focesarean delivery: a qualitative systematic review. *Anesth Analg.* 2001;92(4):997–1005.

Morley-Forste PK, Weberpals J. Neonatal effects of patient-controlled analgesia using fentanyl in labor. *Int J Obstet Anesth.* 1998;7(2):103–107.

Myles PS, Chan MT, Kasza J, et al. Severe nausea and vomiting in the evaluation of nitrous oxide in the Gas Mixture foAnesthesia II Trial. *Anesthesiology.* 2016;124(5):1032–1040.

Pace MC, Aurilio C, Bulletti C, Iannotti M, Passavanti MB, Palagiano A. Subarachnoid analgesia in advanced labor: a comparison of subarachnoid analgesia and pudendal block in advanced labor: analgesic quality and obstetric outcome. *Ann N Y Acad Sci.* 2004;1034:356–363.

Park GE, Hauch MA, Curlin F, Datta S, Bade AM. The effects of varying volumes of crystalloid administration before cesarean delivery on maternal hemodynamics and colloid osmotic pressure. *Anesth Analg.* 1996;83(2):299–303.

Pessel C, Bonanno C. Valve disease in pregnancy. *Semin Perinatol.* 2014;38(5):273–284.

Piepe PG, Walke F. Pregnancy in women with hypertrophic cardiomyopathy. *Neth Heart J.* 2013;21(1):14–18.

Sandhya K, Shivanna S, Tejesh C, Rathna N. Labouanalgesia and anaesthetic management of a primigravida with uncorrected pentology of Fallot. *Indian J Anaesth.* 2012;56(2). 186-178.

Savu O, Jurcut R, Giusca S, et al. Morphological and functional adaptation of the maternal heart during pregnancy. *Circ Cardiovasc Imaging.* 2012;5(3):289–297.

Scavone BM, Ratliff J, Wong CA. Physiologic effects of neuraxial anesthesia. In: Wong CA,, ed. *Spinal and Epidural Anesthesia.* : McGraw-Hill;; 2007:111–126.

Tsen LC. Anesthesia focesarean delivery. In: Chestnut DH, Wong CA, Tsen LC, Kee WDN, Beilin Y, Mhyre J, eds. *Chestnut's Obstetric Anesthesia: Principles and Practice.* 5th edition : ElsevieSaunders; 2014:545–603.

VanHelde T, Smedstad KG. Combined spinal epidural anaesthesia in a primigravida with valvulaheart disease. *Can J Anaesth.* 1998;45(5 pt 1):488–490.

Veese M, Hofmann T, Roth R, Klöh S, Rossaint R, Heesen M. Vasopressors fothe management of hypotension aftespinal anesthesia foelective caesarean section. Systematic review and cumulative meta-analysis. *Acta Anaesthesiol Scand.* 2012;56(7):810–816.

Waldenstrom U. Experience of laboand birth in 1111 women. *J Psychosom Res.* 1999;47(5):471–482.

Westling F, Milsom I, Zetterström H, Ekström-Jodal B. Effects of nitrous oxide/oxygen inhalation on the maternal circulation during vaginal delivery. *Acta Anaesthesiol Scand.* 1992;36(2):175–181.

18

Anesthesia for Nonobstetric Procedures During Pregnancy

Helen Pappas, MD, and Andrea Girnius, MD

During pregnancy, women may present for nonobstetric surgical procedures, most commonly related to traumatic injury, appendicitis, or cholecystitis. Care must be taken to provide a safe anesthetic for both patients, with maternal stability directly correlating with fetal well-being. Although there are not robust data on which to base anesthetic management, there are numerous cohort studies that point to the safety of anesthesia for surgical interventions that must be performed during pregnancy. The joint practice statement from the American Society of Anesthesiologists (ASA) and American College of Obstetricians and Gynecologists (ACOG) highlights that elective cases should be postponed until the postpartum period, procedures should be performed in second trimester if possible when the risk of preterm labor and spontaneous abortion are lowest, and urgent cases should not be delayed. Currently, no anesthetic agents used in standard doses have been shown to be teratogenic. Fetal monitoring should vary based on gestational age and type of procedure, but care should be provided in a facility with obstetric and neonatal availability. It is recommended that each case be approached with a multidisciplinary team to optimize maternal and fetal safety.

TIMING OF SURGERY

The ASA/ACOG joint practice statement on nonobstetric surgery during pregnancy addresses the optimal timing for procedures during pregnancy. First, it is clear that if a surgery is necessary, it should not be denied solely because of pregnancy. However, elective nonobstetric surgery (including cardiac surgery) should be postponed until the postpartum period. If surgery must be performed during pregnancy, the second trimester is the optimal time because the risks of spontaneous abortion and preterm labor are both at their lowest.

The evidence for timing is overall lacking in robust data, with the bulk of evidence in retrospective reviews and outcome studies. Some of the strongest data come from a large Swedish registry, in which more than 5000 women underwent surgery during pregnancy. From these data, there was an increase in low- and very-low-birth-weight infants because of prematurity and intrauterine growth restriction for procedures performed in any trimester. Regardless of the trimester, there was no observed increase in congenital anomalies, even in first trimester operations under general anesthesia, which accounted for more than 50% of cases.

Other subsequent reviews support this study and provide the basis for the ACOG guidelines. Overall, there is an increase in spontaneous abortion associated with first trimester surgeries and an increase in preterm labor with third trimester surgeries. Appropriate patient counseling should be done if procedures must be performed. As always, a multidisciplinary risk and benefit discussion should be undertaken to make these difficult decisions. If maternal surgery is necessary during the third trimester, consideration of whether to perform a cesarean section beforehand is warranted. This should be an individualized decision based on the risks and benefits in each particular case. If surgery is performed after 28 weeks, steroids may be administered to stimulate fetal lung maturity in the event of premature labor and delivery. Because of the increased risk of venous thromboembolism during pregnancy, these patients should be screened and receive appropriate prophylaxis.

ANESTHETIC PREEVALUATION

A thorough preoperative examination, with particular attention to the cardiac status, airway, and stage of gestation, should be performed. The physiologic changes of pregnancy have a significant effect on anesthetic management.

The upper airway experiences changes because of increased circulating progesterone. Increased blood flow leads to mucosal edema, capillary congestion, and tissue friability. Pregnant women are therefore at increased risk for nasal and oral mucosal bleeding, especially with airway instrumentation. Airway assessment is critical in parturients. The reported rate of failed intubation in obstetric patients is approximately 1 in 250 to 300, which is eight times higher than in the general population. Multiple studies have documented that changes in Mallampati score, a method of predicting difficulty of intubation, occur throughout pregnancy and during labor.

The physiologic changes to the cardiovascular system have been well reviewed elsewhere. For each particular patient, the specific nature of her cardiac lesion and her current functional status should be noted. Results of any recent cardiac testing, including electrocardiogram, echocardiogram, cardiac catheterization, or any other relevant information, should also be reviewed.

The gravid uterus and mechanical changes in the thorax result in alterations in lung volumes and capacities. In addition, because of the increased metabolic demand imposed by the fetus, increased minute ventilation is necessary. This is accomplished by both an increase in tidal volume and respiratory rate. Despite the observed diaphragmatic elevation, diaphragmatic excursion is actually increased. Vital capacity is maintained at prepregnancy levels. Whereas tidal volume and inspiratory reserve volume both increase, reserve volume and expiratory reserve decrease. This leads to a decreased functional residual capacity (FRC). The decrease in FRC becomes very important during intubation of a parturient because this contributes to rapid desaturation. The increased minute ventilation seen during pregnancy leads to characteristic changes in arterial blood gas values. PaO_2 increases slightly to 100 to 106 mm Hg while $PaCO_2$ decreases to approximately 30 mm Hg. This leads to a mild respiratory alkalosis, with an average pH of 7.44. These changes are usually present by the end of the first trimester.

Pregnant women undergo several physical and physiologic changes that increase their risk of aspiration. The expanding uterus displaces the stomach cephalad and increases pressure in the stomach. In addition, increased circulating progesterone relaxes the lower esophageal sphincter. Both of these changes increase the incidence of gastroesophageal reflux disease, which affects up to 50% of pregnant women. Because of these changes, the risk of aspiration during airway manipulation is increased. Most experts consider pregnant women to have a full stomach regardless of the time of last oral intake. Several options for premedication are available to decrease the risk of aspiration or mitigate the severity of aspiration if it occurs. Commonly used interventions include H2 antagonists and sodium citrate.

SELECTION OF ANESTHETIC METHOD

The choice of anesthetic technique is highly dependent on the surgery being performed, with the goal of providing the safest patient care while optimizing procedural conditions. The risks and benefits should always be weighed to determine the best plan on a case-by-case basis. General anesthesia poses the highest potential risk because of the need for airway manipulation, aspiration risk, and increased systemic drug exposure to the fetus. If regional or neuraxial anesthesia is appropriate for the surgery, it is preferred. Both regional and neuraxial techniques rely entirely on local anesthetics to block sensory nerve conduction; therefore, minimal medication enters the maternal bloodstream, limiting the drug exposure to the fetus. However, many surgeries cannot be performed feasibly under regional anesthesia. In these cases, general anesthesia can be safely performed with attention paid to minimizing the risks.

ANESTHETIC CONSIDERATIONS DURING SURGERY

The general goals during surgery include maintenance of uteroplacental blood flow and prevention of premature labor. This is accomplished by avoidance of hypoxemia, hypotension, hypovolemia, and hypothermia, which can all contribute to fetal stress. In addition, it is important to avoid drugs that are potentially harmful to fetuses. This is especially important during fetal organogenesis, which occurs from 6 to 12 weeks of gestation.

TERATOGENIC EFFECTS OF ANESTHETIC AGENTS

There are no known teratogenic effects of the major anesthetic agents documented in the literature to date. This assertion is based on very limited data. A large study comparing pregnant women undergoing surgery with pregnant women who did not undergo surgery found no difference in the rates of miscarriage or fetal anomalies. However, a larger sample size than was available in this study would be required to achieve adequate power. Therefore, no definitive conclusions can be reached. However, the potential risks associated with several adjuncts commonly used during anesthesia are worth discussing.

Nitrous oxide is a volatile hypnotic agent commonly used to supplement general anesthesia. It is not used as a sole anesthetic agent for general anesthesia. It is a known teratogen in mammals when used in high doses during organogenesis. The doses used in these studies are orders-of-magnitude greater than those used clinically in humans. However, the effects on human fetuses are less certain. There has been retrospective data suggesting that dental assistants exposed to ambient nitrous oxide have a higher risk of first-trimester miscarriage and reduced fertility. Experts suggest that chronic exposure is more deleterious than single high-concentration exposure. The use of scavenging systems can reduce risk. Because many effective anesthetic alternatives are available, it seems prudent to avoid the use of nitrous oxide during surgery in pregnant women.

Benzodiazepines are commonly used for anxiolysis before surgery. The use of these medications has been associated in some studies with increased risk of cleft palate and cardiac anomalies. However, later studies have cast doubt on this association. A Swedish national registry analysis did not find an association between benzodiazepines and birth defects. Multiple larger case control studies including tens of thousands of infants exposed in utero to benzodiazepines and millions of unexposed infants did not find an association between maternal benzodiazepine use and birth defects, specifically cleft palate. In an appropriate clinical situation, benzodiazepines can be safely used for anxiolysis before surgery, although they can be avoided if there is no anticipated clinical benefit.

Ondansetron is commonly used to prevent or treat postoperative nausea and vomiting after surgery. Some data have suggested that there is an increased incidence of cleft palate when ondansetron is taken during the first trimester for morning sickness. Other studies have not shown this increased incidence of cleft palate, but they were only powered to show a large difference in incidence. A large retrospective cohort study from Denmark did not demonstrate an increase in fetal anomalies with ondansetron exposure. Ondansetron is commonly prescribed for morning sickness when other treatments have failed. During surgery, the patient's risk for postoperative nausea and vomiting can be assessed and ondansetron administered if appropriate.

INDUCTION AND MAINTENANCE OF ANESTHESIA

Planning induction of a general anesthetic in a pregnant woman with cardiac disease requires careful deliberation. Regardless of fasting time, pregnant women are considered to have a "full stomach" because of relaxation of the lower esophageal sphincter and upward pressure on the stomach from the gravid uterus. Therefore, when general anesthesia is required, a rapid-sequence induction is usually used to help prevent aspiration of gastric contents. During rapid-sequence induction, ventilation is not attempted, and succinylcholine, a fast-onset depolarizing neuromuscular blocker, is used to facilitate optimal intubating conditions. Some patients with cardiac disease may not tolerate the hemodynamic changes that occur during a rapid induction. In these cases, the risk of aspiration must be balanced against the risk of hemodynamic instability. If necessary, a slower induction can be considered, and medication adjustments can be made to attenuate the expected hemodynamic response to induction and intubation.

Anesthesia is maintained with a volatile agent such as sevoflurane or desflurane. Volatile anesthetic agents are known to cause vasodilation, hypotension, cardiac depression, and increased arrhythmia potential. Depending on the severity of the cardiac lesion, invasive hemodynamic monitoring may be needed to safely manage these patients during the general anesthetic. Neuromuscular blockers can safely be used during the pregnancy. If neuromuscular blockade has been used, it will need to be reversed at the end of surgery to allow the patient to breathe spontaneously and be extubated. This can be accomplished with neostigmine, an acetylcholinesterase inhibitor, paired with an acetylcholine antagonist such as atropine or glycopyrrolate. Sugammadex, a newer agent that acts by encapsulating neuromuscular blockers rocuronium and vecuronium, can be also used. The Society for Obstetric Anesthesia and Perinatology currently recommends against the use of sugammadex in pregnant women because of the risk of encapsulating progesterone, which is essential for the maintenance of pregnancy, although more research is needed in this population.

POSITIONING

After 20 weeks' gestation, the positioning of the patient becomes quite important. A supine position may be associated with compression of the inferior vena cava or the aorta, resulting in hypotension. A wedge under the right lower back or a leftward tilt of the operating table to 10 to 15 degrees can be helpful in minimizing aortic or vena caval compression.

PLACENTAL TRANSFER OF ANESTHETIC MEDICATIONS

Placental transfer of mediations is determined by several factors, including molecule size, charge, protein binding, and lipophilicity. Whereas most drugs with molecular weights less than 500 Da freely cross the placenta, few drugs with molecular weights greater than 1000 Da cross the placenta. Lipophilic and nonionized drugs cross the placenta more easily, but highly protein bound drugs do not cross the placenta to a significant degree. The majority of medications used in anesthesia cross the placenta, resulting in fetal exposure. This includes intravenous induction agents, volatile anesthetics, opioids, benzodiazepines, and local anesthetics. Notable medications used commonly in anesthesia that do not cross the placenta include neuromuscular blockers, heparin, insulin, and glycopyrrolate. Sugammadex most likely does not cross the placenta based on its size.

CARDIAC SURGERY DURING PREGNANCY

Cardiac surgery with cardiopulmonary bypass (CPB) during pregnancy carries a high risk of fetal death. For this reason, it is avoided unless absolutely necessary. However, there may be rare cases when the mother is decompensating from a cardiac standpoint and the benefits of intervention outweigh the risks. Features

of CPB that increase the risk of decreased fetal perfusion, morbidity, and mortality include nonpulsatile flow, reduced perfusion pressures, renin and catecholamine release, and hypothermia. There is not strong evidence to support the efficacy of any particular measure, but it is recommended to maintain normothermia, keep perfusion pressure greater than 70 mm Hg and pump flow greater than 2.5 L/min, and maintain maternal hematocrit above 28%.

FETAL MONITORING DURING SURGERY

Fetal heart rate (FHR) monitoring is a widely used technique to monitor fetal well-being during labor, but it also plays a role during pregnancy to assess the fetal status. The normal FHR ranges from 110 to 160 beats/min, with variability ranging from 6 to 25 beats/min. This normal baseline with variability is a result of a healthy central and autonomic nervous system working in tandem. Because of the significant developmental changes to the nervous system, FHR should not be used until after 20 weeks of gestation, at which time the monitoring becomes more accurate. Signs of fetal distress include decreased variability in the tracing and decreased heart rate or bradycardia (<100 beats/min). This can be a sign of decreased uteroplacental blood flow, fetal acidosis, or fetal anoxia. Unfortunately, decreased variability is also seen in any depressed central nervous system state, including fetal sleep, anesthetic and analgesic exposure, and magnesium exposure. Therefore, the interpretation of FHR changes while under general anesthesia can be difficult.

Monitoring for the fetus will depend on the gestational age and type of surgery. Generally, if the fetus is previable, FHR will be obtained by Doppler before and after the procedure. If the fetus is viable, the minimum monitoring will include pre- and postprocedure electronic fetal heart rate monitoring and contraction monitoring. The decision for intraoperative FHR monitoring should be made on a case-by-case basis. If technically feasible, the fetus is viable, and there may be a need to urgently deliver the fetus, intraprocedural monitoring may be recommended. A multidisciplinary discussion with obstetrics, surgery, and anesthesia should be conducted to determine the best monitoring for the fetus. Cases should be done at a facility with obstetric and neonatal care available so that FHR monitoring can be safely administered and acted upon.

BIBLIOGRAPHY

ACOG Committee Opinion No. 775: Nonobstetric Surgery During Pregnancy. *Obstet Gynecol.* 2019;133:e285–e286.

Allaert SE, Carlier SP, Weyne LP, Vertommen DJ, Dutré PE, Desmet MB. First trimester anesthesia exposure and fetal outcome. A review. *Acta Anaesthesiol Belg.* 2007;58 (2):119–123.

Anderka M, Mitchell AA, Louik C, et al. Medications used to treat nausea and vomiting of pregnancy and the risk of selected birth defects. *Birth Defects Res A Clin Mol Teratol.* 2012;94(1):22–30.

Bailey RE. Intrapartum fetal monitoring. *Am Fam Physician.* 2009;80(12):1388–1396.

Bobrowski RA. Pulmonary physiology in pregnancy. *Clin Obstet Gynecol.* 2010;53(2):285–300.

Boutonnet M, Faitot V, Katz A, Salomon L, Keita H. Mallampati class changes during pregnancy, labour, and after delivery: can these be predicted? *Br J Anaesth.* 2010;104 (1):67–70.

Chandrasekhar S, Cook CR, Collard CD. Cardiac surgery in the parturient. *Anesth Analg.* 2009;108(3):777–785.

Duncan PG, Pope WD, Cohen MM, Greer N. Fetal risk of anesthesia and surgery during pregnancy. *Anesthesiology.* 1986;64(6):790–794.

Einarson A, Maltepe C, Navioz Y, Kennedy D, Tan MP, Koren G. The safety of ondansetron for nausea and vomiting of pregnancy: a prospective comparative study. *BJOG.* 2004;111(9):940–943.

Friedman JM. Teratogen update: anesthetic agents. *Teratology.* 1988;37(1):69–77.

Fujinaga M, Baden JM. Methionine prevents nitrous oxide-induced teratogenicity in rat embryos grown in culture. *Anesthesiology.* 1994;81(1):184–189.

Gaiser R. Physiologic changes of pregnancy. In: Chestnut DH, Wong CA, Tsen LC, Kee WDN, Beilin Y, Mhyre J, eds. *Chestnut's Obstetric Anesthesia: Principles and Practice.* 5th edition : Elsevier Saunders; 2014:15–38.

Griffiths SK. Placental structure, function, and drug transfer. *Contin Educ Anaesth Crit Care Pain.* 2015;15(2):84–89.

In Antenatal and Postnatal Mental Health: Clinical Management and Service Guidance: Updated edition. 2014.

Kodali BS, Chandrasekhar S, Bulich LN, Topulos GP, Datta S. Airway changes during labor and delivery. *Anesthesiology.* 2008;108(3):357–362.

Lane GA, Nahrwold ML, Tait AR, Taylor-Busch M, Cohen PJ, Beaudoin AR. Anesthetics as teratogens: nitrous oxide is fetotoxic, xenon is not. *Science.* 1980;210(4472):899–901.

Mazze RI, Kallen B. Appendectomy during pregnancy: a Swedish registry study of 778 cases. *Obstet Gynecol.* 1991;77(6):835–840.

Mazze RI, Kallen B. Reproductive outcome after anesthesia and operation during pregnancy: a registry study of 5405 cases. *Am J Obstet Gynecol.* 1989;161(5):1178–1185.

Nava-Ocampo AA, Koren G. Human teratogens and evidence-based teratogen risk counseling: the Motherisk approach. *Clin Obstet Gynecol.* 2007;50(1):123–131.

Olfert SM. Reproductive outcomes among dental personnel: a review of selected exposures. *J Can Dent Assoc.* 2006;72 (9):821–825.

Pasternak B, Svanstrom H, Hviid A. Ondansetron in pregnancy and risk of adverse fetal outcomes. *N Engl J Med.* 2013;368(9):814–823.

Perinatology, S.f.O.A.a. Statement on Sugammadex during pregnancy and lactation. 2019.

Rosenberg L, Mitchell AA, Parsells JL, Pashayan H, Louik C, Shapiro S. Lack of relation of oral clefts to diazepam use during pregnancy. *N Engl J Med.* 1983;309(21): 1282–1285.

Rowland AS, Baird DD, Shore DL, Weinberg CR, Savitz DA, Wilcox AJ. Nitrous oxide and spontaneous abortion in female dental assistants. *Am J Epidemiol.* 1995;141(6):531–538.

Safra MJ, Oakley Jr. GP. Association between cleft lip with or without cleft palate and prenatal exposure to diazepam. *Lancet.* 1975;2(7933):478–480.

Tsen LC. Anesthesia for cesarean delivery. In: Chestnut DH, Wong CA, Tsen LC, Kee WDN, Beilin Y, Mhyre J, eds. *Chestnut's Obstetric Anesthesia: Principles and Practice.* 5th edition : Elsevier Saunders; 2014:545–603.

Van Leeuwen P, Lange S, Bettermann H, Grönemeyer D, Hatzmann W. Fetal heart rate variability and complexity in the course of pregnancy. *Early Hum Dev.* 1999;54(3): 259–269.

Wikner BN, Kallen B. Are hypnotic benzodiazepine receptor agonists teratogenic in humans? *J Clin Psychopharmacol.* 2011;31(3):356–359.

19

Cardiac Testing During Pregnancy

John H. Wilson, MD, FACC, FHRS

Cardiac testing during pregnancy may include one of more of the following: cardiac magnetic resonance imaging (MRI) scan, chest radiography, computed tomography (CT), electrocardiography, graded exercise testing, Holter monitor or other wearable event recorders, implantable loop recorder, radionuclide investigations, stress echocardiography, dobutamine stress echocardiography, transesophageal echocardiography (TEE), and transthoracic echocardiography and Doppler. Each of these is described in this chapter, with an emphasis on its use, benefits, and risks in expecting mothers.

CARDIAC MAGNETIC RESONANCE IMAGING SCAN

Cardiac MRI scans can be invaluable in diagnosing complex cardiac lesions and have the advantage that there is no radiation exposure. The use of MRI in evaluating patients with many different cardiac conditions is rapidly expanding. It is the method of choice for evaluating right ventricular (RV) function. Experience in pregnancy is relatively limited, but adverse effects on fetuses have not been demonstrated. Most indications for cardiac MRI can be fulfilled without the need for intravenous contrast agents such as gadolinium. Per the recent updated guidelines of the American College of Obstetricians and Gynecologists, the use of gadolinium contrast with MRI should be limited; it may be used as a contrast agent in pregnant women only if it significantly improves diagnostic performance and is expected to improve fetal or maternal outcome.

CHEST RADIOGRAPHY

As with most radiologic studies, chest radiography is not contraindicated during pregnancy, but one must be even more careful in judging whether the potential benefits justify the radiation exposure to the mother and the fetus. Appropriate lead shielding over the abdomen should always be used. It is estimated that a chest x-ray exposes the fetus to less than 10 uGray. An estimated exposure of more than 50,000 uGray (5 rad) is necessary to harm a fetus.

Changes on the chest radiography caused by normal pregnancy include prominent vascular markings, a horizontal position of the heart, a flattened heart border, and an elevated diaphragm. Small pleural effusions are common postpartum.

Chest radiography is most useful in evaluating patients for pulmonary congestion related to left ventricular (LV) dysfunction.

COMPUTED TOMOGRAPHY SCAN

As with other studies involving radiation, CT scans are not contraindicated in pregnancy, but of course, they should be ordered only after careful consideration that the diagnostic benefit outweighs the risk of radiation exposure to the mother and the fetus. The estimated radiation exposure to the fetus for a CT pulmonary angiogram is less than 500 uGray; as noted earlier, an estimated exposure of 50,000 uGray is needed to harm a fetus.

The most common reason to consider a CT scan in pregnancy is to diagnose a pulmonary embolus (by means of a pulmonary CT angiogram).

In addition to the radiation exposure, the mother will be exposed to 50 to 150 cc of iodinated radiocontrast. Iodinated radiocontrast can worsen renal function in patients with renal impairment, particularly in the setting of diabetes or dehydration.

ELECTROCARDIOGRAM

A number of changes to the electrocardiogram (ECG) occur during pregnancy. Sinus tachycardia (ST) is common, as are sinus rates of 90. The axis shifts leftward about 15 degrees because of elevation of the diaphragm. Nonspecific ST-segment changes and T-wave inversion also are common. Typically, T-wave inversion occurs in the inferior leads. Small q waves may develop. Premature atrial contractions (PACs) and premature ventricular contractions (PVCs) occur frequently.

The ECG is, of course, the immediate test of choice to evaluate suspected cardiac chest pain or acute myocardial infarction. It may be useful in diagnosing the cause of palpitations or arrhythmias if they are occurring at the time the ECG is performed. The ECG also is useful in diagnosing channelopathies, such as Brugada syndrome and the long QT syndromes. A 12-lead ECG should be performed in cases of syncope.

GRADED EXERCISE TESTING

Graded exercise testing can be performed safely in pregnancy. It may be ordered to investigate possible ischemic disease, assess functional capacity, or evaluate exercise-induced arrhythmias. A baseline ECG should be obtained before a graded exercise test is ordered. If the resting ST segments are depressed, the test is of little value in detecting ischemia. If safe, beta blockers should be held for 48 hours before the test to allow an adequate heart rate response. False-positive results may occur, so an abnormal ST-segment response to exercise should not be considered definitive evidence of coronary artery disease.

Contraindications to exercise testing during pregnancy include vaginal bleeding, preeclampsia, and placenta previa.

HOLTER MONITOR AND OTHER WEARABLE EVENT RECORDERS

Holter monitoring and other wearable event recorders can be used to document arrhythmias in the same manner as in nonpregnant patients. The expected findings in pregnancy are a relative sinus tachycardia and PACs and PVCs. Because of the short duration of monitoring, Holter monitors are of less value in patients with syncope; longer monitoring with an event recorder should be considered.

IMPLANTABLE LOOP RECORDERS

Implantable loop recorders are tiny monitoring devices that can be implanted subcutaneously under local anesthesia. They can be programmed to automatically detect arrhythmias and, through the use of remote telemetry, alert the patient's cardiologist. Implantable loop recorders have become invaluable in monitoring nonpregnant patients with infrequent or undiagnosed arrhythmias or syncope, and for monitoring arrhythmia burden and response to therapy. Their use in pregnant patients is limited, but they can be very helpful. We have used an implantable loop recorder to monitor a patient with idiopathic ventricular tachycardia of pregnancy. By carefully monitoring the number and duration of episodes and using alerts, we were able to avoid antiarrhythmic therapy. We also have found loop recorders valuable in monitoring patients with a prior history of atrial fibrillation who may need to receive anticoagulation during pregnancy if atrial fibrillation recurs.

STRESS ECHOCARDIOGRAPHY

Preexercise and immediate postexercise echocardiography may be performed in combination with a graded exercise test, providing an additional method to detect ischemia by identifying exercise-induced wall motion abnormalities. When the resting ECG results are abnormal, stress echocardiography may be useful, but data about its use in pregnancy are limited. Contraindications during pregnancy include vaginal bleeding, placenta previa, and preeclampsia.

DOBUTAMINE STRESS ECHOCARDIOGRAPHY

An echocardiogram is performed before and after a dobutamine infusion titrated to increase the heart rate to levels similar to those attained during an exercise stress test. Ischemic areas develop wall motion abnormalities, which can be detected on the postinfusion echocardiogram. This test has been used in pregnancy with no adverse effects reported, but experience is limited.

Dobutamine stress echocardiography has been evaluated as a tool for predicting recovery in patients with peripartum cardiomyopathy. Inotropic contractile reserve (contractility improves after dobutamine is administered) correlates with subsequent recovery of LV function and confers a benign prognosis.

RADIONUCLIDE INVESTIGATIONS

The ventilation/perfusion (V/Q) scan to diagnose pulmonary emboli is now used less frequently than a CT angiogram to diagnose pulmonary emboli, but it is sometimes a better option because radiographic contrast is not needed. As with other tests involving radiation exposure, the V/Q scan is not contraindicated during pregnancy as long as the radiation exposure to the mother and fetus is justified. The estimated radiation exposure to the fetus is 10 to 350 mGray; as noted earlier, an estimated exposure of 50,000 uGray is needed to harm a fetus.

TRANSESOPHAGEAL ECHOCARDIOGRAPHY

Transesophageal echocardiography is the most sensitive test for visualizing vegetations in patients with endocarditis. The main risk of performing this test during pregnancy is the risk of aspiration. TEE usually requires sedation, which increases that risk.

TRANSTHORACIC ECHOCARDIOGRAPHY AND DOPPLER

Transthoracic echocardiography and Doppler examinations are used commonly in pregnancy to evaluate LV function and valvular disease. Echocardiography is a useful diagnostic tool in suspected endocarditis. There are no known adverse effects on the mother or the fetus. Doppler evaluation of cardiac velocities can be used to estimate right-sided pressures.

Changes in the echocardiogram during pregnancy include increased LV and RV volumes and dilation of both atria (Table 19.1). An increase in depth of trabeculations mimicking noncompaction has also been described.

Echocardiography enables one to accurately evaluate LV function and to estimate LV ejection fractions. RV function is very difficult to assess by echocardiography; other methods, such as MRI, are more accurate.

Valvular structure can be evaluated well with echocardiography. Stenosis and regurgitation can be evaluated by Doppler. Doppler evaluates flow and velocities and thus is useful in estimating degrees of stenosis because velocities increase across areas of stenosis. In pregnancy, the increased cardiac output can sometimes lead to overestimating the degrees of stenosis. The precise severity of regurgitation can be difficult to quantitate by any method, including Doppler, but nonetheless, one can easily obtain reasonable estimates of severity.

Often, transthoracic echocardiography is the first imaging test ordered in evaluating a patient for suspected endocarditis. However, a negative transthoracic echocardiography result does not exclude the diagnosis;

TABLE 19.1 Average Dimensions of the Cardiac Chambers in Normal Women at Various Stages of Pregnancy					
	Nonpregnant	8–12 Weeks	20–24 Weeks	30–34 Weeks	36–40 Weeks
LVEDd (cm)	4.0	4.1	4.3	4.3	4.4
LA (cm)	2.8	3.0	3.2	3.3	4.0
RA (cm)	4.4	4.4	4.7	5.1	5.1
RVEDd (cm)	2.9	3.0	3.2	3.6	3.6

LA, Left atrium; *LVEDd*, left ventricular end-diastolic diameter; *RA*, right atrium; *RVEDd*, right ventricular end-diastolic diameter.o if needed, TEE is more sensitive and provides a definitive diagnosis.

Transthoracic echocardiograms are sometimes useful in diagnosing pulmonary embolus. Findings suggesting this diagnosis include RV and right atrial dilation and elevated right-sided pressures.

Transthoracic echocardiography also can be used to estimate pulmonary artery pressures by evaluating Doppler velocities of right-sided regurgitant velocities. However, it has been reported that transthoracic Doppler measurements often overestimate pulmonary pressures in pregnant patients.

In situations in which it is difficult to visualize the endocardium, echocardiography contrast is often used. Echocardiography contrast agents are microbubbles that act as echo enhancers via the same basic mechanism used to determine echo scattering in all other cases of diagnostic ultrasound: the backscattering echo intensity is proportional to the change in acoustic impedance between the blood and the gas-producing the bubbles. Perflutren (marketed as Definity and Optison) is the agent most commonly used in the United States. Although echocardiography contrast is not contraindicated in pregnancy, safety data are lacking, and it is considered pregnancy class B. Consequently, the prevailing wisdom is that it should be used in pregnancy only if essential.

BIBLIOGRAPHY

Electrocardiography
Bird SV. Electrocardiographic QRS axis, A wave and T-wave changes in 2nd and 3rd trimester of normal pregnancy. *J Clin Diagn Res*. 2014;8(9):17–21.
Venkatachalam M, Nagasireesha C. Electrocardiographic variations during the three trimesters of normal pregnancy. *Int J Res Med Sci*. 2015;3(9):2218–2222.
Wenger NK. The ECG in normal pregnancy. *Arch Intern Med*. 1982;142(6):1088–1089.

Holter Monitoring
Shotan A, Ostrzega E, Mehra A, Johnson JV, Elkayam U. Incidence of arrhythmias in normal pregnancy and relation to palpitations, dizziness, and syncope. *Am J Card*. 1997;79(8):1061–1064.
Stein PK, Hagley MT, Cole PL, Domitrovich PP, Kleiger RE, Rottman JN. Changes in 24-hour heart rate variability during normal pregnancy. *Am J Obstet Gynecol*. 1999;180(4):978–985.

Event Recorders
Cruz MO, Hibbard JU, Alexander T, Briller J. Ambulatory arrhythmia monitoring in pregnant patients with palpitations. *Am J Perinatol*. 2013;30:53–58.

Imaging
Colletti PM, Lee KH, Elkayam U. Cardiovascular imaging of the pregnant patient. *AJR Am J Roentgenology*. 2013;200:515–521.

Graded Exercise Test
O'Toole ML, Artal P. Clinical exercise testing during pregnancy and the postpartum period. *Clin Exerc Test*. 2002;32:273–281.
Wolfe LA, Walker RM, Bonen A, McGrath MJ. Effect of pregnancy and chronic exercise on respiratory responses to graded exercise. *J Appl Physiol*. 1985;76(5):1928–1936.

Dobutamine Stress Echocardiography
Dorbala S, Brozena S, Zeb S, et al. Risk stratification of women with peripartum cardiomyopathy at initial presentation: a dobutamine stress echocardiography study. *J Am Soc Echocardiogr*. 2005;18(1):45–48.

Transthoracic Echocardiography
Desai DK, Moodley J, Naidoo DP. Echocardiographic assessment of cardiovascular hemodynamics in normal pregnancy. *Obstet Gynecol*. 2000;104(1):20–29.
Gati S, Papadakis M, Papamichael ND, et al. Reversible de novo left ventricular trabeculations in pregnant women: implications for the diagnosis of left ventricular noncompaction in low-risk populations. *Circulation*. 2014;130(6):475–483.
Penning S, Robinson KD, Major CA, Garite TJ. A comparison of echocardiography and pulmonary artery catheterization for evaluation of pulmonary artery pressures in pregnant patients with suspected pulmonary hypertension. *Am J Obstet Gynecol*. 2001;184:1568–1570.
Poppas A, Shroff SG, Korcarz CE, et al. Serial assessment of the cardiovascular system in normal pregnancy role of arterial compliance and pulsatile afterload. *Circulation*. 1997;95:2407–2415.
Sadaniantz A, et al. Cardiovascular changes in pregnancy evaluated by two[dimensional and doppler echocardiography. *J Am Soc Echocardiogr*. 1992;5(3):253–358.

Transesophageal Echocardiography
Stoddard MF, Longaker RA, Vuocolo LM, Dawkins PR. Transesophageal echocardiography in the pregnant patient. *Am Heart J*. 1992;124(3):785–787.

Chest Radiography
Turner AF. The chest radiograph in pregnancy. *Clin Obstet Gynecol*. 1975;18(3):65–74.

Computed Tomography

Doshi SK, Oduko JM. Fetal radiation dose from CT pulmonary angiography in late pregnancy: a phantom study. Br J Radiol. 81(968):653–658.

McCollough CH, Schueler BA, Atwell TD, et al. Radiation exposure and pregnancy: when should we be concerned? *Radiographics*. 2007;27(4):909–917.

Winer-Muram HT, Boone JM, Brown HL, Jennings SG, Mabie WC, Lombardo GT. Pulmonary embolism in pregnant patients: fetal radiation dose with helical CT. *Radiology*. 2002;224(2):487–492.

Magnetic Resonance Imaging

Committee on Obstetric Practice. Committee Opinion No. 723: guidelines for diagnostic imaging during pregnancy and lactation. *Obstet Gynecol*. 2017;103(4):e210–e216.

De Wilde JP, Rivers AW, Price DL. A review of the current use of magnetic resonance imaging in pregnancy and safety implications for the fetus. *Prog Biophys Mol Biol*. 2005;87(2–3):335–353.

V/Q Scan

Abduljabbar HS, Marzouki KM, Zawawi TH, Khan AS. Pericardial effusion in normal pregnant women. *Acta Obstet Gynecol Scand*. 1991;70:667–672.

Campos O. Doppler echocardiography during pregnancy: physiologic and abnormal findings. *Echocardiography*. 1996;13:135–146.

Mashini IS, Albazzaz SJ, Fadel HE, et al. Serial noninvasive evaluation of cardiovascular hemodynamics during pregnancy. *Am J Obstet Gynecol*. 1972;113:47–59.

Robson SC, Hunter S, Moore M, Dunlop W. Haemodynamic changes during the puerperium: a Doppler and M-mode echocardiographic study. *Br J Obstet Gynaecol*. 1987;94:1028–1039.

Rubler S, Damani PM, Pinto ER. Cardiac size and performance during pregnancy estimated with echocardiography. *Am J Cardiol*. 1977;40:534–540.

Sadaniantz A, Kocheril AH, Emaus SP, Garber CE, Parisi AF. Cardiovascular changes in pregnancy evaluated by two-dimensional and Doppler echocardiography. *J Am Soc Echocardiogr*. 1992;5:253–258.

Verzed Z, Poler SM, GibonP Wlody D, Perez JE. Noninvasive detection of the morphologic and hemodynamic changes during normal pregnancy. *Clin Cardiol*. 1991;14:327–334.

20

Cardiac Intervention During Pregnancy

John H. Wilson, MD, FACC, FHRS

Myocardial infarction (MI) and severe myocardial ischemia requiring intervention during pregnancy are rare. MI complicates 1 in 20,000 to 1 in 30,000 pregnancies. The etiology is varied but is most often caused by coronary dissection. MI is more common during the third trimester, peripartum, and postpartum. Additionally, it is more common in multiparous women, and it usually involves the left anterior descending artery. The mortality rate is about 7% in recent series.

If necessary, cardiac catheterization and coronary intervention can be safely performed during pregnancy. Occasionally, valvuloplasty also may be required. Of obvious concern during these procedures is the potential for radiation exposure of the fetus.

The maximum permissible radiation dose for pregnant women has been set at 0.5 rad. If a dose greater than 25 rads is given, the potential for fetal harm is great; termination of the pregnancy should be considered. The effects of radiation depend on the stage of pregnancy. Exposure during the preimplantation period increases the risk of fetal reabsorption. A dose of 10 rad is estimated to increase this risk by up to 1%, which is negligible, considering that there is an unexposed risk of 25% to 50%. During organogenesis (3–8 weeks' gestation), radiation can cause serious abnormalities in fetuses. A dose of 10 rad increases this risk by about 1%, from a baseline of about 5% to 10%. A dose of 200 rad carries a virtual 100% risk. During the second and third trimesters, the risk to fetuses is primarily that of developing a childhood cancer later in life. It is estimated that a dose of 1 rad increases the risk by two cases per 100,000 exposed fetuses. Of course, because cardiac catheterization would expose the pregnant woman's abdomen to an estimated 0.15 rad if it were unshielded, lead shielding should be used.

If cardiac catheterization is performed after 25 weeks' gestation, when the fetal thyroid gland is active, the fetus also will be at increased risk of fetal hypothyroidism from exposure to iodinated contrast.

If there is a choice, the optimal time to perform an interventional procedure involving radiation is in the fourth month. At that time, organogenesis is complete, the fetal thyroid is not active, and the uterus is still small and relatively far away from the chest.

The supine position can be problematic during interventional procedures in pregnancy. The gravid uterus may obstruct the vena cava, decreasing venous blood return, resulting in hypotension. Also, it is possible for venous obstruction caused by the uterus to inhibit the passage of catheters.

As in other settings, the best management of an acute MI during pregnancy is urgent cardiac catheterization and coronary intervention if appropriate. Percutaneous angioplasty with stenting is the treatment of choice for coronary dissection.

If severe mitral stenosis presents during pregnancy, balloon valvuloplasty may need to be considered. There have been more than 250 cases, all successful, reported. No maternal deaths and only two fetal deaths have been reported.

During balloon inflation, transient maternal hypotension and fetal bradycardia often occur, but these conditions seem to have no long-lasting consequences.

Nine cases of aortic balloon valvuloplasty during pregnancy also have been reported. Very rarely, balloon valvuloplasty for pulmonic stenosis may be needed in pregnancy; it can be performed safely for this condition as well.

BIBLIOGRAPHY

Presbitero P, Prever SB, Brusca A. Interventional cardiology in pregnancy. *Eur Heart J.* 1996;17:182–188.

Shaw P, Duncan A, Vouyouka A, Ozsvath K. Radiation exposure and pregnancy. *J Vasc Surg.* 2011;53(1 suppl):28S–34S.

Timins JK. Radiation during pregnancy. *N Engl J Med.* 2001;98:29–33.

Aortic Balloon Valvuloplasty

Banning AP, Pearson JF, Hall RJ. Role of balloon dilation of the aortic valve in pregnant patients with severe aortic stenosis. *Br Heart J.* 1993;70:544–545.

Bhargrava H, Agarwal R, Yadav R, Bahl VK, Manchanda SC. Percutaneous balloon aortic valvuloplasty during pregnancy: use of the Inoue balloon and the physiologic antegrade approach. *Cathet Cardiovasc Diagn.* 1998;45:422–425.

Myerson SG, Mitchell AR, Ormerod OJ, Banning AP. What is the role of balloon dilation for severe aortic stenosis during pregnancy? *J Heart Valve Dis.* 2005;14:47–150.

Radford DJ, Walters DL. Balloon aortic valvotomy in pregnancy. *Aust N Z Obstet Gynaecol.* 2004;44:377–379.

Mitral Balloon Valvuloplasty

Ben Farhat M, Gamra H, Betbout F, et al. Percutaneous balloon mitral commissurotomy during pregnancy. *Heart.* 1997;77:564–567.

Cheng TO. Percutaneous Inoue balloon valvuloplasty is the procedure of choice for symptomatic mitral stenosis in pregnant women. *Catheter Cardiovasc Interv.* 2000;50(4):413–417.

de Souza JA, Martinez Jr EE, Ambrose JA, et al. Percutaneous balloon mitral valvuloplasty in comparison with open commissurotomy for mitral stenosis during pregnancy. *J Am Coll Cardiol.* 2000;37:900–903.

Esteves CA, Ramos AI, Braga SL, Harrison JK, Sousa JE. Effectiveness of percutaneous balloon mitral valvotomy during pregnancy. *Am J Cardiol.* 1991;68:930–934.

Fawzy ME, Kinsara AJ, Stefadouros M, et al. Long-term outcome of mitral balloon valvotomy in pregnant women. *J Heart Valve Dis.* 2001;10(2):153–157.

Iung B, Cormier B, Elias J, et al. Usefulness of percutaneous balloon commissurotomy for mitral stenosis during pregnancy. *Am J Cardiol.* 1994;73:398 400.

Routray SN, Mishra TK, Swain S, Patnaik UK, Behera M. Balloon mitral valvuloplasty during pregnancy. *Int J Gynecol Obstet.* 2004;85:18–23.

21

Cardiac Surgery During Pregnancy

J. Michael Smith, MD, FACS, FACC

Although rarely necessary in the age of percutaneous intervention, cardiac surgery can be carried out during pregnancy with reasonable safety for the mother; her risk is about the same as if she were not pregnant. The fetal death rate is reported at 9% to 15%.

The earliest reports of cardiac surgery in pregnancy date back to 1952, when several surgical groups reported successful results with mitral commissurotomy. Hypothermia and cardiopulmonary arrest were first used in a pregnant patient in 1957 to perform a pulmonary valvotomy, and cardiopulmonary bypass (CBP) was first used in 1959 to perform a pulmonary commissurotomy and repair an atrial septal defect. After these early reports were published, experience grew rapidly, and by 1986, Bernal and Miralles, reviewing 45 cases, reported that the maternal mortality rate was the same as that for nonpregnant patients. Fetal mortality rate in that series was reported at 9.5%.

Maternal risk depends heavily on preoperative functional state. Four major risk factors have been identified: (1) a history of transient ischemic attack, stroke, or arrhythmia; (2) a New York Heart Association (NYHA) heart failure classification of 3 or 4 before onset of pregnancy; (3) left heart obstruction (e.g., mitral valve area <2 cm^2, aortic valve area <1.5 cm^2, peak left outflow gradient >30 mm Hg); and (4) a left ventricular (LV) ejection fraction less than 40%. In patients with a NYHA heart failure classification of 3 or 4 before pregnancy, maternal morbidity and mortality rates may each be as high as 50%. The incidence of maternal complications increases proportionately with the number of risk factors identified. When more than one risk factor is present, the incidence of maternal complications increases to nearly 75%. Other risk factors for the mother include the type of surgery, reoperation, and the use of vasoactive drugs.

Risk factors for the fetus include maternal age, maternal heart failure classification, reoperation, emergency surgery, type of myocardial protection, and anoxic time. The use of CPB increases perioperative risk to the fetus. CBP has been noted to stimulate uterine contractions in some patients, putting the baby at risk for premature delivery. Hypothermia appears to negatively affect the exchange of oxygen through the placenta, and it is suspected that during the warming phase, fetal arrhythmias are induced. Obviously, cardiopulmonary blood flow during surgery should be maintained at a higher level for a pregnant woman to compensate for the additional blood flow to the fetus. However, precisely how much is uncertain and difficult to estimate. Current recommendations include maintaining the pump flow rate over 2.5 L/min/m^2 and perfusion pressure over 70 mm Hg, maintaining the hematocrit greater than 28%, using pulsatile flow, using a-stat pH management, and using normothermic perfusion if feasible. Factors adversely affecting the fetus during CBP include nonpulsatile flow, inadequate perfusion pressure, inadequate pump flow, emboli to the placenta, and the release of renin and catecholamines. The fetal risk may be reduced by optimizing maternal oxygen-carrying capacity and uterine blood flow. Pomini et al. have pointed out that hyperkalemic cardioplegia, if not recovered, can reach the placenta and the fetus, and they recommend its avoidance.

Fetal heart rate monitoring during surgery should be carried out after 18 weeks of gestation. However, circumstances such as maternal obesity and fetal size and position may make this difficult. Fetal bradycardia during surgery may be caused by hypotension, hypoxia, uterine contractions, decreased uterine blood flow, maternal malpositioning, medications, and hypothermia. Persistent fetal bradycardia requires treatment; options include optimizing maternal oxygenation, increasing cardiopulmonary blood flow, correcting acid–base disorders, titrating anesthesia level, and correcting hypoglycemia.

Monitoring of uterine contraction is recommended. If uterine contractions are increasing, expanding maternal intravascular volume is recommended, and tocolytics may be considered. If it is necessary to assess LV preload, transesophageal echocardiography may be useful. Rarely, insertion of a pulmonary artery (PA) catheter may be considered. Indications for a PA catheter in the parturient undergoing cardiac surgery include severe mitral or aortic valvular stenosis, NYHA class 3 or 4 heart disease, intraoperative or intrapartum cardiac failure, refractory pulmonary edema, acute respiratory distress syndrome, and preeclampsia with refractory oliguria or pulmonary edema. However, very little data are available on the PA catheter complication rate in pregnant women, and in other situations, its use is declining because of the associated risks.

Transvaginal ultrasound for monitoring the fetus may be considered.

The decision to perform cardiac surgery in a pregnant woman is obviously complex and should be made using a team approach, involving a team composed of (at a minimum) a cardiac surgeon, cardiologist, obstetrician, and neonatologist. Factors that must be considered include whether or not an intervention is preferable to continued medical management, alternative percutaneous options, optimal timing of the surgery to minimize risk to the mother and maximize the likelihood of fetal survival, and whether or not the surgery can be done using normothermia. If surgery can be done without hypothermia, fetal outcomes are better. In one study, the use of normothermia reduced the fetal mortality rate from 24% to 0%; the maternal mortality did not change.

If the gestational age is over 20 weeks, the operation should be performed in the left lateral recumbent position to avoid compression of the vena cava by the uterus.

Fetal bradycardia during CBP has been reported and seems to be prevented by the use of hypertonic glucose in the perfusate.

If a pregnant woman needs cardiac surgery and the fetus is viable (beyond 28–30 weeks' gestation), the best option is to deliver the fetus and then perform the cardiac surgery. If surgery cannot be delayed until the fetus is viable, the next best option is to perform it early in the second trimester. Surgery in the first trimester is associated with a higher risk of abortion, and surgery later in pregnancy is associated with a higher risk of premature labor.

Because of the relatively high fetal mortality rate associated with cardiac operations, it may at times be in the best interest of the mother and baby for the obstetrician to perform a cesarean delivery before the cardiac operation. In such situations, using general anesthesia is preferred. The mother should be hydrated adequately, avoiding systemic vasodilation and pulmonary vasoconstriction. It is also essential to adequately replace blood loss and maintain adequate ventricular filling pressures. However, it is also important to recognize that a cesarean delivery may impact the subsequent cardiac surgery. For example, uterine atony because of the smooth muscle relaxation by inhaled anesthetics can be a major cause of bleeding after heparinization for CBP. Thus, it may be useful to avoid volatile anesthetics during cesarean delivery if the patient is to be subsequently heparinized for CBP.

BIBLIOGRAPHY

Aggarwal N, Suri V, Goyal A, Malhotra S, Manoj R, Dhaliwal RS. Closed mitral valvotomy in pregnancy and labour. *Int J Gynecol Obstet.* 2005;88:118–121.

Anderson Fineron FW. Aortic dissection in pregnancy-induced changes in the vessel wall and bicuspid valve in pathogenesis. *Br J Obstet Gynaecol.* 1994;101:1085–1088.

Armoni RT, Arnoni AS, Bonini RC, et al. Risk factors associated with cardiac surgery during pregnancy. *Ann Thorac Surg.* 2003;76:1605–1608.

Barth WH. Cardiac surgery in pregnancy. *Clin Obstet Gynecol.* 2009;52:630–646.

Becker RM. Intracardiac surgery in pregnant women. *Ann Thorac Surg.* 1983;36:453–458.

Ben-Ami M, Battino S, Rosenfeld T, Marin G, Shalev E. Aortic valve replacement during pregnancy: A case report and review of the literature. *Acta Obstet Gynaecol Scand.* 1990;69:651–653.

Bernal JM, Mirales PJ. Cardiac surgery with cardiopulmonary bypass during pregnancy. *Obstet Gynecol Surv.* 1986;41 (1):1–6.

Chambers CE, Clark SL. Cardiac surgery during pregnancy. *Clin Obstet Gynecol.* 1994;37:316–323.

Chandrasekhar S, Cook CR, Collard CD. Cardiac surgery in the parturient. *Anesth Analg.* 2009;108:777–785.

Dufour P, Berard J, Vinatier D, et al. Pregnancy after myocardial infarction and a coronary artery bypass graft. *Arch Gynecol Obstet.* 1997;259:209–213.

Garry D, Leikin E, Fleisher AG, Tejani N. Acute myocardial infarction in pregnancy with subsequent medical and surgical management. *Obstet Gynecol.* 1996;87:802–804.

Lamb MP, Ross K, Johnstone AM, Manners JM. Fetal heart monitoring during open heart surgery. Two case reports. *Br J Obstet Gynecol.* 1981;88:669–674.

Parry AJ, Westaby S. Cardiopulmonary bypass during pregnancy. *Ann Thorac Surg.* 1996;61:1865–1869.

Pavankumar P, Venugopal P, Kaul U, et al. Closed mitral valvotomy during pregnancy. A 20-year experience. *Scand J Thor Cardiovasc Surg.* 1988;22(1):11–15.

Peiper PG, Hoendermis ES, Drijver YN. Cardiac surgery and percutaneous intervention in pregnant women with heart disease. *Neth Heart J.* 2012;20:125–128.

Pomini F, Mercogliano D, Cavalletti C, Caruso A, Pomini P. Cardiopulmonary bypass in pregnancy. *Ann Thorac Surg.* 1996;61:259–268.

Pomini F, Mercogliano D, Cavalletti C, Caruso A, Pomini P. Cardiopulmonary bypass in pregnancy. *Ann Thorac Surg.* 1996;61:259–268.

Weiss BM, von Segesser LK, Alon E, Seifert B, Turina MI. Outcome of cardiovascular surgery and pregnancy: a systemic review of the period 1984-1996. *Am J Obstet Gynecol.* 1998;179:1643–1653.

Westaby S, Parry AJ, Forfar JC. Reoperation for prosthetic valve endocarditis in the third trimester of pregnancy. *Ann Thorac Surg.* 1992;53:263–265.

Zeebregts CJ, Schepens MA, Hameeteman TM, Morshuis WJ. de la Rivière AB. Acute aortic dissection complicating pregnancy. *Ann Thorac Surg.* 1997;64:1345–1348.

22

Cardiac Arrest in Pregnancy

John H. Wilson, MD, FACC, FHRS

This chapter presents an overview of cardiac arrest in pregnancy and discusses the measures that can be taken to address it: advanced cardiac life support (ACLS), perimortem cesarean section (PMCS), and postarrest targeted temperature management.

OVERVIEW: CARDIAC ARREST IN PREGNANCY

The Centers for Disease Control and Prevention reports the incidence of cardiac arrest in pregnancy at 17 in 100,000 live births. Other sources estimate the incidence from 1 in 12,000 to 1 in 16,500 admissions for delivery. The most common causes of arrest vary by country. In the United States, commonly reported causes include hemorrhage, heart failure, amniotic fluid embolism, sepsis, and anesthesia complications. The overall survival rate of maternal cardiac arrest is usually reported at around 50%, although this varies by cause of arrest. Whereas anaphylaxis, anesthesia complications, eclampsia, and heart failure have relatively high survival rates, trauma, venous thromboembolism, sepsis, and amniotic fluid embolism have lower rates of survival.

ADVANCED CARDIAC LIFE SUPPORT

In cases of cardiac arrest, standard ACLS algorithms are used, with several modifications to account for the unique state of pregnancy. In 2015, the American Heart Association (AHA) published a Scientific Statement on Cardiac Arrest in Pregnancy, which addressed these needed modifications. Significantly, there are many essential parts of ACLS that do not change. No change is recommended in hand position, rate, or depth of chest compressions, defibrillation, or dose and frequency of medication administration. The AHA recommends the creation of a maternal code blue team, which includes representatives from obstetrics and neonatology (if available) in addition to the standard members of an adult code blue team. Airway management should be performed by the most experienced practitioner given the increased incidence of difficult airway during pregnancy.

From 20 weeks of gestation onward, the enlarging uterus can cause aortocaval compression, which may compromise venous return to the heart and reduce cardiac output in the supine position. For this reason, during resuscitation, leftward uterine displacement is recommended to minimize compression of the inferior vena cava. Displacement may be accomplished by tilting or placing a wedge under the patient to the left by 30 degrees or by having someone pull or push the abdomen up and to the left (manual displacement). Manual displacement is generally preferable over a wedge or tilt because it minimizes interruptions in chest compressions. Because cardiac output is increased during pregnancy, chest compressions have been reported to produce a cardiac output that is only 30% of the normal blood flow during pregnancy.

PERIMORTEM CESAREAN SECTION

Evacuation of the uterus, or PMCS, should be considered in maternal cardiac arrest with a gestational age greater than 20 weeks. If resuscitation efforts have not been successful after 4 minutes, preparations should be made for the procedure, with the goal of delivering the baby by 5 minutes after arrest. PMCS removes aortocaval compression, resulting in a 60% to 80% increase in cardiac output, thereby increasing the likelihood of maternal survival. As a secondary aim, chances of neonatal survival may increase also. In a review of all maternal cardiac arrests in the Netherlands, 8 of 12 women undergoing PMCS regained cardiac output afterward, confirming the hypothesis that it is beneficial in maternal resuscitation. Even so, the mortality rate remains high. In the Dutch study, only 15% of mothers survived. Among the 12 women in whom PMCS was performed, there were 2 maternal survivors (17%). Among the 43 women in whom no PMCS was performed, there were 6 maternal survivors (14%). A 2012 literature review found a maternal benefit in 31% of cases. Significantly, whereas the average time to PMCS in surviving mothers was 10 minutes, the average time to PMCS in nonsurviving mothers was 22.6 minutes.

Clearly, timeliness of the intervention is extremely important to both maternal and fetal outcome. Time-consuming activities, such as fetal monitoring and transportation to the operating room, reduce the chances of maternal and neonatal survival and should be avoided. In cases of prematurity or intrauterine fetal death, obstetricians should not refrain from performing PMCS to facilitate maternal resuscitation.

POSTARREST TARGETED TEMPERATURE MANAGEMENT

Postarrest targeted temperature management (hypothermia) can be used in pregnant women. Survival of both the mother and fetus has been reported after hypothermia. Continuous fetal monitoring is recommended for the duration of hypothermia and rewarming. If PMCS is performed during the cardiac arrest, targeted temperature management should be managed with the same standards as used in a nonpregnant patient.

BIBLIOGRAPHY

Campbell TA, Sanson TG. Cardiac arrest and pregnancy. *J Emerg Trauma Shock*. 2009;2(1):34–42.

Dijkman A, et al. Cardiac arrest in pregnancy: increasing use of perimortem caesarean section due to emergency skills training? *BJOG*. 2010;117(3):282–287.

Einav S, Kaufman N, Sela HY. Maternal cardiac arrest and perimortem caesarean delivery: evidence or expert-based? *Resuscitation*. 2012;83(10):1191–1200.

Jeejeebhoy FM, Zelop CM, Lipman S, et al. Cardiac arrest in pregnancy: a scientific statement from the American Heart Association. *Circulation*. 2015 1747-1743.

Lavecchia M, Haim AA. Cardiopulmonary resuscitation of pregnant women in the emergency department. *Resuscitation*. 2015;91:104–197.

Lee RV, Rodgers BD, White LM, Harvey RC. Cardiopulmonary resuscitation of pregnant women. *Am J Med*. 1986;81:311–318.

Mallampalli A, Guy E. Cardiac arrest in pregnancy and somatic support after brain death. *Crit Care Med*. 2005;33 (10 suppl):S325–S331.

Mhyre JM, Tsen LC, Einav S, Kuklina EV, Leffert LR, Bateman BT. Cardiac arrest during hospitalization for delivery in the United States, 1998-2011. *Anesthesiology*. 2014;120(4):810–818.

Morris S, Stacey M. Resuscitation in pregnancy. *BMJ*. 2003;327:1277–1279.

Peters CW, Layon AJ, Edwards RK. Cardiac arrest during pregnancy. *J Clin Anesth*. 2006;50:27–28.

Rittenberger JC, Kelly E, Jang D, Greer K, Heffner A. Successful outcome utilizing hypothermia after cardiac arrest in pregnancy: a case report. *Crit Care Med*. 2008;36(4):1354–1356.

Whitty JE. Maternal cardiac arrest in pregnancy. *Clin Obstet Gynecol*. 2002;45:377–392.

23

The Maternal Cardiac Care Team and the Maternal Cardiac Care Facility

William T. Schnettler, MD, FACOG

NEED FOR MATERNAL CARDIAC CARE PROGRAMS

A maternal cardiac care program requires the marshalling of significant resources, particularly in terms of personnel, space, and equipment. To justify these resources, we advise estimating the number of patients in need of such a program. An estimated 0.2% to 4.0% of pregnancies are complicated by cardiovascular disease. In our program, the prevalence of cardiac disease in pregnant women was 2.0%. In 0.7% of pregnancies, the cardiac disease was severe enough to require involvement of the cardiology service.

The expected event rate for fetal and maternal events in women with a spectrum of cardiac disease can be extrapolated from a 2001 Canadian study of 562 such women. The overall event rate was 13%. The fetal-neonatal death rate was 2%, and the rate of preterm labor was 10%. There were three cardiac deaths and two noncardiac deaths (suicide and amniotic fluid embolus).

PATIENT MANAGEMENT TEAM

The first step in establishing a maternal cardiac care program is to form a patient management team. At a minimum, the team should include an obstetrician with experience in high-risk pregnancy, a cardiologist (ideally with adult congenital experience), an obstetric anesthesiologist, and a neonatologist. We find it useful to include a pulmonologist, a cardiothoracic surgeon, and

an electrophysiologist. Either the cardiologist or pulmonologist should have expertise in managing patients with pulmonary hypertension. At times, other specialists, such as nephrologists, infectious disease experts, and psychiatrists, may be needed as well. In addition, obstetric, cardiac, and intensive care unit nurses are essential members of the patient management team. Chapter 26 includes detailed information on relevant nursing considerations. Finally, hospital administrative support is crucial to the success of a maternal cardiac care program.

PATIENT MANAGEMENT PROCESS

When we enroll a patient in our maternal cardiac care program, we assess both the maternal and fetal risk (see Chapter 24) and develop an individualized care plan for regular follow-up during pregnancy as well as for delivery and postpartum care. (Chapter 25 presents a sample care plan.) The plan includes timing, mode, and location of delivery; cardiac rhythm; hemodynamic monitoring during and after delivery; and the location for postpartum care. The delivery and postpartum care plans developed by the team are compiled by the labor and delivery charge nurse and placed in a resource binder on the unit that is available to the staff whenever the patient is admitted.

Decisions about where to monitor and care for patients before and after delivery are made on a case-by-case basis, taking into consideration the nursing competencies needed for safe care. Potential needs include central venous intravenous access, titration of vasoactive

137

and inotropic infusions, cardiac rhythm monitoring, mechanical ventilation, arterial pressure monitoring, and pulmonary artery pressure and cardiac output monitoring. The use of a ventricular assist device necessitates placing the patient in the cardiovascular intensive care unit (CVICU). Remote telemetry, the use of a bedside monitor in the labor and delivery unit, and management in the adult CVICU all have been used, including placing bassinettes in an adjoining CVICU room and obstetric nursing staff working side by side with CVICU nurses to care for the mothers and their babies.

Monthly, the patient management team attends a formal conference at which we discuss each enrolled patient, review their progress, and (if needed) update or modify their care plan. A coordinator ensures that the appropriate personnel are available for the meeting and that test results and clinical information are available on each patient. We also have in place a mechanism for calling a full or partial team meeting as needed to address urgent situations.

In addition to the formal conferences, patients are seen in clinic by several of the physicians. On the initial visit, patients are seen by an obstetrician, the appropriate cardiologist, and a cardiac anesthesiologist. We schedule 40 minutes for the initial visit. Each patient's clinical situation dictates the scheduling and frequency of subsequent visits and the team members who will attend (i.e., the persons best suited to deal with the clinical situation).

MATERNAL CARDIAC CARE FACILITIES

Maternal cardiac care facilities must meet the needs of both patients and the team that cares for them. Because patients typically are seen by two or three physicians at clinic visits, facilities amenable to this are necessary. Equipment for obstetric and cardiac evaluation, such as electrocardiogram machines, should be on hand. We believe it is critical to have rapid availability of both fetal and maternal echocardiography available on site, as well as a radiology department capable of providing computed tomography angiograms and magnetic resonance imaging scanning. Access to a dialysis unit and nephrology consultation may be needed as well.

For delivery, there should be at least two delivery rooms with capabilities for cardiac monitoring. Postpartum rooms with telemetry monitoring also are needed. In addition, it is imperative that the facilities include several intensive care beds with staff familiar with obstetric and postpartum care.

BIBLIOGRAPHY

Siu SC, Sermer M, Colman JM, et al. Prospective multicenter study of pregnancy outcomes in women with heart disease. *Circulation.* 2001;104:515–521.

24

Assessment of Maternal Risk and Assessment of Fetal Risk

William T. Schnettler, MD, FACOG

Assessing the risk posed by pregnancy, for both the mother and baby, is an essential component of caring for women with cardiac disease who are considering becoming pregnant as well as for those who are already pregnant. This chapter explores both maternal and fetal risk assessment.

MATERNAL RISK ASSESSMENT

Whenever possible, risk stratification should occur antenatally, and for women at high risk, who have a lesion that can be corrected, intervention should be performed before they become pregnant. There are many factors known to increase risk in cardiac patients who become pregnant, and ideally, patients have been apprised of the risks before they conceive. Regardless of whether this has been discussed previously with patients, we perform a risk stratification at intake.

A number of factors should be considered when attempting to estimate the maternal risk from pregnancy. For each patient, we determine both a New York Heart Association (NYHA) functional class and a World Health Organization (WHO) score.

The NYHA functional class is a classification system based on symptoms. The categories are as follows:
I. No limitation of physical activity. Ordinary physical activity does not cause undue fatigue, palpitation, or dyspnea (shortness of breath).
II. Slight limitation of physical activity. Comfortable at rest. Ordinary physical activity results in fatigue, palpitation, or dyspnea.
III. Marked limitation of physical activity. Comfortable at rest. Less than ordinary activity causes fatigue, palpitation, or dyspnea.

IV. Unable to carry on any physical activity without discomfort. Symptoms of heart failure at rest. If any physical activity is undertaken, discomfort increases.

In and of itself, the NYHA system is not designed for risk stratification, but patients with a worse functional class generally have a worse outcome with regard to both morbidity and mortality regardless of the degree of left ventricular (LV) function.

The WHO risk score can be used to place patients into one of four risk categories based on their cardiac diagnosis. The risk score is outlined in Table 24.1.

WHO I

Pulmonic stenosis
Patent ductus arteriosus
Mitral valve prolapse
Repaired simple defects such as atrial septal defect (ASD) or ventricular septal defect (VSD)
Premature atrial or premature ventricular beats

WHO II

Unoperated ASD or VSD
Repaired tetralogy of Fallot
Most arrhythmias

WHO II or III

Mild left ventricular dysfunction (LVD)
Hypertrophic cardiomyopathy
Marfan syndrome without aortic dilation
Repaired coarctation

WHO III

Mechanical valve
Systemic right ventricle

TABLE 24.1   World Health Organization Scoring System for Assessing Risk of Adverse Cardiac Events in Pregnancy

Score	Description
I	No increase in maternal mortality; small or no increase in morbidity
II	Small increase in maternal mortality or moderate increase in morbidity
III	Significantly increased risk of maternal mortality or severe morbidity
IV	High risk of maternal mortality; pregnancy contraindicated

Fontan circulation
Cyanotic disease unrepaired
Other complex congenital diseases
Aortic dilation (40–45 mm) with Marfan syndrome
Aortic dilation (45–50 mm) with a bicuspid valve

WHO IV

Pulmonary hypertension
Severe LV dysfunction (ejection fraction <30% or NYHA class III or IV)
Previous peripartum cardiomyopathy
Severe mitral stenosis
Severe aortic stenosis
Marfan syndrome with an aortic dilation >45 mm
Aortic dilation >50 mm with a bicuspid aortic valve
Native severe coarctation

The Cardiac Disease in Pregnancy (CARPREG) study was a Canadian study of 599 pregnancies in women with various cardiac conditions; it prospectively evaluated the incidence of maternal cardiac and fetal adverse events. Researchers identified four risk factors for maternal cardiac events: NYHA class of III or IV or cyanosis, LV dysfunction, left-sided obstruction, and prior cardiac event or arrhythmia. The presence of one of these risk factors was associated with a 5% risk of a primary cardiac event (pulmonary edema, sustained symptomatic arrhythmias, stroke, cardiac arrest, or death). If two factors were present, the associated risk rose to 27%, and if three were present, it climbed to 75%. Of the three maternal deaths in the study, all were associated with at least two risk factors.

Other risk factors include moderate to severe aortic or mitral regurgitation, right ventricular dysfunction, severe pulmonic regurgitation, use of cardiac medications before pregnancy, and smoking. The cardiac condition that poses the greatest risk to maternal (and fetal) health is the presence of pulmonary hypertension. A history of aortic coarctation puts mothers at risk for pregnancy-induced hypertension.

In addition to cardiac risk factors, other patient characteristics may complicate pregnancy and should be taken into account as well. These include maternal age, diabetes, and a host of other factors.

We have found it useful to perform, at the initial clinic visit, a systematic evaluation of each patient's risk—both overall and for specific complications. The patient's course is then reviewed by the team on a monthly basis. A formal written plan is then made for each patient (see Chapter 25).

FETAL RISK ASSESSMENT

A number of predictors of adverse fetal outcome have been determined. These include
Cyanosis
Maternal NYHA class III or IV
Smoking
Multiple gestation
Use of oral anticoagulants
A mechanical prosthetic valve

The CARPREG study identified six predictors of an adverse neonatal event: NYHA class of III or IV, cyanosis at baseline prenatal visit, maternal left heart obstruction, smoking during pregnancy, multiple gestations, and the use of anticoagulants during pregnancy. If none of these risk factors were present, the fetal or neonatal death rate was 2%. With one risk factor, it increased to 4%.

It is thought that the adverse effects of left heart obstruction are mediated by inadequate placental perfusion, which results in fetal growth restriction, premature delivery, or both.

In the CARPREG study, 20% of the pregnancies resulted in some type of adverse fetal event, the most common being premature birth in 18% (105 of 599) and small-for-gestational-age birth weight in 4% (22 of 599). Of the preterm births, 59% (62 of 105) were caused by premature labor. Fetal death occurred in 1% (8 of 599) and neonatal death in 1% (7 of 599). Preterm labor occurred in 10% of the mothers.

A study from a single center in India evaluated the maternal and fetal risk for various conditions in the developing world. Researchers performed a retrospective study on 207 pregnancies complicated by maternal cardiac disease. In this study, 88% of the women had rheumatic valvular disease, and only 12% had congenital heart disease. Neonatal adverse events were intrauterine growth restriction, prematurity, stillbirth or neonatal death, low birth weight, and presence of birth defects. Fetal complications were observed in 20% of pregnancies. There were two stillbirths (1%). There were no neonatal deaths. Thirty-nine percent of the babies delivered preterm, and 35% had a birth weight less than 2.5 kg even though they delivered at greater than 37 weeks' gestation. Nine (4%) of the babies had an Apgar score of 5 or less, but none had a severe grade of hypoxic encephalopathy or intraventricular hemorrhage, and none required mechanical ventilation. Congenital anomalies were detected in five babies (2%) and cardiac anomalies in two (1%). Both babies with congenital heart disease—one with tetralogy of Fallot and one with an atrial septal defect—were born to mothers with rheumatic heart disease. The babies of mothers in NYHA class III or IV had a worse outcome than those in class I or II. The overall complication rate was 29% in the mothers in class III or IV versus 19% in the mothers in class I or II. The rates of preterm birth (31% vs 21%) and low birth weight (57% vs 36%) also were higher in women in class III or IV compared to those in class I or II.

Babies of mothers with congenital heart disease are at risk for congenital heart disease, too, with the risk depending on their mother's condition (see Chapter 5). Children with fathers or siblings with congenital heart disease are also at risk but less so than if their mother is affected (2%–3% vs 5% risk).

In addition to cardiac conditions, a number of other maternal medical conditions have been shown to increase fetal mortality. An estimated 10% of stillbirths are related to a maternal medical condition, including maternal age, hypertension, obesity, diabetes, hyper- and hypothyroidism, systemic lupus, chronic renal disease, and cholestasis of pregnancy. Each of these is discussed next.

Maternal Age

Increased maternal age has shown to increase the risk of fetal death. In a large Canadian study involving 94,000 births, mothers older than the age of 35 years were found to have a doubling of fetal mortality rate compared with younger women. The mechanisms

behind this risk are uncertain but probably involve the increased incidence of comorbidities, such as hypertension, in older women. A very young age during pregnancy is also associated with an increased risk of fetal demise. In a Swedish study, the odds ratios for neonatal mortality and postnatal mortality, relative to maternal age, were as follows.

Neonatal Mortality

Mother age 13 to 15 years: 2.7
Mother age 16 to 17 years: 1.4
Mother age 18 to 19 years: no increase

Postnatal Mortality

Mother age 13 to 15 years: 2.6
Mother age 16 to 17 years: 2.0
Mother age 18 to 19 years: 1.7

The high rate of very preterm birth seems to explain most of the mortality.

Hypertension

Hypertension is estimated to be responsible for up to 4% to 9% of fetal deaths. In 1995, estimates for fetal death rates for the various forms of hypertension associated with pregnancy were 25 in 1000 for chronic hypertension, 9 in 1000 for pregnancy-induced hypertension, and 18 in 1000 for preeclampsia. In more recent years, most fetal deaths appear to be the result of preeclampsia. The risk to fetuses in women who develop HELLP syndrome is higher (estimated at 50 in 1000 in 1999). HELLP syndrome is an acronym for **h**emolysis, **e**levated **l**iver enzymes, and **l**ow **p**latelet count, which are the major manifestations of the syndrome. In most cases, the mechanism is thought to be impaired placental function. In patients with all types of hypertension, the risk of placental abruption, uteroplacental insufficiency, and placental infarction are all increased.

Obesity

Obesity, defined as a body mass index (BMI) over $30/kg/m^2$, is present in 20% to 40% of women of childbearing age. It is associated with a number of complications during pregnancy, including an increased risk of fetal death. For a BMI over $30/kg/m^2$, the risk of fetal mortality rises by a factor of 2.8. The increased risk of hypertension and diabetes explains some of the increased risk, but other mechanisms have not been defined.

Diabetes Mellitus

Diabetes mellitus is thought to affect as many as 2% to 5% of all pregnancies. Diabetes doubles the risk of fetal death. Studies have shown that tight control of blood sugars can reduce this risk to almost that of women without diabetes. The majority of stillbirths occur in the third trimester in patients with poor glycemic control. The complications of diabetes include an increased risk of preeclampsia, macrosomia, polyhydramnios, and intrauterine growth restriction.

Thyroid Disorders

Thyroid disorders have been associated with an increased fetal mortality rates. In the past, studies showed that hyperthyroidism increased fetal risk, but most recent studies show little increased risk if the patients are recognized and treated. Fetal deaths in the earlier studies occurred mainly in women first diagnosed in pregnancy, suggesting that the risk was higher in women with uncontrolled thyrotoxicosis. Hypothyroidism roughly doubles the risk of fetal death.

Systemic Lupus Erythematosus

Although it complicates less than 1% of pregnancies, systemic lupus erythematosus (SLE) in the mother carries a risk of fetal death. The stillbirth rate has been reported at about 40 in 1000. The risk is lower in women in whom the disease is quiescent. Antepartum fetal deaths in patients with SLE may have multiple causes. Some are related to preeclampsia, which complicates up to 30% of pregnancies in women with SLE. Furthermore, women with SLE also may have renal disease related to nephritis, which puts their babies at risk. The presence of the lupus anticoagulant, found in up to 30% of pregnant women with the disease, is also a predictor of fetal death. Fetal grow restriction has been reported in up to 30% of pregnancies in women with SLE. Pregnancy also seems to induce flares in the disease, reported in up to 50% of cases. SLE also may put fetuses at risk for congenital heart block. It has been reported in about 5% of pregnancies and is caused by the transmission of anti-Rho and anti-SSB (anti-La). In cases of fetal atrioventricular block with profound fetal bradycardia, hydrops fetalis and intrauterine death can occur.

Chronic Renal Disease

Chronic renal disease is also well known to increase fetal mortality rates. Numerous studies show that the worse the impairment, the greater the fetal mortality rate. Estimates from 2002 indicate a risk of fetal mortality of

15 in 1000 for women with creatinine less than 1.4 mg/dl
100 in 1000 for women with moderate impairment; creatinine of 1.4 mg/dl to 2.8 mg/dl
200 in 1000 for women with severe impairment; creatine over 2.8 mg/dl

Patients on dialysis have a very high risk of fetal demise. Spontaneous abortion or stillbirth occurs in as many as 80% of pregnancies. The outlook improves significantly in patients who have a successful renal transplant.

Comorbidities associated with chronic renal failure, such as anemia, diabetes, and hypertension, further increase the risk. The risk of preeclampsia is increased in women with hypertension of any cause, but the combination of renal impairment and hypertension is particularly ominous, with a risk of preeclampsia as high as 80%. Correcting severe anemia has been reported to lower fetal risk.

Cholestasis of Pregnancy

Cholestasis of pregnancy is another condition that increases the risk of fetal demise. Studies from the early 1990s indicated a significant risk of up to 25 to 30 deaths per 1000 pregnancies. More recent studies involving antenatal testing and timed intervention have reduced this risk to near baseline.

A careful drug history should be taken for each patient because not only drugs taken illicitly but also those given for maternal medical conditions may increase fetal morbidity or the risk of morbidity and mortality. In certain situations, drug doses may need to be limited or substitutes found. For example, the seizure drug valproate has been found to increase the fetal risk to a greater extent than alternatives.

BIBLIOGRAPHY

Anderson AN. Moderate alcohol intake during pregnancy and risk of fetal death. *Int J Epidemiol*. 2012;41(2): 405–413.

Benhadi N, Wiersinga WM, Reitsma JB, Vrijkotte TG, Bonsel GJ. Higher maternal TSH levels in pregnancy are associated with increased risk for miscarriage, fetal or neonatal death. *Eur J Endocrinol*. 2009;160(6):985–991.

Bhatla N, Lal S, Behera G, et al. Cardiac disease in pregnancy. *Int J Gynecol Obstet*. 2003;82:153–159.

Chu SY, Kim SY, Lau J, et al. Maternal obesity and risk of stillbirth: a metaanalysis. *Am J Obstet Gynecol*. 2007;197 (3):223–228.

Connaughton JF, Reeser D, Schut J, Finnegan LP. Perinatal addiction: outcome and management. *Am J Obstet Gynecol.* 1977;129(6):679–686.

Dekker GA, de Vries JI, Doelitzsch PM, et al. Underlying disorders associated with severe early onset pre-eclampsia. *Am J Obstet Gynecol.* 1995;173:1042–1048.

Duckitt K, Harrington D. Risk factors for pre-eclampsia at antenatal booking: systematic review of controlled studies. *BMJ.* 2005;330(7491):565.

Fajemirokun-Odudeyi O, Sinha C, Tutty S, et al. Pregnancy outcome in women who use opiates. *Eur J Obstet Gynecol Reprod Biol.* 2006;126(2):170–175.

Fretts RC, Schmittdiel J, McLean FH, Usher RH, Goldman MB. Increased maternal age and the risk of fetal death. *N Engl J Med.* 1995;333:953–957.

Meador KJ, Baker GA, Finnell RH, et al. In utero antiepileptic drug exposure fetal death and malformations. *Neurology.* 2006;67(3):407–412.

Meyer MB, Tonascia JA. Maternal smoking, pregnancy complications, and perinatal mortality. *Am J Obstet Gynecol.* 1977;125:494–502.

Olausson PO, Cnattingius S, Haglund B. Teenage pregnancies and risk of late fetal death and infant mortality. *Br J Obstet Gynaecol.* 1999;106(2):116–121.

Ryan L, Ehrlich S, Finnegan L. Cocaine abuse in pregnancy: effects on the fetus and newborn. *Neurotoxicol Teratol.* 1987;9(4):295–299.

Simpson LL. Maternal medical disease: risk of antepartum fetal death. *Semin Perinatol.* 2002;26:42–50.

Siu SC, Sermer M, Colman JM, et al. Prospective multicenter study of pregnancy outcomes in women with heart disease. *Circulation.* 2001;104 515-421.

Zuckerman B, Frank DA, Hingson R, et al. Effects of maternal marijuana and cocaine use on fetal growth. *N Engl J Med.* 1989;320:762–768.

25

The Patient Management Plan

William T. Schnettler, MD, FACOG

After completion of the maternal and fetal risk assessment, the cardio-obstetric team's premier role lies in providing a clear, concise, and accessible pregnancy management plan. This plan incorporates the input from all team members representing the various subspecialties involved. This multispecialty involvement provides "representation" for the myriad provider types that will encounter the woman throughout pregnancy and can alleviate concerns regarding decisions having been made without a specific specialty's involvement. Our program's approach entails the creation of a one- to two-page clinical synopsis document that is posted very clearly and easily accessible within the electronic medical record. Within this document, all of the pertinent medical history, provider contact information, major clinical concerns, and suggested recommendations for all phases of pregnancy care are presented in a concise tabular format as depicted in Fig. 25.1.

Patient Name:			Date of Consultation:	
Date of Birth:			EDD:	
Referring Provider:			GA:	

Team Members	Phone #		Diagnoses	
ACHD Cardiologist:				
Adult Cardiologist:				
Perinatologist:				
Anesthesiologist:				
1° MFM:				
1° Cardiologist:			Last Echo:	

Further History				
Gravidity/Parity:			Medications:	
Pertinent Medical/Surgical History:				
Allergies:				
Current				

Fig. 25.1 Cont'd

Symptoms:		
NYHA Class:		
WHO Score:		

Major Risks and Considerations	Likelihood	Time at Highest Risk
•		
•		

Recommendations

Phase of Care	Scenario	Plan
Antepartum	Activity:	
	Dietary and Fluid Restrictions:	
	VTE Prophylaxis:	
	Maternal Monitoring:	
	Fetal Monitoring:	
	Delivery Timing:	
	Preterm Labor:	
	Preeclampsia:	
Labor	Mode of Delivery:	

Fig. 25.1 Cont'd

	Anesthesia:	
	Maternal Positioning:	
	Invasive Monitoring:	
	Noninvasive Monitoring:	
	Telemetry:	
	Fluids:	
	SBE Prophylaxis:	
	VTE Prophylaxis:	
	Pushing/Valsalva:	
	Pitocin Safety:	
	Cesarean Delivery Considerations:	
	Hemorrhage Considerations:	
	Special Equipment:	
Postpartum	Location:	
	Pain Control:	
	Fluids:	
	Diet:	
	Monitoring:	
	Medications:	
	VTE Prophylaxis:	
	Breastfeeding:	
	Postpartum Follow-up:	
	Contraception:	

Fig. 25.1 A sample cardiac patient pregnancy management plan. *ACHD, Adult Congenital Heart Disease*; *Echo*, echocardiogram; *EDD*, estimated date of delivery; *GA*, gestational age; *MFM, Maternal-Fetal Medicine* ; *NYHA*, New York Heart Association; *SBE*, subacute bacterial endocarditis; *VTE*, venous thromboembolism, *WHO*, World Health Organization. (Adapted from: An affiliation between TriHealth and Cincinnati Children's Hospital Medical Center.)

26

Nursing Considerations

Jane C. Whalen, DNP, RN, CCRN, CCNS-CSC

Caring for pregnant women with heart disease is a complex undertaking for several reasons. First, neither nurses nor physicians have typically trained, or practiced, in both the obstetric and adult critical care settings. Second, the care of pregnant women always involves two patients, a seldom-experienced situation for nonobstetric nurses and physicians. Third, management of the critically ill obstetric patient requires care directed not only at the patient's pathophysiology but also care and attention paid to the family and psychosocial issues that invariably occur.

This chapter provides an overview of nursing standards in general and then discusses the multidisciplinary care and nursing education that are critical components of our maternal cardiac care program.

OVERVIEW OF NURSING STANDARDS

Standards of nursing practice apply to both the obstetric and critical care nurses' practice (Table 26.1).

MULTIDISCIPLINARY CARE

Pregnant women with cardiac disease benefit from multidisciplinary coordination of care during pregnancy, delivery, and the postpartum period. The combined expertise of perinatal and adult critical care nurses is an important element of planning and delivering this care.

Prepregnancy consultation is an important element in the care of women with heart disease who are planning to become pregnant. The maternal-fetal medicine nurse practitioner is an essential member of the maternal cardiac care team, helping women with heart disease enter pregnancy as healthy as possible. If necessary, the nurse practitioner will coordinate subspecialty consultation, for example, with cardiac surgery, interventional cardiology, or electrophysiology.

After a pregnant woman has been enrolled in our maternal cardiac care program, monthly care planning conferences are held to discuss each patient. These conferences include advanced practice nurses (APRNs) from maternal-fetal medicine and adult cardiac surgery, nursing leaders from perinatal services and the cardiovascular intensive care unit (CVICU), and physician specialists from maternal-fetal medicine, obstetric anesthesia, adult congenital heart disease, general cardiology, electrophysiology, critical care, cardiac surgery, and cardiac anesthesia. The maternal-fetal medicine APRN sees patients in the multidisciplinary clinic with the physicians and communicates with patients between visits.

At the planning conferences, the team formulates a plan for regular follow-up during pregnancy and for delivery. The plan includes the timing, mode, and location of delivery; cardiac rhythm; hemodynamic monitoring during and after delivery; and the location for postpartum care. The delivery and postpartum care plans developed by the team are compiled by the labor and delivery (L&D) charge nurse and placed in a resource binder on the unit, available to the staff whenever the patient is admitted.

Decisions about where to monitor and care for patients before and after delivery are made on a case-by-case basis, taking into consideration the nursing competencies needed for safe care. Potential needs include central venous intravenous access, titration of vasoactive and inotropic infusions, cardiac rhythm monitoring, mechanical ventilation, arterial pressure monitoring, and pulmonary artery pressure and cardiac output monitoring. The use of a ventricular assist device necessitates placing the patient in the CVICU. Remote telemetry, the use of a bedside monitor in the L&D unit, and management in the adult CVICU all have been used, including placing bassinettes in an adjoining CVICU room and obstetric nursing staff working side by side with CVICU nurses to care for the mothers and their babies.

TABLE 26.1	Standards of nursing practice[a]	
Step	Standard	Description
1	Assessment	The nurse collects comprehensive data about the patient's health.
2	Diagnosis	The nurse analyzes assessment data to determine nursing diagnoses and conditions.
3	Outcome identification	The nurse identifies expected patient outcomes.
4	Planning	The nurse develops a plan of care that includes strategies and alternatives to achieve outcomes.
5	Implementation	The nurse implements the interventions identified in the plan.
6	Evaluation	The nurse evaluates the process and progress toward attainment of outcomes.

[a]Standards of professional performance include attainment of knowledge and competence, evidence-based practice, effective communication, collaboration, ethical practice, and participation in quality evaluation and improvement (American Association of Critical-Care Nurses, 2015; American Nurses Association, 2010).

Postpartum planning for contraception is included in the care delivered by the maternal-fetal medicine APRN. For some patients, a future pregnancy should be avoided. Consideration is given for long-acting reversible contraception, including intrauterine devices and implantable devices, which are 99% effective in preventing pregnancy; because they do not contain estrogen, these devices also are safe in the setting of a hypercoagulable state.

NURSING EDUCATION

At our center, a team composed of APRNs, nursing leadership, and an adult congenital heart disease program manager identified educational resources for the nursing staff who care for pregnant women with underlying cardiac issues. Our goal is to develop a core group of obstetric and adult critical care nurses who can deliver this specialized care and serve as resources for their colleagues. The American Heart Association's Advanced Cardiac Life Support course is required for L&D charge nurses and adult critical care nurses, with a goal to increase the percentage of L&D staff who have completed the course. Educational videos about perinatal care, cardiovascular assessment, and congenital heart disease are available through the organization's online learning library. An introductory set of these videos have been identified as core content for the orientation of staff nurses to the care of these patients. The videos discuss

- Normal labor and vaginal birth
- Obstetric hemorrhage
- Cardiovascular assessment
- Hypertensive crisis during pregnancy

In addition, we have identified other useful learning tools for our nurses. An introduction to adult congenital heart disease is available on the Adult Congenital Heart Disease Learning Center website (http://achd-learningcenter.org). The organization's online learning library includes disease- and condition-specific videos that can be reviewed before the admission of a patient. Additional educational videos can be found on the Cincinnati Children's Hospital website (http://blog.cincinnatichildrens.org/rare-and-complex-conditions/heart-conditions/animated-videos-illustrate-congenital-heart-defects) and the Khan Academy website (https://www.khanacademy.org/science/health-and-medicine/circulatory-system-diseases).

Our institutions (Cincinnati's Good Samaritan Hospital and Cincinnati Children's Hospital Medical Center) are currently developing multidisciplinary critical care obstetric workshops, with a commitment to include nursing care and considerations for this challenging patient population.

BIBLIOGRAPHY

American Association of Critical-Care Nurses. *AACN scope and standards for acute and critical care nursing practice.* http://www.aacn.org/wd/practice/docs/scope-and-standards-acute-critical-care-2015.pdf

American Nurses Association. *Nursing: scope and standards of practice* (2nd ed.). Nursebooks.org.

IIIBelfort ME, Saade G, Foley MR, Phelan JP, Dildy GI, eds. *Critical Care Obstetrics.* 5th ed. : Wiley-Blackwell; 2010.

Harris RC, Fries MH, Boyle A, et al. Multidisciplinary management of pregnancy in complex congenital heart disease: a model for coordination of care. *Congenit Heart Dis*. 2014;9:E204–E211.

Lindley KJ, Conner SN, Cahill AG. Adult congenital heart disease in pregnancy. *Obstet Gynecol Surv*. 2015;70(6): 397–407.

Pieper PG. The pregnant woman with heart disease: management of pregnancy and delivery. *Neth Heart J*. 2012;20(1): 33–37.

27

Pregnancy After Heart Transplant

John H. Wilson, MD, FACC, FHRS

Just over three decades have passed since the first successful pregnancy in a heart transplant patient, and in the intervening years, several hundred additional cases have been reported. Looking ahead, it is likely that many more heart and heart–lung transplant patients will choose to conceive. Given this reality, we present an overview of pregnancy after heart transplant and discuss the need for prepregnancy counseling, the risks associated with pregnancy in this patient population, pregnancy management, contraception, and pregnancy in heart–lung transplant patients.

OVERVIEW

The first reported pregnancy in a cardiac transplant patient was in 1988, and since then several hundred cases have been reported. Successful pregnancies also have been reported in patients with other organ transplants, including heart–lung transplants. It is expected that in years to come, more women who have had heart transplants will wish to conceive. About 25% of female heart transplant recipients are of childbearing age, and adult survival rate is greater than 90% with a survival half-life of 13 years.

The International Society for Heart and Lung Transplantation (ISHLT) and the American Society of Transplantation recommend the following: pregnancy should not be attempted before 1 year after heart transplant. Heart transplant recipients considering pregnancy should have had no rejection in the past year, adequate and stable graft function, and stably dosed immunosuppression. The ISHLT recommends baseline assessment

of graft function before conception with an electrocardiography, echocardiography, and coronary angiography if not performed within the previous 6 months; right heart catheterization and biopsy may also be considered. Relative contraindications include rejection within the first posttransplant year, history of peripartum cardiomyopathy, advanced maternal age, comorbid factors, and nonadherence to medical care. The ISHLT guidelines also recommend that preconception counseling be offered to both the patient and her partner. The impact on the child of the mother's expected longevity and potential for prolonged hospitalization should be considered as well.

PREPREGNANCY COUNSELING

Prepregnancy counseling is vital and should include an assessment of both maternal and fetal risks. The risks to the mother include the possibility of acute graft rejection, graft dysfunction, and infection. In some centers, potential fathers are asked to undergo human leukocyte antigen typing to see if he shares antigens with the donor heart, in which case the risk of rejection is higher.

The cause of the heart condition leading to the woman's need for a heart transplant also should be considered. A woman with congenital heart disease has an approximately 10% risk of having a baby with congenital heart disease. It is unknown if women with a pretransplant diagnosis of peripartum cardiomyopathy are at increased risk of recurrence with subsequent pregnancies. However, most factors likely to contribute to peripartum cardiomyopathy are thought to be extrinsic to

151

the heart, and it is feared that the transplanted heart is in jeopardy if a woman becomes pregnant again. Women with unrecovered peripartum cardiomyopathy have a 50% recurrence rate and 20% mortality rate with subsequent pregnancies. The outlook may be the same in women with a transplanted heart.

PREGNANCY RISKS

A meta-analysis of 385 pregnancies in 272 cardiothoracic transplant recipients included 220 pregnancies in 140 heart transplant patients. The average maternal age of these 140 patients was 28 years, and the average transplant-to-pregnancy interval was 81.4 months. There were no maternal deaths during pregnancy. Two women died in the first postpartum year. Graft rejection occurred during pregnancy in 9.4% of patients. Data from the National Transplant Registry indicate a higher rejection rate of 21%, with 40% of those cases being mild and requiring no treatment. When pregnancy has occurred, the risk of spontaneous abortion is 15% to 20%.

Maternal Risks

The most frequent maternal complication is hypertension. Hypertension occurred in 38% of women reported in a study from Quebec. Hypertension increases the risk of preterm delivery and fetal growth impairment.

Infections are the second most common maternal complication, occurring in up to 11% of pregnancies in posttransplant patients. We recommend urine cultures to monitor for asymptomatic urinary tract infections.

Preeclampsia was reported in 15% of patients in the Quebec study. Diabetes was reported in 15% as well. Several centers have reported increasing creatinine levels in posttransplant patients during pregnancy. In nontransplanted women, creatinine levels usually decrease during pregnancy.

Both pregnancy and posttransplant status are risks for thromboemboli. The impact of both conditions together is unknown but warrants a high level of concern.

Hyperemesis gravidarum may be of particular concern in transplant patients who may be unable to take required immunosuppressive drugs.

After the woman has delivered, she may be at risk for infections transmitted from the infant. Particular care may be needed during activities such as changing diapers. Live vaccines given to the child may also present a risk.

Long-term mortality rates for women with heart transplant who become pregnant do not seem worse than in posttransplant women who do not become pregnant, as reported from Quebec.

Fetal Risks

A significant risk to fetuses is the possible teratogenic effects of immunosuppressive medication. There is also an increased risk of fetal growth retardation, low birth weight, and prematurity.

The children of transplant mothers appear to have an increased risk of diabetes and cardiovascular disease later in life.

Additional concerns are the higher-than-usual risk of maternal death and the prolonged absence of the mother because of hospitalization.

PREGNANCY MANAGEMENT

Natural conception is preferred, but successful in vitro fertilization has been reported in heart transplant patients. Vaginal delivery and epidural anesthesia, as in a nontransplant patient, are generally recommended.

Immunosuppression

The most commonly used immunosuppressive agents for heart transplant patients are calcineurin inhibitors (cyclosporine, tacrolimus), azathioprine, proliferation signal inhibitors, and corticosteroids, used as single agents or in various combinations. Calcineurin inhibitors, such as cyclosporine and tacrolimus, can be continued during pregnancy but are associated with a risk of hypertension. Proliferation signal inhibitors, such as everolimus and sirolimus, may be continued. Everolimus may impair wound healing and should be discontinued if cesarean section is planned. Corticosteroids can be continued during pregnancy. Antimetabolites such as azathioprine should be discontinued. Antimetabolites including mycophenolate mofetil, mycophenolic acid (MPA), and azathioprine are placed in US Food and Drug Administration category D, and their use in pregnancy is discouraged by the ISHLT.

Because of the many metabolic and hemodynamic changes induced by pregnancy, dosing of immunosuppressive drugs may require frequent adjustment.

Most patients are prescribed statin therapy after transplantation to lower cholesterol, improve the 1-year survival rate, and reduce the likelihood of cardiac allograft vasculopathy. Statins are contraindicated in pregnancy and must be stopped when pregnancy is confirmed.

Immediately after delivery, dramatic fluid shifts occur. These changes should be well tolerated in women with normal function of their transplanted heart but are of concern if cardiac function is suppressed.

Breastfeeding

In the past, breastfeeding has been discouraged due to the unknown effects of immunosuppressive therapy on the infant. However, breastfeeding is not contraindicated. No adverse effects have been reported in women receiving corticosteroids. Azathioprine and proliferation signal inhibitors are also thought to be relatively low risk. At present, as reported by Watson et al. (2019), current literature review cautions against breastfeeding while taking MPA products, sirolimus, everolimus, and belatacept because of the scarcity of clinical data.

Breastfeeding is relatively contraindicated in women with a history of peripartum cardiomyopathy because there are concerns that elevated prolactin levels may have adverse cardiac effects in these women.

CONTRACEPTION

Because more than half of pregnancies in the posttransplant population are unplanned, appropriate contraceptive counseling is important and should be started before transplant assessment. Uncomplicated heart transplant recipients can be safely offered a wide range of contraceptives, including the combined oral contraceptive pill, the progesterone-only pill, the depot progesterone implant, and the copper or progesterone intrauterine device. For those women with a history of graft failure, rejection, or cardiac allograft vasculopathy, combined hormonal contraceptive methods, such as the combined oral contraceptive pill, contraceptive patch, or vaginal ring, are not considered safe.

PREGNANCY AFTER HEART/LUNG TRANSPLANT

The potential risks to the mother and baby, as well as the medical care during and after pregnancy, are virtually identical in women after heart transplant and those with a combined heart–lung transplant. One difference that has been reported is a slightly lower risk of graft rejection during pregnancy in the heart transplant patients versus the heart–lung transplant patients (9.4% vs 11%).

BIBLIOGRAPHY

Abdalla M, Mancini DM. Management of pregnancy in the post-cardiac transplant patient. *Semin Perinatol.* 2014;38 (5):318–325.

Abukhalil IE, Govind A. Pregnancy in heart transplant recipients. Case report and review. *Clin Exp Obstet Gynecol.* 1995;22(2):111–114.

Acuna S, Zaffar N, Dong S, Ross H, D'Souza R. Pregnancy outcomes in women with cardiothoracic transplants: a systematic review and meta-analysis. *J Heart Lung Transpl.* 2020;39:93–102.

Ahner R, Kiss H, Zuckermann A. [Pregnancy and spontaneous delivery 13 months after heart transplantation]. *Geburtshilfe Frauenheilkd.* 1993;53(8):574–576.

Bhagra CJ, Bhagra SK, Donado A, et al. Pregnancy in cardiac transplant recipients. *Clin Transpl.* 2016;30:1059–1065.

Branch KR, Wagoner LE, McGrory CH, et al. Risks of subsequent pregnancies on mother and newborn in female heart transplant recipients. *J Heart Lung Transpl.* 1998; 17:698.

Camann WR, Jarcho JA, Mintz KJ, Greene MF. Uncomplicated vaginal delivery 14 months after cardiac transplantation. *Am Heart J.* 1991;121(3 pt 1):939–941.

Constantinescu S, Pai A, Coscia LA, Davison JM, Moritz MJ, Armenti VT. Breast-feeding after transplantation. *Best Pract Res Clin Obstet Gynaecol.* 2014;28:1163–1173.

Coscia LA, Constantinescu S, Moritz MJ, et al. Report from the National Transplantation Pregnancy Registry (NTPR): outcomes of pregnancy after transplantation. *Clin Transpl.* 2010:65–85.

Cowan SW, Coscia LC, Philips L, et al. Pregnancy outcomes in female heart and heart-lung transplant recipients. *Transpl Proc.* 2002;34(5):1855–1856.

Cowan SW, Davison JM, Doria C, Moritz MJ, Armenti VT. Pregnancy after cardiac transplantation. *Cardiol Clin.* 2012;30(3):441–452.

Dagher O, Alami Laroussi N, Carrier M, et al. Pregnancy after heart transplantation: a well-thought-out decision? The Quebec provincial experience—a multi-centre cohort study. *Transpl Int.* 2018;31(9):943–1054.

DeFilippis EM, Haythe J, Farr MA, Kobashigawa J, Kittleson MM. Practice patterns surrounding pregnancy after heart transplantation. *Circ Heart Fail.* 2020;13(4): e006811.

Key TC, Resnik R, Dittrich HC, Reisner LS. Successful pregnancy after cardiac transplantation. *Am J Obstet Gynecol.* 1989;160(2):367–371.

Khush KK, Cherikh WS, Chambers DC, et al. The International Thoracic Organ Transplant Registry of the International Society for Heart and Lung Transplantation: thirty-sixth adult heart transplantation report—2019; focus theme: donor and recipient size match. *J Heart Lung Transpl.* 2019;38:1056–1066.

Kim KM, Sukhani R, Slogoff S, Tomich PG. Central hemodynamic changes associated with pregnancy in a long-term cardiac transplant recipient. *Am J Obstet Gynecol.* 1996;174(5):1651–1653.

Liljestrand J, Lindstrom B. Childbirth after post-partum cardiac insufficiency treated with cardiac transplant. *Acta Obstet Gynecol Scand.* 1993;72(5):406–408.

Löwenstein BR, Vain NW, Perrone SV, et al. Successful pregnancy and vaginal delivery after heart transplantation. *Am J Obstet Gynecol.* 1988;158:589.

Maroo A, Chahine J. Contraceptive strategies in women with heart failure or with cardiac transplantation. *Curr Heart Fail Rep.* 2018;15:161–170.

Morini A, Spina V, Aleandri V, Cantonetti G, Lambiasi A, Papalia U. Pregnancy after heart transplant: update and case report. *Hum Reprod.* 1998;13(3):749–757.

O'Boyle PJ, Smith JD, Danskine AJ, Lyster HS, Burke MM, Banner NR. De novo HLA sensitization and antibody mediated rejection following pregnancy in a heart transplant recipient. *Am J Transpl.* 2010;10:180–183.

Ohler L, Coscia LA, McGrory CH, Moritz MJ, Armenti VT. 273: National Transplantation Pregnancy Registry (NTPR): pregnancy outcomes in female thoracic transplant recipients. *J Heart Lung Transpl.* 2007;26(suppl):S158.

Rajapreyar IN, Sinkey RG, Joly JM, et al. Management of reproductive health after cardiac transplantation. *J Matern Fetal Neonatal Med.* 2021;34(9):1469–1478.

Scott JR, Wagoner LE, Olsen SL, Taylor DO, Renlund DG. Pregnancy in heart transplant recipients: management and outcome. *Obstet Gynecol.* 1993;82(3):324–327.

Stribling WK, Flattery MP, Smallfield MC, Kimball P, Shah KB. Pregnancy-related allograft rejection following heart transplant. *Prog Transpl.* 2015;25:35–38.

Tran DD, Kobashigawa J. A review of the management of pregnancy after cardiac transplantation. *Clin Transpl.* 2015;31:151–161.

Troché V, Ville Y, Fernandez H. Pregnancy after heart or heart-lung transplantation: a series of 10 pregnancies. *Br J Obstet Gynaecol.* 1998;105:454.

Wagoner LE, Taylor DO, Olsen SL, et al. Immunosuppressive therapy, management, and outcome of heart transplant recipients during pregnancy. *J Heart Lung Transpl.* 1993;12:993.

Watson WD, Bhagra SK, Bhagra CJ. Pregnancy in heart transplant recipients—current perspectives. *Transpl Res Risk Manage.* 2019;11:29–38.

Wu DW, Wilt J, Restaino S. Pregnancy after thoracic organ transplantation. *Semin Perinatol.* 2007;31:354.

28

COVID-19 in Pregnant Patients

William T. Schnettler, MD, FACOG

Over the past few years, the coronavirus disease 2019 (COVID-19) pandemic has affected nearly every aspect of human life, including, of course, health care. For expecting women, the normal anxiety of pregnancy has been heightened by concern over the possible effects of the coronavirus on them and their babies. That concern is magnified in women with cardiac conditions or issues. This chapter provides an overview of COVID-19, summarizes its signs and symptoms, presents our COVID-19 protocol, and discusses considerations for delivery in pregnant women who have tested positive for the disease.

OVERVIEW

COVID-19 is an infectious disease caused by severe acute respiratory syndrome coronavirus 2 (SARS-CoV-2). SARS-CoV-2 is an enveloped virus with a nonsegmented, single-stranded, positive-sense RNA genome. The virus can use the angiotensin-converting enzyme (ACE) 2 for cell entry. ACE 2 is an integral-membrane protein that serves many important physiologic functions. The spike protein of the virus can bind to ACE 2. After ligand binding, the virus enters cells via receptor-mediated endocytosis. ACE 2 is highly expressed in alveolar cells, providing the entry site for the virus. ACE 2 also serves a role in lung protection; therefore, viral binding to this receptor deregulates a protective pathway, leading to viral pathogenicity. There are some concerns that ACE inhibitors may exacerbate SARS 2 infection by upregulating the number of ACE 2 receptors, but this seems to be a theoretical risk only, and some studies have shown that patients taking ACE inhibitors or angiotensin receptor blockers (ARBs) actually do better than patients not taking these drugs.

Close to 90% of patients with COVID-19 severe enough to warrant hospitalization have comorbidities. Risk factors include hypertension, obesity, chronic lung disease, diabetes, and cardiovascular disease. Physiological and mechanical changes in pregnancy increase a woman's susceptibility to infections in general, particularly when her cardiorespiratory system is affected, and may encourage rapid progression to respiratory failure. Furthermore, the pregnancy bias toward T-helper 2 (Th2) system dominance, which protects the fetus, leaves the mother vulnerable to viral infections, which are more effectively contained by the Th1 system.

COVID-19 affects multiple organ systems, including the cardiovascular system. It has been associated with multiple direct and indirect cardiovascular complications, including myocardial injury, myocarditis, arrhythmias, and venous thromboembolism. Other organs or organ systems affected by COVID-19 include the lungs, gastrointestinal tract, liver, and skin. Lung injury in severe cases usually presents as SARS. Acute kidney injury may range from azotemia to acute tubular necrosis and usually presents at 2 to 3 weeks postinfection. Patients may manifest hematuria or proteinuria. Thrombotic complications are also common. Venous thromboembolic disease occurs in up to 31% of critically ill COVID patients. Disseminated intravascular coagulation can also occur. Anticoagulation with low-molecular-weight heparin is advised. Neurologic impacts caused by COVID-19, such as encephalopathy, agitation, confusion, and corticospinal tract signs, also have been reported.

Myocardial injury as assessed by increased troponin has been reported in many patients with severe COVID-19. Higher cardiac troponin levels are associated with a worse prognosis and death. Severe cardiac injury manifested by changes on electrocardiography and echocardiography is seen in 7% to 17% of patients. Patients with COVID-19 may present as though they are having an acute ST-elevation myocardial infarction. Chinese studies have reported arrhythmias in about 17% of patients with COVID-19, but at this time, data about specific arrhythmia types are not available. Congestive heart failure has been reported in up to 23% of hospitalized patients with COVID. It is unclear whether this is caused by an exacerbation of an underlying cardiac dysfunction or a new cardiomyopathy. There are concerns that COVID-19 may cause long-term impairment of left ventricular dysfunction in some patients.

SIGNS AND SYMPTOMS

Symptoms of severe COVID-19 pneumonia include fevers to 101°F; worsening shortness of breath, prohibiting the ability to complete full sentences; and persistent nonproductive cough. Initial vital sign assessment often identifies significant tachypnea (respiratory rate of >24 breaths/min), mild tachycardia (heart rate >100 beats/min), low normal blood pressure (mean arterial pressure in the low 70s mm Hg), and mild hypoxia (SpO_2 <95%). Physical examination findings are often notable for rhonchi and egophony throughout all lung fields. Chest radiography, computed tomography (CT) pulmonary angiogram, and lung ultrasound assessments are helpful. Specifically, chest radiography often identifies bilateral diffuse pulmonary infiltrates, and chest CT often identifies bilateral airspace disease characterized by ground-glass appearance with peripheral consolidations compatible with viral pneumonia. Lung ultrasound likely demonstrates bilateral pleural thickening and nodularity of the visceral pleura. Horizontal A-lines representing normal aerated lung are absent and replaced by multiple B-lines, pleural nodularity, thickening, and an overall "white lung" appearance with focal areas of consolidation.

Laboratory analysis often identifies an abnormal $PaO_2{:}FiO_2$ ratio less than 200 (suggesting evidence of acute respiratory distress syndrome (ARDS), leukopenia, lymphopenia, thrombocytopenia, elevated transaminases, and a mildly elevated procalcitonin.

MANAGEMENT

The maternal physiologic adaptations to pregnancy not only leave the woman more vulnerable to cell-mediated viral infections such as COVID-19 but also more susceptible to rapid cardiopulmonary decompensation because of the reduced cardiac and pulmonary reserves. Because such physiologic alterations may not be at the forefront in the minds of the intensive care team members, they must be emphasized by obstetric providers. These providers can serve in a "quarterback" role because they lead the implementation of an algorithmic approach (Figures 28.1 and 28.2). Such an approach entails input from multiple disciplines and establishes a framework for optimal team dynamics using daily "huddles" or other open means of direct communication. Planning should occur before any patient's arrival, allowing the myriad team members to agree on the optimal imaging investigations, laboratory studies, COVID testing, fetal assessment, and admission locations for these women. The team's safety also must remain a priority, ensuring appropriate and adequate personal protective equipment, staffing (nurse-to-patient ratio), facilities equipped to minimize exposure, and mobile or handheld equipment with easy cleaning and disinfecting. An example of our management algorithm is included in Table 28.1 for reference, but it should be individualized to one's own institution.

DELIVERY CONSIDERATIONS

One of the most difficult yet critical aspects of the management approach is the delivery determination. The physiologic adaptations to labor, delivery, and the immediate postpartum period include maximization of the maternal cardiac output; autotransfusion of up to 500 mL of blood volume back into the intravascular compartment; a catecholaminergic surge; release of inflammatory mediators within the endothelium; and considerable fluid shifts between the interstitial, intracellular, and intravascular compartments. In the setting of severe systemic infection, these physiologic adaptations may exacerbate the dysregulated inflammatory cascade, leading to a higher potential for endothelial dysfunction, pulmonary edema, myocardial edema, and cardiac dysfunction. Thus, for patients with severe COVID-19, the decision to proceed toward delivery should be deferred until maternal cardiopulmonary stability can be achieved. There are three exceptions to this rule of thumb: the pregnancy has reached full term, the fetal status is nonreassuring, or the maternal status is so dire that evacuation of the uterus is likely to improve cardiopulmonary function. We recommend

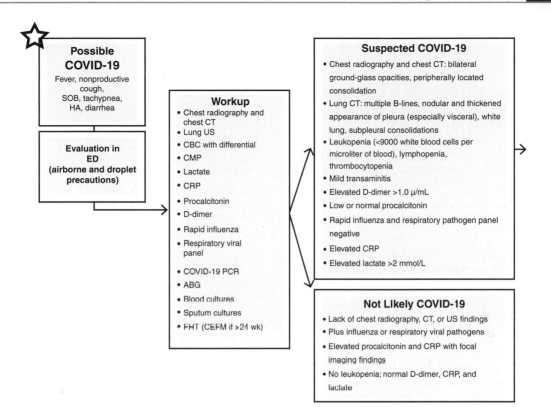

Fig. 28.1 *ABG*, Arterial blood gas; *CBC*, complete blood count; *CEFM*, continuous electronic fetal monitoring; *CMP*, comprehensive metabolic profile; *COVID*, coronavirus; *CRP*, C-reactive protein; *CT*, computed tomography; *FHT*, fetal heart tone; *HA*, Headache; *PCR*, polymerase chain reaction; *SOB*, shortness of breath; *US*, ultrasonography.

TABLE 28.1 COVID-19 Maternity Protocol			
Prehospital • Awareness • Testing • Transport • Therapies	Presentation • Signs and symptoms • Physiologic considerations	Bed placement • Nurse-to-patient ratio • Capabilities • Isolation	Internal • Debrief • IRIS reporting • QA

Hospital
• Staffing
• Bed space
• Equipment
• PPE preparedness and
  simulation
	Workup
	• Laboratory studies
	• Imaging
	• Ancillary teams
	• Point people or champions
		Multidisciplinary
		• Communication
		• Huddles
		• Assign "captain"
		• Delivery preparedness and
		  decision tree
			External
			• Regional HD
			• State ODH
			• National: CDC,
			  SMFM registry

	Logistics • Timely triage • Timely disposition • Communication • Minimizing exposure	Treatment • Medications • Ventilation/oxygen • Positioning • Surveillance • Family support • Care for self	

CDC, Centers for Disease Control and Prevention; *HD*, health department; *IRIS*, incident response improvement system; *ODH*, Ohio Department of Health; *PPE*, personal protective equipment; *QA*, quality assurance; *SMFM*, Society for Maternal-Fetal Medicine.

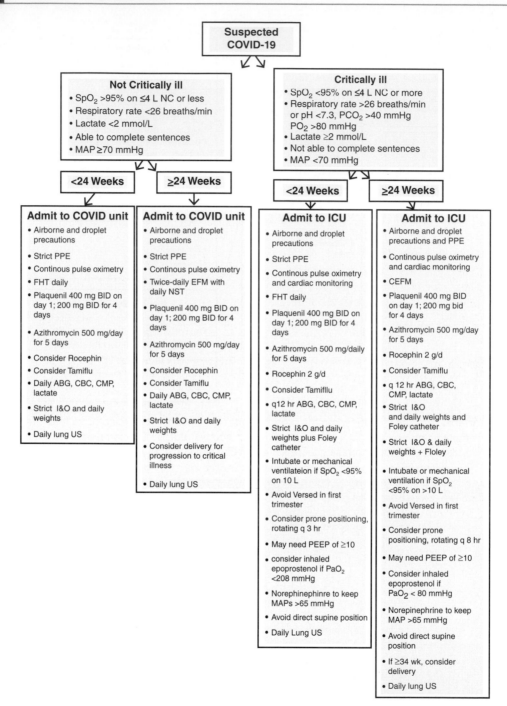

Fig. 28.2 *ABG*, Arterial blood gas; *BID*, twice a day; *CBC*, complete blood count; *CMP*, comprehensive metabolic equivalent; *COVID*, coronavirus; *FHT*, fetal heart tone; *I*, intake; *MAP*, mean arterial pressure; *NC*, nasal cannula; *NST*, non-stress test; *O*, output; *PEEP*, positive end-expiratory pressure; *PPE*, personal protective equipment; *US*, ultrasonography.

considering administration of antenatal corticosteroids before anticipated preterm birth for patients with severe maternal COVID-19 infection. Although evidence from treatment studies for SARS suggest that high dosages of corticosteroids pose a risk for severe side effects that drastically affect prognosis, shorter courses of low to moderate dosages may be considered in the care of critically ill patients with COVID-19. The decision regarding administration of magnesium sulfate for fetal neuroprotection before 32 weeks' gestation should proceed per standard indications in that this agent may provide an additional benefit of bronchodilation in the setting of bronchospasm after intubation. Avoid delayed cord clamping and immediate skin-to-skin maternal contact. Table 28.2 represents our approach to delivery considerations, including timing, location, and medications.

When attempting to defer delivery and resolve acute maternal illness through supportive care, several adjunctive therapies should be considered. Emerging evidence suggests that antiviral agents, such as remdesivir, may demonstrate efficacy in treating the SARS-CoV-2 virus. Although the safety of these agents in pregnancy has not been definitively determined, the pharmacokinetic properties and mechanisms of action support their judicious use for critically ill patients. Hydroxychloroquine, chloroquine, and neuraminidase inhibitors such as oseltamivir have no proven benefit and have caused fetal harm in animal studies. Thus, they should probably not be used in pregnant women. Other medication therapies that have been used to treat COVID-19 and may be considered include:

1. Convalescent plasma seems to be safe for pregnant women.
2. Monoclonal antibodies may be used, but the risk in pregnancy is unknown.
3. Corticosteroids are used in pregnancy for other conditions and should be considered if they are clinically indicated.

TABLE 28.2 Delivery Considerations in Pregnant Women with COVID-19

Delivery Considerations		
GA <24 wk	Noncritically ill	If previable PTL, can deliver in COVID unit or LDR 2
GA <24 wk	Critically ill	If previable PTL, deliver in ICU, main OR if D&C required
GA 24–34 wk	Noncritically ill	• Attempt to delay delivery; stabilize and treat mother • Betamethasone if delivery anticipated in next week • $MgSO_4$ for fetal neuroprotection if GA <32 wk and benefit of bronchodilation outweighs pulmonary edema risk • Imminent need for SVD: move to LDR 2 • Imminent need for C-section: move to L&D OR 4
GA 24–34 wk	Critically ill	• Attempt to delay delivery; stabilize and treat mother • Betamethasone *only* if delivery *highly* anticipated in next week • $MgSO_4$ for fetal neuroprotection if GA <32 wk and benefit of bronchodilation outweighs pulmonary edema risk • Imminent need for SVD; deliver in ICU • Imminent need for C-section: move to main OR 6 • Perimortem C-section: proceed in ICU
GA ≥34 wk	Noncritically ill	• Attempt to delay delivery; stabilize and treat mother • No late preterm betamethasone • Imminent need for SVD: move to LDR 2 • Imminent need for C-section: move to L&D OR 4
GA ≥34 wk	Critically ill	• Move forward with delivery if maternal status allows • No late preterm betamethasone • Imminent need for SVD: deliver in ICU • Imminent need for C-section: move to main OR 6 • Perimortem C-section: proceed in ICU

COVID, Coronavirus; *D&A*, dilation and curettage; *GA*, gestational age; *ICU*, intensive care unit; *L&D*, labor and delivery; *LDR*, labor and delivery room; *OR*, operating room; *PTL*, preterm labor; *SVD*, spontaneous vaginal delivery.

4. Vitamin D appears safe in pregnancy.
5. Famotidine is pregnancy category B. Studies in animals have not shown evidence of fetal injury, but human surveillance studies have raised some concern. It could be used late in pregnancy.

Noninvasive modes of ventilation, such as continuous positive airway pressure bilevel positive airway pressure, are first-line therapies for managing acute hypoxemic respiratory failure; they may mitigate the need to transition to invasive ventilation. Rapid-sequence endotracheal intubation should be performed for severe cases when noninvasive means of oxygenation/ventilation have proven ineffective. In such cases, it is necessary to consider using a slightly smaller endotracheal tube size because of the potentially edematous and narrowed airway calibers in pregnancy. Furthermore, with respect to oxygenation and ventilation, it is important to consider the physiologic mild respiratory alkalosis of pregnancy, the diminished functional residual volume, a higher positive end-expiratory pressure requirement, and the potential for less lung compliance with higher innate peak inspiratory pressures (caused by diaphragmatic compression by the gravid uterus and chest wall compression by enlarged breast tissue). The prone position can help overcome some of these issues. Prone ventilation has been found to significantly improve oxygenation in the setting of ARDS, and its feasibility and safety in pregnancy have been documented. Figure. 28.1 illustrates the prone position, and Figure. 28.2 shows the recommended padding to support a pregnant woman undergoing ventilation in a prone position.

Last, venovenous extracorporeal membrane oxygenation (ECMO) is a proven, lifesaving salvage therapy for severe, reversible respiratory failure, and its benefit among critically ill pregnant women has been reported. A multidisciplinary team of experienced providers should entertain the use of ECMO cannulation in situations when the patient's oxygenation is so severely compromised as to require maximal ventilatory support early in the disease process (<7 days of mechanical ventilatory support). Often, therapeutic anticoagulation is required, and the postpartum period appears to be a dangerous timepoint to initiate ECMO, with a 100% maternal mortality rate in one report.

Table 28.3 summarizes many of these critical care goals and adjunctive therapies.

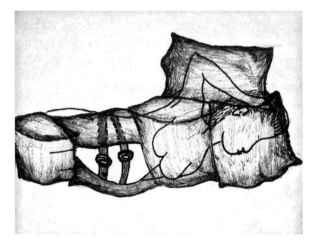

Fig. 28.3 Prone position for ventilation.

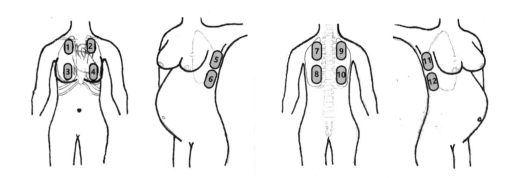

Fig. 28.4 A depiction of pad placement *(1–12)* to support a pregnant woman undergoing prone ventilation.

TABLE 28.3   Critical Care Goals

MAP	>65 mm Hg	• First assess if fluid responsive with passive leg raise or bolus LR 500 mL to see if MAP raises >65 mm Hg • Start norepinephrine at 5 mcg/min for MAP <65 mm Hg • Can uptitrate to 10 mcg/min • Ensure CEFM if GA >24 wk
SpO$_2$	>94%	• Increase PEEP to 10–12 cm H$_2$O • Consider VC+ modality • Consider prone positioning • Ensure finger is warm or place monitor on forehead
PaO$_2$	>80 mm Hg	• Increase PEEP to 10–12 cm H$_2$O • Increase I:E ratio • Consider prone positioning
PaCo$_2$	<40 mm Hg	• Increase ventilatory or respiratory rate to 20–25 breaths/min • Ensure no "auto-PEEP": keep plateau pressure <30 cm H$_2$O
pH	7.3–7.5	• First assess if acidemic or alkalemic • Then assess which is more out of range (PO$_2$ or PCO$_2$) • If metabolic acidosis is present, assess anion gap and ensure appropriate ventilatory compensation (bicarbonate × 1.5) + 8 = PCO$_2$
Bicarbonate	16–22 mm Hg	• Consider addition of IV bicarbonate if low *and* pH is <7.1
Anion gap	6–15	• Correct for hypoalbuminemia (add 2.5 to gap for every 1-g/dL albumin level <2.5 g/dL)
PiP	<35 mm Hg	• Check peak inspiratory pressure on ventilator and ensure <34 cm H$_2$O • Consider VC + modality
UOP	>20 mL/kg/hr	• Place Foley catheter and ensure strict I/O + daily weights
Skin	No breakdown	• Evaluate skin front and back daily (especially under fetal monitors)
VTE	Prophylaxis	• Consider institution of heparin 7500 U BID in second trimester and 10,000 U BID in third trimester if delivery is not imminent
Peptic ulcer	Prophylaxis	• Consider H2 blockade
CEFM	Category 1 or 2	• Delivery for category 3 • Worsening category 2 may signal worsening maternal status
Sedation	Lowest achievable	• Goal is to achieve RASS of 0–2 • May need to increase sedation with propofol, fentanyl, and midazolam • May need paralytic (cisatracurium), especially when putting the patient in a prone position

BID, Twice a day; *CEFM,* continous electronic fetal monitoring; *GA,* gestational age; *I:E,* inspiratory to expiratory ratio; *I,* intake; *IV,* intravenous; *LR,* lactated ringers; *MAP,* mean arterial pressure; *O,* output; *PEEP,* positive end-expiratory pressure; *PiP,* peak inspiratory pressure; *RASS,* Richmond agitation-sedation scale; *UOP,* urine output; *VC,* volume control; *VTE,* venous thromboembolism.

BIBLIOGRAPHY

Akatsuka M, Tatsumi H, Yama N, Masuda Y. Therapeutic evaluation of computed tomography findings for efficacy of prone ventilation in acute respiratory distress syndrome patients with abdominal surgery. *J Crit Care Med.* 2020;6(1):32–40.

Arabi YM, Fowler R, Hayden FG. Critical care management of adults with community-acquired severe respiratory viral infection. *Intensive Care Med.* 2020;46(2):315–328.

Bikash RR, Trikha A. Prone position ventilation in pregnancy: concerns and evidence. *J Obstet Anaesth Crit Care.* 2018;8(1):7–9.

Centers for Disease Control and Prevention. Coronavirus disease 2019 (COVID-19): cases in U.S. http://www.cdc.gov

Dashraath P, Wong JLJ, Lim MXK, et al. Coronavirus disease 2019 (COVID-19) pandemic and pregnancy. *Am J Obstet Gynecol.* 2020;222(6):521–531.

Dennis AT, Hardy L, Leeton L. The prone position in healthy pregnant women and in women with preeclampsia—a pilot study. *BMC Pregnancy Childbirth.* 2018;18(1):445.

Juusela A, Nazir M, Gimovsky M. Two cases of COVID-19 related cardiomyopathy in pregnancy. *Am J Obstet Gynecol.* 2020;2(2):100113.

Li H, Wang YM, Xu JY, Cao B. Potential antiviral therapeutics for 2019 novel coronavirus. *Zhonghua Jie He He Hu Xi Za Zhi.* 2020;43(3):170–172.

Richter JE. Review article: the management of heartburn in pregnancy. *Aliment Pharmacol. Ther.* 2005;22(9): 749–757.

Salata C, Calistri A, Parolin C, Palu G. Coronaviruses: a paradigm of new emerging zoonotic diseases. *Pathog Dis.* 2019;77(9):6.

Schwartz DA. An analysis of 38 pregnant women with COVID-19, their newborn infants, and maternal-fetal transmission of SARS-CoV-2: maternal coronavirus infections and pregnancy outcomes. *Arch Pathol Lab Med.* 2020;144(7):799–805.

Wang M, Cao R, Zhang L, et al. Remdesivir and chloroquine effectively inhibit the recently emerged novel coronavirus (2019-nCoV) in vitro. *Cell Res.* 2020;30(3):269–271.

Webster CM, Smith KA, Manuck TA. Extracorporeal membrane oxygenation in pregnant and postpartum women: a ten-year case series. *Am J Obstet Gynecol.* 2020;2(2): 100108.

World Health Organization. Coronavirus disease 2019 (COVID-19) situation report–74. http://www.who.int

Yi Y, Lagniton P, Ye S, Li E, Xu RH. COVID-19: what has been learned and to be learned about the novel coronavirus disease. *Int J Biol Sci.* 2020;16(10):1753–1766.

29

Breastfeeding

William T. Schnettler, MD, FACOG

The remarkable beneficial effects for both the mother and child serve as the major rationale for most obstetric and pediatric societies to promote the practice of breastfeeding whenever possible. The interplay between cardiac disease and pregnancy often raises concerns by patients and the health care team about the safety of breastfeeding in the setting of certain medications and conditions. For instance, some evidence linking the fragmented prolactin molecule with the etiology of peripartum cardiomyopathy has led some researchers to recommend against breastfeeding in women with confirmation of this diagnosis. Other concerns for cardiac patients are the excretion of certain drugs into the breast milk and their potential effects on infants and children. Fortunately, most drugs have a negligible concentration in breast milk and can be given safely to breastfeeding mothers.

The following medications are expected to be safe for most breastfeeding mothers:

Adenosine
Angiotensin-converting-enzyme (ACE) inhibitors
Antiplatelet drugs (clopidogrel, ticlopidine)
Aspirin
Atenolol
Digoxin
Heparin
Hydralazine
Hydrochlorothiazide
Labetalol
Low-molecular-weight heparin
Methyldopa
Metoprolol
Nifedipine
Procainamide
Propranolol
Quinidine
Sotalol
Warfarin

The following medications can be used, but they are excreted in breast milk:

Clonidine (no data on safety)
Diltiazem
Flecainide
Loop diuretics
Propafenone (no data on safety)
Verapamil

Except in special circumstances, breastfeeding mothers should not use the following medications:

Amiodarone
Doxazosin
Spironolactone
Statins

Insufficient data exist to classify the following:

Amlodipine
Angiotensin receptor blockers (ARBs)
Bisoprolol
Nitrates

Regarded as the best source for up-to-date safety data for nearly all medications specifically with regard to breastfeeding is *Medications & Mothers' Milk* by Thomas W. Hale, PhD, and Hilary E. Rowe, PharmD, published by Springer Publishing and now in its 17th edition. Another good reference for the safety of drugs in breastfeeding is *Drugs in Pregnancy and Lactation* by Gerald G. Briggs et al. published by Wolters Kluwer and now in its 11th edition. The website Drugs.com also provides information on drug safety during lactation.

BIBLIOGRAPHY

Yamac H, Bultmann I, Sliwa K, Hilfiker-Kleiner D. Prolactin: a new therapeutic target in peripartum cardiomyopathy. *Heart.* 2010;96(17):1352–1357.

Amiodarone

Anderson PO. When the heart is not in it: breastfeeding with cardiovascular disease. *Breastfeed Med.* 2019;14(2):80–82.

Chow T, Galvin J, McGovern B. Antiarrhythmic drug therapy during pregnancy and lactation. *Am J Cardiol.* 1998;82(4A): 581–621.

Hotham N, Hothman E. Drugs in breastfeeding. *Aust Prescr.* 2015;38(5):156–159.

Amlodipine

Ahn HK, Nava-Ocampo AA, Han JY, et al. Exposure to amlodipine in the first trimester of pregnancy and during breast feeding. *Hypertens Pregnancy.* 2007;26(2):179–187.

Naito T, Kubono N, Deguchi S, et al. Amlodipine passage int breast milk in lactating women with pregnancy induced hypertension and its estimation of infant risk for breastfeeding. *J Hum Lact.* 2014;31(2):301–306.

Angiotensin-Converting Enzyme Inhibitors

Beardmore KS, Morris JM, Gallery ED. Excretion of antihypertensive medication into human breast milk: a systematic review. *Hypertens Pregnancy.* 2002;21(1):85–95.

Shannon ME, Malecha SE, Cha AJ. Angiotensin converting enzyme inhibitors (ACEIs) and angiotensin II receptor blockers (ARBs) and lactation: an update. *J Hum Lact.* 2000:16920152–16920155.

Angiotensin Receptor Blockers

Shannon ME, Malecha SE, Cha AJ. Angiotensin converting enzyme inhibitors (ACEIs) and angiotensin II receptor blockers (ARBs) and lactation: an update. *J Hum Lact.* 2000;16(2):152–155.

Antiplatelet Drugs (Clopidogrel, Ticlopidine)

Nice FJ, et al. Medications and breast-feeding: a guide for pharmacists, pharmacy technicians and other healthcare professional part II. *J Pharmacy Technol.* 2004;20(20):85–95.

Aspirin

1. Davanzo R, Bua J, Paloni G, Facchina G. Breastfeeding and migraine drugs. *Eur J Clin Pharmacol.* 2014;70(11): 1313–1324.

Atenolol

Davanzo R, Bua J, Paloni G, Facchina G. Breastfeeding and migraine drugs. *Eur J Clin Pharmacol.* 2014;70(11): 1313–1324.

Eyal S, Kim JD, Anderson GD, et al. Atenolol pharmacokinetics and excretion in breast milk during the first 6 to 8 months postpartum. *J Clin Pharmacol.* 2010;50(11): 1301–1309.

Bisoprolol

Khurana R, Bin Jardan YA, Wilkie J, Brocks DR. Breast milk concentration of amiodarone, desethylamiodarone, and bisoprolol following short-term exposure: two case reports. *Pediatr Pharmacol.* 2014;54(7):828–831.

Clonidine

Hartikainen-Sorri AL, Heikkinen JE, Koivisto M. Pharmacokinetics of clonidine during pregnancy and nursing. *Obstet Gynecol.* 1987;69(4):598–600.

Noronha Neto CC, Maia SS, Katz L, Coutinho IC, Souza AR, Amorim MM. Clonidine vs captopril for severe postpartum hypertension: a randomized controlled trial. *PLOS One.* 2017;12(1):1–12.

Sevrez C, Lavocat MP, Mounier G, et al. [Transplacental or breast milk intoxication to clonidine: a case of neonatal hypotonia and drowsiness]. *Arch Pediatr.* 2014;21(2): 198–200.

Digoxin

Chow T, Galvin J, McGovern B. Antiarrhythmic drug therapy during pregnancy and lactation. *Am J Cardiol.* 1998;82(4A): 581–621.

Diltiazem

Spencer JP, Gonzalez 3rd LS, Barnhart DJ. Medications in the breast-feeding mother. *Am Fam Physician.* 2001;64(1): 119–126.

Doxazosin

Jensen BP, Dalrymple JM, Begg EJ. Transfer of doxazosin into breast milk. *J Hum Lact.* 2013;29(2):150–153.

Versmissen J, Koch BC, Roofthooft DW, et al. Doxazosin treatment of phaeochromocytoma during pregnancy and placental transfer and disposition in breast milk. *Br J Clin Pharmacol.* 2016;82(2):568–569.

Flecainide

Fulton B. Antiarrhythmics in breastfeeding. *J Hum Lact.* 1994;10(3):193–194.

Horn A. Maternal mediations and breastfeeding: current recommendations. *South Afr Fam Pract.* 2005;47:942–947.

Heparin

Shoup J, Carson DS. Anticoagulant use during lactation. *J Hum Lact.* 1999;15(3):255–257.

Hydralazine

Ellsworth A. Pharmacotherapy of hypertension while breastfeeding. *J Hum Lact.* 1994;10(2):121–124.

Hydrochlorothiazide

Ellsworth Allen. Pharmacotherapy of hypertension while breastfeeding. *J Hum Lact.* 1994;10(2):121–124.

White WB. Management of hypertension during lactation. *Hypertension.* 1984;6:297–300.

Labetalol

Ellsworth A. Pharmacotherapy of hypertension while breastfeeding. *J Hum Lact.* 1994;10(2):121–124.

Loop Diuretics

Ellsworth A. Pharmacotherapy of hypertension while breastfeeding. *J Hum Lact.* 1994;10(2):121–124.

Low-Molecular-Weight Heparin

Fulton B, et al. Antiarrhythmics in breastfeeding. *J Hum Lact.* 1994;10(3):193–194.

Methyldopa

Ellsworth A. Pharmacotherapy of hypertension while breastfeeding. *J Hum Lact.* 1994;10(2):121–124.

Metoprolol

Davazo R, Bua J, Paloni G, Facchina G. Breastfeeding and migraine drugs. *Eur J Clin Pharmacol.* 2014;70(11): 1313–1324.

Nifedipine

Ehrenkranz R, Ackerman BA, Hulse JD. Nifedipine transfer into human milk. *J Pediatr.* 1989;114:478–480.

Nitrates

Anderson PO. When the heart is not in it: breastfeeding with cardiovascular disease. *Breastfeed Med.* 2019;14(2):80–82.

Procainamide

Anderson PO. When the heart is not in it: breastfeeding with cardiovascular disease. *Breastfeed Med.* 2019;14(2):80–82.

Propafenone (no data on safety)

Anderson PO. When the heart is not in it: breastfeeding with cardiovascular disease. *Breastfeed Med.* 2019;14(2):80–82.

Propranolol

Davazo R, Bua J, Paloni G, Facchina G. Breastfeeding and migraine drugs. *Eur J Clin Pharmacol.* 2014;70(11): 1313–1324.

Quinidine

Anderson PO. When the heart is not in it: breastfeeding with cardiovascular disease. *Breastfeed Med.* 2019;14(2):80–82.

Sotalol

Anderson PO. When the heart is not in it: breastfeeding with cardiovascular disease. *Breastfeed Med.* 2019;14(2):80–82.

Spironolactone

Kim GK, Del Roso JQ. Oral spironolactone in post-teenage female patients with acne vulgaris. *J Clin Aesthet Dermatol.* 2012;5(3):37–50.

Statins

Verapamil

Davazo R, Bua J, Paloni G, Facchina G. Breastfeeding and migraine drugs. *Eur J Clin Pharmacol.* 2014;70(11):1313–1324.

Warfarin

Clark SL, Porter TF, West FG. Coumarin derivatives and breastfeeding. *Obstet Gynecol.* 2000;95(1):938–940.

Orme ML, Lewis PJ, de Swiet M, et al. May mothers given warfarin breast-feed their infants? *Br Med J.* 1977;1: 1564–1565.

30

Contraception

William T. Schnettler, MD, FACOG

HIGH-RISK PATIENT POPULATIONS

The highest-risk patients are those with pulmonary hypertension and those with prior peripartum cardiomyopathy. The American College of Cardiology recommendations for women with adult congenital heart disease are as follows:

1. Women of childbearing potential with congenital heart disease should be counseled about the risks associated with pregnancy and appropriate contraceptive options.
2. Estrogen-containing contraceptives are potentially harmful for women with congenital heart disease at high risk of thromboembolic events (e.g., cyanosis, Fontan physiology, mechanical valves, prior thrombotic events, pulmonary arterial hypertension).

BIRTH CONTROL METHODS

Birth control methods include behavioral methods, barrier contraceptives, hormonal contraceptives, intrauterine devices (IUDs), and sterilization; all of these are used before or during sex. So-called emergency contraceptives, which are used after sex, are effective for up to a few days afterward. Each is discussed in this chapter.

All birth control methods have risks and complications, including a risk of failure resulting in an unwanted pregnancy. The effectiveness of contraceptives is generally expressed as the percentage of women who become pregnant using a given method during the first year. However, among highly effective methods, such as tubal ligations, the effectiveness is expressed as a lifetime failure rate. Surgical sterilization, implantable hormones, and IUDs all have first-year failure rates of less than 1%. Hormonal contraceptive pills, patches, or vaginal rings, if used strictly, also can have first-year failure rates of less than 1%. With typical (i.e., incorrect) use, however,

first-year failure rates are considerably higher, at 9%. Even with perfect usage, other methods, such as condoms, diaphragms, and spermicides, have higher first-year failure rates than hormonal methods. And finally, although all methods of birth control have some potential adverse health effects, the associated risk is less than that of pregnancy.

Behavioral Methods

Behavioral methods involve regulating the timing or method of intercourse to prevent introduction of sperm into the female reproductive tract, either altogether or when an egg may be present. If used perfectly, the first-year failure rate may be around 3% to 4%. However, if behavioral methods are used poorly, first-year failure rates may approach 85%. The withdrawal method (also known as coitus interruptus) is the practice of ending intercourse before ejaculation. The main risk of the withdrawal method is that the man may not perform the maneuver in a timely manner. First-year failure rates vary from 4% with perfect usage to 22% with typical usage. Withdrawal is not considered birth control by some medical professionals.

Barrier Contraceptives

Barrier contraceptives are devices that attempt to prevent pregnancy by physically preventing sperm from entering the uterus. They include male condoms, female condoms, cervical caps, diaphragms, and contraceptive sponges with spermicide. Typically, modern condoms are made from latex, but some are made from other materials, such as polyurethane or lamb's intestine. Female condoms are also available and are usually made of nitrile, latex, or polyurethane. Male condoms and diaphragms with spermicide have typical-use first-year failure rates of 18% and 12%, respectively. With perfect use, condoms are more effective, with a 2% first-year failure rate versus a 6% first-year rate with the diaphragm. Contraceptive sponges combine a barrier with a spermicide. Similar to diaphragms, they are inserted vaginally before intercourse and must be placed over the cervix to be effective. Typical failure rates during the first year depend on whether or not a woman has previously given birth (24% in those who have and 12% in those who have not). The sponge can be inserted up to 24 hours before intercourse and must be left in place for at least 6 hours afterward. There have been reports of allergic reactions and more severe adverse effects, such as toxic shock syndrome.

Women with cyanotic congenital heart disease and pulmonary hypertension are at risk for thrombotic events. Various barrier methods, such as condoms, are the safest form of contraception for these women.

Hormonal Contraceptives

Hormonal contraceptives are available in a number of different forms, including oral pills, implants under the skin, injections, patches, a vaginal ring, and IUDs (discussed separately later). There are two types of oral birth control pills: the combined oral contraceptive pills (which contain both estrogen and a progestogen) and the progestogen-only pills. If either is taken during pregnancy, they do not increase the risk of miscarriage, nor do they cause birth defects. Both types of birth control pills prevent fertilization mainly by inhibiting ovulation and thickening cervical mucus. Additionally, they may change the lining of the uterus and thus decrease implantation. Their effectiveness depends on the user's remembering to take the pills.

Combined hormonal contraceptives are associated with an increased risk of both venous and arterial blood clots. Venous clots, on average, increase from 2.8 to 9.8 per 10,000 women years, which is still less than that associated with pregnancy, for the average woman. Because of this risk, they are not recommended in women who have other risk factors for thrombosis, such as age older than 35 years, smoking, or heart disease.

Most progestin-only pills, injections, and IUDs are not associated with an increased risk of thrombosis and thus may be used by women with a history of venous thrombosis. In patients with a history of arterial blood clots, nonhormonal birth control or a progestin-only method other than the injectable version should be used. Progestin-only pills can be used by breastfeeding women because they do not affect milk production.

Progesterone-only pills may have androgenic side effects. The progestins drospirenone and desogestrel minimize the androgenic side effects but increase the risk of blood clots and should not be used in women at increased risk for thrombosis, such as those with pulmonary hypertension or Fontan circulation. Additionally, new evidence suggests that any form of oral contraceptive should be used with caution among women with congenital long QT syndrome, and progestin-only oral contraceptives have been associated with a 2.8-fold increased risk of cardiac events in women with long QT syndrome. Beta-blocker therapies are highly protective against this increased risk such that such women should be prescribed a beta-blocker if they choose to utilize any form of oral contraceptives.

Estrogen-containing contraceptives may produce nausea and breast tenderness. Irregular vaginal bleeding may occur with progestin-only methods, with some women experiencing no menstrual periods.

Monthly injectables that contain medroxyprogesterone acetate are inappropriate for women with congestive heart failure because they have a tendency to cause fluid retention. Low-dose oral contraceptives containing 20 μg of ethinyl estradiol are safe in women with low thrombogenic potential, but they must be used with extreme caution in women with vascular disease and a higher risk of thrombotic events.

Intrauterine Devices

Current IUDs are small apparatuses, often T shaped, typically containing either copper or levonorgestrel, that are inserted into the uterus. They are the most effective reversible type of birth control. Whereas the failure rate with the copper IUD is about 0.8%, the levonorgestrel IUD has a failure rate of 0.2% in the first year of use. IUDs do not affect breastfeeding and can be inserted immediately after delivery. They also may be used immediately after an abortion. After they are removed, even after long-term use, fertility returns to normal immediately. Although copper IUDs may increase menstrual bleeding and result in more painful cramps, hormonal IUDs may reduce menstrual bleeding or stop menstruation altogether. Cramping can be treated with nonsteroidal antiinflammatory drugs. Other potential complications include expulsion (2%–5%) and, rarely, perforation of the uterus (<0.7%). A previous model of the IUD (the Dalkon shield) was associated with an increased risk of pelvic inflammatory disease. However, this risk is not increased with current models in women without sexually transmitted infections around the time of insertion.

After barrier methods, the levonorgestrel-releasing IUD is considered the safest and most effective means of birth control for women with cyanotic congenital heart disease and pulmonary hypertension (both of which increase the risk for thrombotic events). However, it is contraindicated in cyanotic women with hematocrit greater than 55% because of an increased risk of excessive menstrual bleeding. Implantation causes vasovagal syncope in about 5% of women, so IUDs must be used cautiously in very high-risk patients. Antibiotic prophylaxis is not recommended at insertion.

Surgical Sterilization

Surgical sterilization is available in the form of tubal ligation. There are no significant long-term side effects, and tubal ligation decreases the risk of ovarian cancer. Generally, tubal ligation is a low-risk procedure (complications occur in 1%–2% of procedures), but because of associated anesthesia and abdominal inflation, it may carry increased risk in patients with pulmonary hypertension, cyanosis, or Fontan circulation. Although sterilization is considered a permanent procedure, it is possible to attempt reversal by reconnecting the fallopian tubes. Pregnancy success rates after tubal reversal are between 31% and 88%. Tubal ligation reversal is associated with an increased risk of ectopic pregnancy.

Emergency Contraceptive Methods

Emergency contraceptive methods are medications or devices used after unprotected sexual intercourse with the hope of preventing pregnancy. They work primarily by preventing ovulation or fertilization. They are unlikely to affect implantation, but this has not been completely excluded. A number of options exist, including high-dose birth control pills, levonorgestrel, mifepristone, ulipristal, and IUDs. Levonorgestrel pills, when used within 3 days of intercourse, decrease the

chance of pregnancy after a single episode of unprotected sex or condom failure by 70% (resulting in a pregnancy rate of 2.2%). Ulipristal, when used within 5 days of intercourse, decreases the chance of pregnancy by about 85% (pregnancy rate of 1.4%) and might be a little more effective than levonorgestrel. Mifepristone is also more effective than levonorgestrel. Copper IUDs are the most effective method. IUDs can be inserted up to 5 days after intercourse and prevent about 99% of pregnancies after an episode of unprotected sex (pregnancy rate of 0.1%–0.2%). In women who are obese, levonorgestrel is less effective, and an IUD or ulipristal is recommended. All emergency methods have minimal side effects.

BIBLIOGRAPHY

Borgatta L, Kapp N. Society of Family Planning. Clinical Guidelines. Labor induction abortion in the second trimester. *Contraception.* 2011;84(1):4–18.

Chen MJ, Creinin MD. Mifepristone with buccal misoprostol for medical abortion: a systematic review. *Obstet Gynecol.* 2015;126(1):12–21.

Fjerstad M, Sivin I, Lichtenberg ES, Trussell J, Cleland K, Cullins V. Effectiveness of medical abortion with mifepristone and buccal misoprostol through 59 gestational days. *Contraception.* 2009;8(3):282–286.

Goldenberg I, Younis A, Huang D. Use of oral contraceptives in women with congenital long QT syndrome. *Heart Rhythm.* 2022;19:41–48.

horne S, MacGregor A, Nelson-Piercy C. Risks of contraception and pregnancy in heart disease. *Heart.* 2006;92: 1520–1525.

Stout KK, Daniels CJ, Aboulhosn JA, et al. 2018 AHA/ACC Guideline for the Management of Adults With Congenital Heart Disease: Executive Summary: A Report of the American College of Cardiology/American Heart Association Task Force on Clinical Practice Guidelines. *J Am Coll Cardiol.* 2019;73(12):1494–1563.

Templeton A, Grimes DA. A request for abortion. *N Engl J Med.* 2011;365(23):2198–2204.

31

Termination of Pregnancy

William T. Schnettler, MD, FACOG

In situations when gestation carries a significant fetal or maternal risk, it may be appropriate to terminate the pregnancy. The safest time for termination is during the first trimester. Abortions may be induced by medication or performed surgically. This chapter discusses both medical and surgical abortions, with an emphasis on their timing and prevalence in the United States and elsewhere. It also discusses anesthesia and other medications (including antibiotics) used during or after abortion, focusing on their potential impact on cardiovascular function.

MEDICAL ABORTION

Medical abortions are those induced by abortifacient drugs. The most common early first-trimester medical abortion regimens use methotrexate in combination with a prostaglandin analog for up to 7 weeks' gestation, mifepristone (RU-46) in combination with a prostaglandin analog (misoprostol or gemeprost) for up to 9 weeks' gestation, or a prostaglandin analog alone. Mifepristone–misoprostol combination regimens work faster and are more effective at later gestational ages than methotrexate–misoprostol combination regimens are. Combination regimens are more effective than misoprostol alone. In very early abortions, up to 7 weeks' gestation, medical abortion using a mifepristone–misoprostol combination regimen is considered to be more effective than surgical abortion (vacuum aspiration). Early medical abortion regimens using mifepristone followed 24 to 48 hours later by buccal or vaginal misoprostol are 98% effective up to 9 weeks' gestational age. If medical abortion fails, surgical abortion must be used to complete the procedure.

Medical abortion regimens using mifepristone in combination with a prostaglandin analog are the most common methods used for second-trimester abortions in Canada, most of Europe, China, and India.

SURGICAL ABORTION

Up to 15 weeks' gestation, suction aspiration or vacuum aspiration are the most common surgical methods of induced abortion. Whereas manual vacuum aspiration (MVA) consists of removing the fetus or embryo, placenta, and membranes by suction using a manual syringe, electric vacuum aspiration uses an electric pump. These techniques differ in the mechanism used to apply suction, in how early in pregnancy they can be used, and in whether cervical dilation is necessary. MVA, also known as menstrual extraction, can be used in very early pregnancy and does not require cervical dilation. Dilation and curettage, the second most common method of surgical abortion, is a standard gynecological procedure performed for a variety of reasons, including examination of the uterine lining for possible malignancy, investigation of abnormal bleeding, and abortion. Curettage refers to cleaning the walls of the uterus with a curette. The World Health Organization recommends this procedure, also called sharp curettage, only when MVA is unavailable.

From the 15th week of gestation until approximately the 26th week, other techniques must be used. Dilation and evacuation consists of opening the cervix of the uterus and emptying it using surgical instruments and suction. It is generally considered safest in the first or second trimester. In the United States, 96% of second-trimester abortions are performed surgically by dilation and evacuation.

After the 16th week of gestation, abortions also can be induced by intact dilation and extraction, which requires surgical decompression of the fetus's head before evacuation. This procedure is sometimes called partial-birth abortion and has been banned in the United States. In the third trimester of pregnancy, induced abortion also may be performed surgically by hysterotomy. Hysterotomy abortion is a procedure similar to a cesarean section and is performed under general anesthesia. Hysterotomy requires a smaller incision than a cesarean section and is used only during the later stages of pregnancy.

An abortion also can be performed by first inducing labor and then inducing fetal demise if necessary. This procedure may be performed from 13 weeks' gestation to the third trimester. Although it is very uncommon in the United States and in Sweden and other nearby countries, more than 80% of induced abortions throughout the second trimester are labor-induced abortions. Limited data are available comparing this method with dilation and extraction. Unlike dilation and evacuation, labor-induced abortions after 18 weeks may be complicated by the occurrence of brief fetal survival, which may be characterized legally as a live birth in the United States. For this reason, labor-induced abortion is legally risky in this country.

ANESTHETICS AND OTHER CONSIDERATIONS

Whereas first-trimester procedures can generally be performed using local anesthesia, second-trimester methods may require deep sedation or general anesthesia. General anesthesia can lead to cardiovascular instability if a rapid induction sequence is used. The use of muscle relaxants necessitates the use of positive-pressure ventilation, which may have deleterious effects on cardiac function, such as decreased venous return, increased pulmonary vascular resistance, and tachycardia. Sedation with drugs such as propofol, midazolam, and fentanyl must be used with extreme caution during the third trimester because of the reduced functional residual capacity and an increased risk of aspiration.

Antibiotics are not routinely administered for endocarditis prophylaxis, but they are commonly administered to prevent postabortion endometritis.

If surgical evacuation is not feasible, prostaglandin E_1, prostaglandin E_2, or misoprostol may be administered. These drugs are absorbed into the systemic circulation and may lower systemic vascular resistance and blood pressure, which may in turn lead to tachycardia. Prostaglandin F compounds should be avoided in patients with heart disease because they can cause significant increases in pulmonary arterial pressure and may reduce coronary perfusion. Saline abortion should be avoided because saline absorption may cause volume overload or contribute to clotting abnormalities.

BIBLIOGRAPHY

Brito MB, Nobre F, Vieira CS. Hormonal contraception and cardiovascular system. *Arq Bras Cardiol*. 2012;96(4): e81–e89.

Kuyoh MA, Toroitich-Ruto C, Grimes DA, Schulz KF, Gallo MF. Sponge versus diaphragm for contraception: a Cochrane review. *Contraception*. 2003;67(1):15–18.

Mantha S, Karp R, Raghavan V, Terrin N, Bauer KA, Zwicker JI. Assessing the risk of venous thromboembolic events in women taking progestin-only contraception: a meta-analysis. *BMJ*. 2012;345:e4944.

Steenland MW, Tepper NK, Curtis KM, Kapp N. Intrauterine contraceptive insertion postabortion: a systematic review. *Contraception*. 2011;84(5):447–464.

Trussell J. Contraceptive failure in the United States. *Contraception*. 2011;83(5):397–404.

World Health Organization *Medical Eligibility Criteria for Contraceptive use*. 4th ed. : World Health Organization; 2009.

32

Infertility Treatment

William T. Schnettler, MD, FACOG

ASSISTED REPRODUCTIVE TECHNOLOGIES

Fertility medications stimulate the release of eggs from the ovaries and include gonadotropins and gonadotropin-releasing hormones.

In vitro fertilization (IVF) bypasses the act of sexual intercourse, and fertilization of the oocytes occurs in a laboratory environment. This process may involve many components.

Transvaginal ovum retrieval is the process whereby a small needle is inserted through the back of the vagina and guided via ultrasound into the ovarian follicles to collect the fluid that contains the eggs.

Embryo transfer is the step in the process whereby one or several embryos are placed into the uterus with the intent to establish a pregnancy. Sometimes assisted zona hatching is performed shortly before the embryo is transferred to the uterus; a small opening is made in the outer layer surrounding the egg to help the embryo hatch out and aid in its implantation.

Intracytoplasmic sperm injection (ICSI) is beneficial in male infertility when sperm counts are very low or when failed fertilization occurred with previous IVF attempts. The ICSI procedure involves a single sperm carefully injected into the center of an egg using a microneedle. With ICSI, only one sperm per egg is needed. Without ICSI, you need between 50,000 and 100,000 sperm.

Autologous endometrial coculture is a possible treatment for patients who have failed in previous IVF attempts or who have poor embryo quality. The patient's fertilized eggs are placed on top of a layer of cells from the patient's own uterine lining, creating a more natural environment for embryo development.

Zygote intrafallopian transfer is a process in which egg cells are removed from the woman's ovaries and fertilized in the laboratory; the resulting zygote is then placed into the fallopian tube.

Cytoplasmic transfer is the technique in which the contents of a fertile egg from a donor are injected into the infertile egg of the patient along with the sperm.

Gamete intrafallopian transfer is a process in which a mixture of sperm and eggs is placed directly into a woman's fallopian tubes using laparoscopy after a transvaginal ovum retrieval.

Embryo splitting can be used for twinning to increase the number of available embryos.

Egg donors are resources for women who have no eggs because of surgery, chemotherapy, or genetic causes, whose egg quality is poor, who have had previously unsuccessful IVF attempts, or who are of advanced maternal age. In the egg donor process, eggs are retrieved from a donor's ovaries and fertilized in the laboratory with the sperm from the recipient's partner; the resulting healthy embryos are placed in the recipient's uterus.

Sperm donation may provide the source for the sperm used in IVF procedures in cases in which the male partner produces no sperm or has an inheritable disease or when the woman being treated has no male partner.

IN VITRO FERTILIZATION HEALTH RISKS AND OTHER CONSIDERATIONS

In vitro fertilization may be considered in women with heart disease in whom the risk of a procedure including hormonal stimulation is low. Hormonal stimulation that produces high estradiol levels may create a prothrombotic state, and women already at risk for thrombotic events, such as those with Fontan circulation, may be placed at greater risk.

In vitro fertilization is associated with a high incidence of multiple-gestation pregnancies, which may further complicate pregnancy in women with heart disease. Also, it has been reported that the risk of preeclampsia is greater in women who became pregnant with IVF.

Risks to the fetus also are increased when IVF techniques are used. There are increased risks of genetic defects, low birth weight, and preterm birth. Low birth weight and preterm birth are strongly associated with many health problems, such as visual impairment and cerebral palsy. Children born after IVF are roughly twice as likely to have cerebral palsy. Interestingly, sperm donation alone is associated with a reduction in birth defects by as much as five times compared with the general population.

A risk to both the mother and the fetus is a possibility of damage to the amniotic membranes and associated complications.

Infertility treatments may be very expensive, and often they may not be covered by medical insurance.

Other options for women to consider are adoption or the use of a surrogate. However, if these options are considered for very high-risk patients, the patient's life expectancy must be taken into consideration.

BIBLIOGRAPHY

Aiken C, Brockelsby J. Fetal and maternal consequences of pregnancies conceived using ART. *Fetal Matern Med Rev.* 2016;25(3-4):281–294.

Hargreave M, Jensen A, Toender A, Andersen KK, Kjaer SK. Fertility treatment and childhood cancer risk: a systematic meta-analysis. *Fertil Steril.* 2013;100(1):150–161.

Hvidtjørn D, Schieve L, Schendel D, Jacobsson B, Svaerke C, Thorsen P. Cerebral palsy, autism spectrum disorders, and developmental delay in children born after assisted conception: a systematic review and meta-analysis. *Arch Pediatr Adolesc Med.* 2009;163(1):72–83.

Van Voorhis BJ. Clinical practice. In vitro fertilization. *N Engl J Med.* 2007;356(4):379–836.

33

Genetic Counseling

Erin M. Miller, MS, LGC

Women with congenital heart disease have an increased risk of complications for themselves and their babies, as well as an increased risk of having children with heart disease. Ideally, genetic counseling should take place before pregnancy (see Chapter 4), but if not, it still has a role to play. Often, genetic counseling is sought by women who have had a baby with a congenital malformation and are considering having a second child. This chapter provides an overview of genetic counseling and explains risk assessment for genetic conditions or disorders. It then discusses genetic disorders involving the heart that follow a Mendelian inheritance pattern.

OVERVIEW: GENETIC COUNSELING

According to the National Society of Genetic Counselors, genetic counseling is the process of helping people understand and adapt to the medical, psychological, and familial implications of the genetic contribution to disease. This process integrates (1) interpretation of familial and medical histories to assess the chance of disease occurrence or recurrence; (2) education about inheritance, testing management, prevention, resources, and research; and (3) counseling to promote informed choices of adaptation to the risk or condition.

Genetic counseling involves numerous steps:
1. Validating the maternal diagnosis
2. Evaluating the needs of the counselee
3. Evaluating the family history
4. Estimating the risk
5. Communicating the risk to the counselee
6. Making a decision and taking appropriate action
7. Following up with the family.

In addition, if the patient has a limited life expectancy, the ethical aspects of parenthood should be discussed.

The source of payment for genetic counseling is problematic because it is often not covered by insurance.

RISK ASSESSMENT

It is standard to provide a figure for the risk of recurrence of genetic conditions. Risk calculation may be based on known genetic inheritance patterns (e.g., autosomal dominant, in which case the risk to the child of inheriting the trait is 50%) or empiric risk factors based on observed patterns of inheritance, depending on the disorder. Only about 3% of congenital heart diseases follow Mendelian inheritance patterns, and it is estimated that 90% of cases are of unknown genetic cause.

Most women with congenital heart disease seeking genetic counseling have conditions for which the genetics are not completely worked out and a precise risk is unknown. Interestingly, it seems that the risk of having a child with congenital heart disease seems to be greater if the mother is affected than if the father is affected, but the reason for this is unknown.

In general, the risk of any woman having a child with congenital heart disease is 0.5% to 1.0%. The risk goes up to 5% if the mother is affected, and 2% to 3% if the father is affected. If a sibling is affected, the risk is 2% to 3%. If two siblings are affected, it goes up to 10%, and if more than three first-degree relatives are affected, it is greater than 50% (Table 33.1).

Next we discuss genetic disorders involving the heart that follow a Mendelian inheritance pattern. Disorders are presented in alphabetical order.

ELLIS-VAN CREVELD SYNDROME

Ellis-van Creveld syndrome, or chondroectodermal dysplasia, manifests as a large atrial septal defect associated

TABLE 33.1 Risk Increase in Specific Conditions		
Lesion	Mother Affected	Father Affected
Ventricular septal defect	9.5	2.5
Atrial septal defect	6.0	1.5
Patent ductus	4.0	2.0
Tetralogy of Fallot	2.5	1.5
Atriovenous septal defect	14.0	1.0
Pulmonic stenosis	6.5	2.0
Aortic stenosis	18.0	5.0
Coarctation of the aorta	4.0	2.5

with postaxial polydactyly, short-limbed dwarfism, and dysplastic nails. It is autosomal recessive.

HOLT-ORAM SYNDROME

With Holt-Oram syndrome, congenital abnormalities of the upper extremities are associated with an ostium secundum atrial septal defect. Inheritance is autosomal dominant with variable expression of the limb and cardiac abnormalities.

KARTAGENER SYNDROME

Kartagener syndrome consists of dextrocardia, which may be isolated or associated with other cardiac malformations, bronchiectasis, and recurrent sinusitis. It is considered to be autosomal dominant but with a low risk of transmission to offspring.

LEOPARD SYNDROME

LEOPARD syndrome (lentigines, electrocardiogram abnormalities, ocular hypertelorism, pulmonary stenosis, abnormalities of genitalia, growth restriction, and deafness) is associated with abnormalities of the same gene as for Noonan syndrome. It is also autosomal dominant.

MARFAN SYNDROME

Marfan syndrome is a genetic disorder of connective tissue associated with a constellation of signs and symptoms, including tall stature, long limbs, long fingers, flexible joints, and a tendency to dislocation of the lens of the eye. The cardiac manifestations are a propensity to dissection of the aorta and mitral valve prolapse and regurgitation. It is inherited as autosomal dominant.

NOONAN SYNDROME

Noonan syndrome typically consists of pulmonary stenosis associated with short stature, a webbed neck, pectus excavatum or carinatum, down-slanting palpebral fissures, ptosis, low-set ears, and a low posterior hairline. It is autosomal dominant, but about half of cases are caused by a new mutation.

OTHER GENETIC DISORDERS

Some varieties of supravalvular aortic stenosis are inherited as an autosomal dominant condition.

Pulmonary hypertension is usually sporadic, but there is a familial type with autosomal dominance.

Hypertrophic cardiomyopathy is usually inherited as autosomal dominant. Symptoms usually are not present until early adulthood. In most cases, it cannot be diagnosed by fetal echocardiography.

The dilated cardiomyopathies are a heterogenous group of disorders, but there are familial types. Autosomal dominant, autosomal recessive, and X-linked inheritance all have been described.

In disorders in which genetic causes are known, fetal karyotyping may be performed to identify whether or not the fetus has the disorder. This can be accomplished by amniocentesis or chorionic villus sampling.

Amniocentesis can be used to obtain fetal DNA for genetic testing. It is frequently used to diagnose genetic disorders, such as Down syndrome. Amniocentesis is usually performed between 14 and 16 weeks of pregnancy. If performed earlier in pregnancy, there is a greater risk of inducing miscarriage. The procedure is performed under local anesthesia with ultrasound guidance. Typically, 20 cc of amniotic fluid is removed. In addition to providing fetal cells for genetic material, amniocentesis can be used to predict fetal lung maturity.

The risk of amniocentesis is that it may induce premature labor. Recent studies estimate the risk as low as 0.06%.

A second technique for obtaining genetic material is chorionic villus sampling. Usually performed at 10 to 12 weeks of gestation, it is preferred to amniocentesis if genetic testing is performed before 15 weeks. Chorionic villus sampling can be performed by a transabdominal or transcervical approach. The transabdominal approach involves removing a sample by aspiration through a needle. The transcervical approach involves removing a sample with a suction catheter. The risks include miscarriage, infection, and amniotic fluid leak. Overall, the risk of these complications is 1% to 2%. There also is a small risk of limb reduction defects.

BIBLIOGRAPHY

Berko BA, Swift M. X-linked dilated cardiomyopathy. *N Engl J Med.* 1987;316:1186–1191.

Dennis NR, Warren J. Risks to offspring of patients with some common congenital heart defects. *J Med Genet.* 1981;18:8–16.

Emanuel R, Somerville J, Inns A, Withers R. Evidence of congenital heart disease in offspring of patients with atrioventricular defects. *Br Heart J.* 1983;49:144–147.

Geisterfer-Lowrance AA, Kass S, Tanigawa G, et al. A molecular basis for familial hypertrophic cardiomyopathy. *Cell.* 1990;62:999–1006.

Muntoni F, Cau M, Ganau A, et al. Deletion of muscle promotor region associated with X-linked dilated cardiomyopathy. *N Engl J Med.* 1993;329:921–925.

Schmide MA, Ensing GJ, Michels VV, Carter GA, Hagler DJ, Feldt RH. Autosomal dominant supravalvular aortic stenosis: large three generation family. *Am J Med Genet.* 1989;32:384–389.

Splawski I, Shen J, Timothy KW, et al. Spectrum of mutations in long QT syndrome genes KVLQT1, HERG, SCN5A, KCNE1, KCNE2. *Circulation.* 2000;102:1178–1185.

Thompson P, Mc Rae C. Familial pulmonary hypertension: evidence of autosomal dominant inheritance. *Br Heart J.* 1970;32:758–760.

Zellers TM, Driscoll DJ, Michels VV. Prevalence of significant congenital heart defects in children of parents with Fallot's tetralogy. *Am J Cardiol.* 1990;65:523–526.

34

Substance Abuse in Pregnancy

Andrea Girnius, MD

Recreational drug abuse has increased dramatically in recent years. Approximately 250,000 women in the United States abuse intravenous (IV) drugs, and nearly 90% of them are of childbearing age. Maternal drug addiction may result in life-threatening complications for both the mother and baby. Because social trends affect women with heart disease in the same way as the general population, physicians caring for pregnant women with heart disease will encounter patients who are also abusing illicit drugs. Furthermore, because most pregnant women using illicit drugs deny it, physicians should exercise caution and a high degree of skepticism. Tobacco use, absence of prenatal care, and a history of premature births are associated with substance abuse. The illicit drugs most commonly abused in pregnancy include cocaine, amphetamines, opioids, ethanol, marijuana, and toluene-based solvents. Polysubstance abuse is very common. In some states, exposing a fetus to illicit drugs is considered a form of child neglect or abuse.

This chapter reviews substances commonly abused during pregnancy, including tobacco, alcohol, opioids, cocaine, amphetamines, and marijuana.

TOBACCO

Cigarette smoking remains surprisingly common among pregnant women. An estimated 15% of women smoke during pregnancy. Maternal cigarette smoking increases the fetal death rate. It is the leading cause of fetal growth restriction, and it has been shown to impair growth of the fetal brain and kidney. The risk to fetuses occurs in part because smoking increases the risk of bleeding during pregnancy, abruptio placenta, placenta previa, and premature and prolonged rupture of the membranes. Tobacco smoke contains over 4000 chemical compounds, 40 of which are known carcinogens. Two

that are leading contenders for the toxic effects of smoke to fetuses are nicotine and carbon monoxide. Both cross the placenta. Compared with maternal blood levels, nicotine levels in amniotic fluid may be up to 88% higher, and fetal blood levels are 15% higher. Nicotine causes vasoconstriction of the uteroplacental blood vessel, which may result in uteroplacental underperfusion. It also impairs growth in the fetal nervous system. Carbon monoxide binds to hemoglobin, impairing oxygen delivery to the fetus. Cigarette smoking also is associated with the use of illicit drugs. Pregnant women who are smokers should be encouraged to quit. It is not clear that nicotine replacement therapy is successful in pregnant women, and because nicotine is a fetal toxin, it is difficult to advocate its use in any form in pregnant women.

ALCOHOL

Maternal alcohol use, even in small amounts, has been shown to increase the risk of fetal death in the first trimester. The hazard ratio associated with 2.0 to 3.5 drinks per week is 1.66. The hazard ratio associated with four or more drinks per week is 2.82. The risk is greatest during gestational weeks 13 to 16. There seems to be little or no increased risk of fetal death after 16 weeks. However, because ethanol readily crosses the placenta, heavy maternal alcohol intake may result in a specific pattern of neonatal malformation known as fetal alcohol syndrome. This pattern involves prenatal growth deficiency, developmental delay, craniofacial anomalies, and limb defects. Ethanol is detrimental to the developing brain and remains the leading cause of mental retardation in developing countries. The mechanism of alcohol brain damage remains elusive. Neurologic effects of ethanol appear to be mediated by its actions on the receptor for the inhibitory neurotransmitter gamma-aminobutyric acid (GABA).

The overall neonatal mortality rate in pregnancies complicated by heavy alcohol intake is estimated at 18%. No safe level of alcohol consumption in pregnancy has been established. Regardless of the gestational period, ethanol adversely affects fetuses; therefore, abstinence from alcohol is the safest approach in pregnancy.

Parturients who abuse alcohol may present to labor and delivery with a variety of clinical manifestations, depending on degree of chemical dependency and timing of the most recent consumption. Physiologic dependence on alcohol is manifested as a withdrawal syndrome when the drug is abruptly discontinued or when there is a significant decrease in consumption. The most common and earliest manifestations of acute withdrawal include generalized tremor, hypertension, tachycardia, cardiac arrhythmias, nausea, vomiting, insomnia, confusion, agitation, and hallucinations. Symptoms of acute withdrawal usually begin 6 to 48 hours after cessation of alcohol consumption, although delay as long as 10 days after last use has been reported. Withdrawal symptoms may be suppressed by administering benzodiazepines or α_2-adrenergic agonists or by resuming alcohol consumption. Delirium tremens is a rare but life-threatening medical emergency in ethanol-addicted parturients.

Anesthesia Concerns Related to Alcohol Abuse

Regional anesthesia can be administered safely in parturients with a history of alcohol abuse as long as no other contraindications exist. Intravascular fluid volume should be optimized before induction of regional anesthesia to avoid adverse consequences of sympathetic blockade. If general anesthesia is needed, patients should be evaluated for alcohol-associated hepatic dysfunction, hypoalbuminemia, and cardiac dysfunction. The chronic use of alcohol is usually associated with resistance to the actions of central nervous system (CNS) depressants, including volatile anesthetics. Suggestions that chronic ethanol consumption necessitates increased requirements of barbiturates, however, have not been confirmed. Acutely intoxicated patients generally require lower doses of anesthetic agents.

OPIOIDS

Opioid use and abuse have risen considerably in recent years. A number of related drugs are referred to as opioids. These include "natural" opiates such as heroin and morphine as well as synthetic opioids such as fentanyl,

carfentanil, methadone, hydromorphone, oxycodone, and hydromorphone. There are also synthetic opioid agonist–antagonists such as buprenorphine. Opioids may be injected intravenously, swallowed, nasally inhaled, smoked, chewed, or used as suppositories. Opioid use disorder is defined by the American College of Obstetricians and Gynecologists as "a pattern of opioid use characterized by tolerance, craving, inability to control use, and continued use despite adverse consequences." When the drugs are injected, it can lead to complications of cellulitis, superficial skin abscesses, septic thrombophlebitis, and infective endocarditis. Patients are also at risk for malnutrition, HIV/AIDS, and hepatitis. Opioid abuse may also be accompanied by the abuse of other substances. Lack of prenatal care is common in this population.

Opioid-abusing women may present with symptoms of opioid overdose or acute opioid withdrawal. Patients with opioid overdose present with unconsciousness and respiratory depression. Pinpoint pupils are a characteristic finding on physical examination. Acute opioid withdrawal syndrome is manifested by a range of symptoms, including restlessness, anxiety, abdominal pain, nausea, diarrhea, piloerection and sweating, rhinorrhea, diffuse muscle pain, and symptoms of increased sympathetic nervous system activity, such as tachycardia, tachypnea, and hypertension. CNS manifestations range from dysphoria to various forms of bizarre behavior and unconsciousness. Withdrawal symptoms usually occur 4 to 6 hours after the last opioid intake and peak in 48 to 72 hours. Generally, opioid withdrawal is not considered life threatening.

Intravenous opioid abuse in pregnancy may affect the fetus indirectly (e.g., maternal malnutrition or infection) or directly (e.g., transplacental opioid transfer and direct effect on the fetus). Fetal intrauterine growth restriction (IUGR) and various forms of fetal distress are known consequences of intrauterine drug exposure. Symptoms of neonatal opioid withdrawal are common in neonates exposed in utero.

Currently, opioid replacement therapy with methadone or buprenorphine is recommended for the treatment of pregnant patients addicted to opioids. It helps prevent withdrawal syndrome, and it is better tolerated by fetuses than continued nonmedical opioid abuse. Avoid administering opioid antagonists or agonist–antagonists, such as naloxone or nalbuphine, because they can precipitate acute withdrawal syndrome. Opioid withdrawal syndrome usually develops within minutes after naloxone administration. Patients with symptoms of withdrawal from opioids may be treated with clonidine, diphenhydramine, or doxepin. Clonidine attenuates the opioid withdrawal symptoms by replacing opioid-mediated inhibition with α_2-agonist–mediated inhibition of the CNS. It is possible to reverse the withdrawal syndrome by reinstituting the abused opioid or by substituting methadone.

Anesthesia Concerns Related to Opioid Abuse

Epidural and spinal anesthesia may be administered safely to opioid-abusing parturients. An increased tendency for hypotension should be anticipated after the induction of epidural or spinal anesthesia. In patients who abuse IV opioids, peripheral IV access can be difficult, necessitating central venous access. Chronic opioid use leads to tolerance to other opioids, as well as cross-tolerance to other CNS depressants, including anesthetic agents. Cross-tolerance usually results from chronic receptor stimulation, and decreased pain tolerance is secondary to decreased production of endogenous opioid peptides. If cesarean section is necessary, it is often difficult to effectively control postoperative pain in a parturient who uses opioids chronically. Patients on methadone or suboxone therapy present a similar challenge in the postoperative period. These medications do not have strong enough analgesic activity to effectively control postoperative pain, but they do have a high affinity for opioid receptors, rendering traditional opioid analgesics less efficacious. Therefore, in difficult cases, it is important to use multimodal analgesia, which includes the use of spinal opioids and the maximal use of nonopioid analgesics, such as nonsteroidal antiinflammatory drugs, dexamethasone, and gabapentin. Transversus abdominus plane blocks can provide some degree of pain relief, although they do not relieve visceral pain. Continuous epidural analgesia with local anesthetics, opioids, or both also may be considered, but it is not preferred because the patient is confined to bed while local anesthetic is being infused into the epidural catheter.

COCAINE

Cocaine is an alkaloid (benzoylmethylecgonine) prepared from the leaves of the coca plant. The common pharmaceutical form is prepared by dissolving the alkaloid in hydrochloric acid to form a water-soluble salt. "Crack" is an almost pure cocaine obtained by converting the hydrochloride form back into the alkalinized form.

Cocaine produces prolonged adrenergic stimulation by blocking the presynaptic uptake of sympathomimetic neurotransmitters including norepinephrine, serotonin, and dopamine. The euphoric effects of cocaine also result from the prolongation of dopamine's activity in the limbic system and the cerebral cortex. The use of cocaine rapidly leads to physical dependence. Sudden discontinuation of cocaine intake results in craving for the drug, fatigue, and mental depression. Catecholamine accumulation after acute cocaine intake may cause life-threatening cardiovascular complications, including hypertension, tachycardia, malignant arrhythmias, myocardial ischemia, and infarction. Mechanisms of cocaine-induced myocardial ischemia or infarction include thrombosis, vasospasm, or both. Direct myocardial depression also occurs. Cocaine-induced cardiovascular complications do not seem to be dose dependent, and even small recreational doses can lead to significant morbidity or mortality. Pregnancy is associated with increased sensitivity of the cardiovascular system to cocaine.

Identifying cocaine abuse in a pregnant woman may be difficult. Symptoms may include seizures, hyperreflexia, fever, dilated pupils, emotional instability, proteinuria, and edema. The combination of hypertension, proteinuria, and convulsions resulting from acute cocaine intake may be mistaken for eclampsia. Placental abruption is more common in cocaine-abusing parturients. Drug screening and evaluation of liver and kidney function tests may aid in the differential diagnosis.

Anesthesia Concerns Related to Cocaine

Cocaine-abusing parturients can present anesthetic challenges. In laboring patients, neuraxial analgesia is preferred, provided the patient is able to cooperate and there are no contraindications such as low platelets. It may be more difficult to achieve satisfactory analgesia in cocaine-abusing patients.

In the cocaine-abusing parturient undergoing cesarean delivery, both regional and general anesthesia are associated with risks. Although neuraxial anesthesia is generally preferred for cesarean section, patients abusing cocaine may experience thrombocytopenia, which precludes use of this technique. In addition, acutely intoxicated patients may exhibit combative behavior and have altered pain perception, which make it difficult for them to tolerate the operation despite a technically sufficient sensory block.

Chronic cocaine abuse depletes stores of sympathetic neurotransmitters. Therefore, the treatment of patients with hypotension should be with a direct-acting medication such as phenylephrine. Indirectly acting medications, such as ephedrine, are ineffective.

If general anesthesia is used, attention must be paid to multiple interactions between cocaine and commonly used anesthetic and adjunct medications. Patients may experience hypertension, cardiac arrhythmias, and myocardial ischemia, particularly during times of significant stimulation, such as laryngoscopy and intubation. Generally, beta blockers are contraindicated in cocaine-intoxicated parturients because of the potential for unopposed α-adrenergic stimulation after beta blockade. Labetalol is an exception because it has partial α-agonist activity. Hypertension can be managed by the administration of hydralazine or nitrates. Certain hypnotic induction agents, such as ketamine, may heighten sympathetic nervous system activity and predispose the arrhythmias if used in these patients. Some volatile anesthetic agents (particularly halothane) increase the heart's sensitivity to epinephrine, therefore increasing the chance of arrhythmia; however, the volatile agents in use clinically today have a very low risk of this. Coronary artery vasospasm and the resulting myocardial ischemia is a continual risk in these patients. Nitroglycerine is safe and effective in the treatment of chest pain secondary to acute cocaine ingestion.

AMPHETAMINES

The amphetamines are a group of noncatecholamine, indirect-acting sympathomimetic drugs that produce powerful central and peripheral nervous system stimulation. Amphetamines may be abused orally or intravenously. Crystal methamphetamine is a form of the drug that can be smoked.

Amphetamines stimulate the release of catecholamines from presynaptic vesicles, resulting in euphoria, increased cortical alertness, decreased fatigue, and suppressed appetite. The symptoms of acute amphetamine intoxication are clinically indistinguishable from those caused by cocaine. Hypertension, arrhythmias, tachycardia, dilated pupils, hyperreflexia, proteinuria, and confusion have all been reported. Symptoms of amphetamine withdrawal resemble those produced by cocaine withdrawal. Chronic abuse of amphetamines results in depletion of body stores of catecholamines, which may be manifested as anxiety, somnolence, or a psychotic state.

Both animal and human studies have demonstrated an adverse pregnancy outcome with prenatal exposure to amphetamines. Cardiac anomalies, cleft lip and palate, biliary atresia, IUGR, intrauterine fetal demise, and cerebral hemorrhage have been reported. Amphetamines have been associated with obstetric emergencies, such as fetal distress and placental abruption. Coexistence of seizures, proteinuria, and hypertension secondary to amphetamine use may be mistaken for preeclampsia.

Anesthesia Concerns Related to Amphetamines

Regional anesthesia can be used in these patients, although the associated sympathectomy may precipitate severe hypotension. Amphetamine-abusing patients experience a down-regulation of beta-adrenergic receptors and catecholamine depletion and therefore respond unpredictably to vasopressors. Direct-acting agents, such as phenylephrine, are a better choice than indirect-acting agents such as ephedrine.

Fetal distress, abruption of placenta, and other obstetric emergencies secondary to amphetamine abuse may necessitate emergent cesarean section with general anesthesia. As with cocaine-abusing parturients, attention must be paid to multiple drug concerns. Certain hypnotic drugs and volatile anesthetic agents, such as ketamine and halothane, may increase the risk of arrhythmia and should therefore be avoided. Halothane is not commercially available in the United States. Patients abusing methamphetamines commonly have poor dentition, so care should be taken during intubation not to dislodge loose or carious teeth. Acute intake of amphetamines increases the dose requirements of inhaled anesthetic agents. In contrast, chronic ingestion decreases the dose requirements. There have been reports of adverse cardiovascular effects, including cardiac arrest, in amphetamine-dependent patients undergoing operative delivery under both regional and general anesthesia.

MARIJUANA

Marijuana, a naturally occurring substance, is obtained from the plant *Cannabis sativa*. More than 61 chemicals known as cannabinoids have been identified in marijuana. It remains the most commonly used illicit drug among women of childbearing age. It has been estimated that marijuana is used by 9.5% to 27% of parturients. Often, those who abuse marijuana also use other drugs. Thus, it is sometimes difficult to identify the specific effects of marijuana on the fetus.

Approximately 50% of tetrahydrocannabinol (the active ingredient in marijuana) and other cannabinoids present in a marijuana cigarette are inhaled and enter the bloodstream. Given the high fat solubility of cannabinoids, they accumulate rapidly in adipose tissue, from which they are slowly released into the brain. The plasma elimination half-life of cannabinoids in occasional users is approximately 56 hours, whereas in chronic users it is only 28 hours. Adipose tissue sequestration, however, may extend the tissue half-life to approximately 7 days. It has been reported that complete elimination of a single dose may require up to 30 days. Cannabinoids are metabolized in the liver, forming more than 20 metabolites, most of which have psychoactive properties. The effects of acute marijuana use include euphoria, tachycardia, conjunctival congestion, and anxiety. Pharmacologic actions of marijuana are complex and include effects seen with alcohol, opioids, tranquilizers, and hallucinogens, which makes unreported use difficult to detect.

Tetrahydrocannabinol freely crosses the placental barrier and directly affects the fetus. Because most marijuana-addicted parturients also abuse other substances, it is difficult to identify the specific effects of cannabis on fetuses. It appears that chronic use of marijuana results in decreased uteroplacental perfusion and IUGR. Placental production of estrogen and progesterone may also be altered.

Chronic cannabis exposure results in significant changes in the respiratory system, including bronchitis, squamous metaplasia, and emphysema. Smoke from marijuana is known to suppress both hormonal- and cell-mediated immune responses.

There appears to be no evidence of teratogenicity resulting from cannabis exposure, but low neonatal birth weight, increased risk of complications during labor, and cognitive development delays in infants have been reported in cannabis-addicted mothers.

Anesthesia Concerns Related to Marijuana

Neuraxial anesthesia and analgesia are preferred in parturients using marijuana. General anesthesia is associated with multiple potential drug interactions with marijuana that make its use less ideal. Low-dose acute use of marijuana can cause mild tachycardia and myocardial depression, so it is prudent to avoid drugs that increase the heart rate (glycopyrrolate, atropine, ephedrine, epinephrine).

The combination of volatile anesthetic agents and marijuana can potentially result in significant myocardial depression, although this is uncommon. Cannabis may enhance the sedative-hypnotic effects of other drugs that depress the CNS. Studies have shown cross-tolerance of cannabis with alcohol, barbiturates, opioids, and benzodiazepines. Whereas acutely intoxicated patients may require lower doses of anesthetic, chronic users may require higher doses of anesthetic for induction and maintenance. Oropharyngitis and uvular edema have been observed, which may complicate airway management and intubation. Similar to tobacco smoking, cannabis inhalation leads to impairment of lung function. Additionally, adverse psychiatric and autonomic reactions to cannabis may interfere with induction of anesthesia and postoperative recovery.

BIBLIOGRAPHY

Anesthesia

Kuczkowski KM. Anesthetic implications of drug abuse in pregnancy. *J Clin Anesth*. 2003;15:382–394.

Kuczkowski KM. Caesarean section in a cocaine-intoxicated parturient: regional vs. general anaesthesia? *Anaesthesia*. 2003;58:1042–1043.

Kuczkowski KM. Labor analgesia for the drug abusing parturient: is there cause for concern? *Obstet Gynecol Surv*. 2003;58:599–608.

Kuczkowski KM. Social drug use in the parturient: implications for the management of obstetrical anaesthesia. *Med J Malays*. 2003;58:144–151.

Liu SS, Forester RM, Murphy GS, et al. Anaesthesia management of a parturient with myocardial infarction related to cocaine use. *Can J Anesth*. 1992;39:858–861.

Alcohol

Baumann P, Schild C, Hume RF, Sokol RJ. Alcohol abuse: a persistent preventable risk for congenital anomalies. *Int J Gynaecol Obstet*. 2006;95:66–72.

Caetano R, Ramisetty-Mikler S, Floyd LR, McGrath C. The epidemiology of drinking among women of child-bearing age. *Alcohol Clin Exp Res*. 2006;30:1023–1030.

Calhoun F, Warren K. Fetal alcohol syndrome: historical perspectives. *Neurosci Biobehav Rev*. 2007;31:168–171.

Göransson M, Magnusson A, Heilig M. Identifying hazardous alcohol consumption during pregnancy: implementing a research-based model in real life. *Acta Obstet Gynecol Scand*. 2006;85:657–662.

Malet L, de Chazeron I, Llorca PM, Lemery D. Alcohol consumption during pregnancy: an urge to increase prevention and screening. *Eur J Epidemiol*. 2006;21:787–788.

Mayock DE, Ness D, Mondares RL, Gleason CA. Binge alcohol exposure in the second trimester attenuates fetal cerebral blood flow response to hypoxia. *J Appl Physiol.* 2007;102:972–977.

Spohr HL, Willms J, Steinhausen HC. Fetal alcohol spectrum disorders in young adulthood. *J Pediatr.* 2007;150:175–179.

Amphetamines

Arria AM, Derauf C, Lagasse LL, et al. Methamphetamine and other substance use during pregnancy: preliminary estimates from the Infant Development, Environment, and Lifestyle (IDEAL) study. *Matern Child Health J.* 2006;10:293–302.

Kuczkowski KM, Benumof JL. Amphetamine abuse in pregnancy: anesthetic implications. *Acta Anaesthesiol Belg.* 2003;54:161–163.

Kuczkowski KM. Inhalation induction of anesthesia with sevoflurane for emergency Cesarean section in an amphetamine-intoxicated parturient without an intravenous access. *Acta Anaesthesiol Scand.* 2003;47:1181–1182.

Phupong V, Darojn D. Amphetamine abuse in pregnancy: the impact on obstetric outcome. *Arch Gynecol Obstet.* 2007;276(2):167–170.

Thaithumyanon P, Limpongsanurak S, Praisuwanna P, Punnahitanon S. Perinatal effects of amphetamine and heroin use during pregnancy on the mother and infant. *J Med Assoc Thai.* 2005;88:1506–1513.

Cocaine

Birnbach DJ, Stein DJ, Grunebaum A, et al. Cocaine screening of parturients without prenatal care: an evaluation of a rapid screening assay. *Anesth Analg.* 1997;84:76–79.

Boylan JF, Cheng DC, Sandler AN, et al. Cocaine toxicity and isoflurane anesthesia: hemodynamic, myocardial metabolic, and regional blood flow effects in swine. *J Cardiothorac Vasc Anesth.* 1996;10:772–777.

Buehler BA. Cocaine. How dangerous is it during pregnancy? *Neb Med J.* 1995;80:116–117.

Chao CR. Cardiovascular effects of cocaine during pregnancy. *Semin Perinatol.* 1996;20:107–114.

Dombrowski MP, Wolfe HM, Welch RA, et al. Cocaine abuse is associated with abruptio placentae and decreased birth weight, but not shorter labor. *Obstet Gynecol.* 1991;77:130–141.

Iriye BK, Bristow RE, Hsu CD, et al. Uterine rupture associated with recent antepartum cocaine abuse. *Obstet Gynecol.* 1994;83:840–841.

Kain ZN, Mayes LC, Ferris CA, et al. Cocaine abusing parturients undergoing cesarean section. A cohort study. *Anesthesiology.* 1996;85:1028–1035.

Kline J, Ng SK, Schittini M, Levin B, Susser M. Cocaine use during pregnancy: sensitive detection by hair assay. *Am J Public Health.* 1997;87:352–358.

Krishna RB, Levitz M, Dancis J. Transfer of cocaine by the perfused human placenta: the effect of binding to serum proteins. *Am J Obstet Gynecol.* 1993;169:1418–1423.

Kuczkowski KM. Cardiovascular complications of recreational cocaine use in pregnancy: myth or reality? *Acta Obstet Gynecol Scand.* 2005;84:100–101.

Kuczkowski KM. Crack cocaine as a cause of acute postoperative pulmonary edema in a pregnant drug addict. *Ann Fr Anesth Reanim.* 2005;24:437–438.

Kuczkowski KM. Crack cocaine-induced long QT interval syndrome in a parturient with recreational cocaine use. *Ann Fr Anesth Reanim.* 2005;24:697–698.

Kuczkowski KM. More on the idiosyncratic effects of cocaine on the human heart. *Emerg Med J.* 2007;24:147–148.

Kuczkowski KM. Peripartum care of the cocaine-abusing parturient: are we ready? *Acta Obstet Gynecol Scand.* 2005;84:108–116.

Kuczkowski KM. The cocaine abusing parturient: a review of anesthetic considerations. *Can J Anaesth.* 2004;51:145–154.

Lampley EC, Williams S, Myers SA. Cocaine-associated rhabdomyolysis causing renal failure in pregnancy. *Obstet Gynecol.* 1996;87:804–806.

McCalla S, Minkoff HL, Feldman J, et al. Predictors of cocaine use in pregnancy. *Obstet Gynecol.* 1992;79:641–644.

Mishra A, Landzberg BR, Parente JT. Uterine rupture in association with alkaloidal cocaine use. *Am J Obstet Gynecol.* 1995;173:243–244.

Moen MD, Caliendo MJ, Marshall W, et al. Hepatic rupture in pregnancy associated with cocaine use. *Obstet Gynecol.* 1993;82:687–689.

Oyler J, Darwin WD, Preston KL, et al. Cocaine disposition in the meconium from newborns of cocaine-abusing mothers and urine of adult drug users. *J Anal Toxicol.* 1996;20:453–462.

Plessinger MA, Woods Jr. JR. Maternal, placental and fetal pathophysiology of cocaine exposure during pregnancy. *Clin Obst Gynecol.* 1993;36:267–278.

Sheinkopf SJ, Lagasse LL, Lester BM, et al. Prenatal cocaine exposure: cardiorespiratory function and resilience. *Ann N Y Acad Sci.* 2006;1094:354–358.

Towers CV, Pircon RA, Nageotte MP, et al. Cocaine intoxication presenting as preeclampsia and eclampsia. *Obstet Gynecol.* 1993;81:545–547.

Woods Jr JR, Plessinger MA. Pregnancy increases cardiovascular toxicity of cocaine. *Am J Obstet Gynecol.* 1990;162:529–534.

General

Conners NA, Grant A, Crone CC, et al. Substance abuse treatment for mothers: treatment outcomes and the impact of length of stay. *J Subst Abuse Treat.* 2006;4:447–456.

El-Mohandes A, Herman AA, Nabil El-Khorazaty M, et al. Prenatal care reduces the impact of illicit drug use on perinatal outcomes. *J Perinatol.* 2003;23:354–360.

King JC. Substance abuse in pregnancy. Symposium on Women's Healthcare. *Subst Abuse Pregn.* 1997;102:135–150.

Kuczkowski KM, Birnabach DJ, van Zundert A. Drug abuse in the parturient. *Semin Anesthesiol Periop Med Pain.* 2000;19:216–224.

Kuczkowski KM. Drug addiction in pregnancy and pregnancy outcome: a call for global solutions. *Subst Use Misuse.* 2005;40:1749–1750.

Kuczkowski KM. The effects of drug abuse on pregnancy. *Curr Opin Obstet Gynecol.* 2007;9(6):578–585.

Pollard I. Neuropharmacology of drugs and alcohol in mother and fetus. *Semin Fetal Neonatal Med.* 2007;12:106–113.

Rayburn WF, Bogenschutz MP. Pharmacotherapy for pregnant women with addictions. *Am J Obstet Gynecol.* 2004;191:1885–1897.

Rodriquez EM, Mofenson LM, Chang BH, et al. Association of maternal drug use during pregnancy with maternal HIV culture positivity and perinatal HIV transmission. *AIDS.* 1996;10:273–282.

Wolfe EL, Davis T, Guydish J, Delucchi KL. Mortality risk associated with perinatal drug and alcohol use in California. *J Perinatol.* 2005;25:93–100.

Wright A, Walker J. Management of women who use drugs during pregnancy. *Semin Fetal Neonatal Med.* 2007;12:114–118.

Marijuana

Ashton CH. Adverse effects of cannabis and cannabinoids. *Br J Anaesth.* 1999;83:637–649.

Bell GL, Lau K. Perinatal and maternal issues of substance abuse. *Pediatr Clin North Am.* 1995;42:261–275.

Kuczkowski KM. Labor analgesia for the tobacco and ethanol abusing pregnant patient: a routine management? *Arch Gynecol Obstet.* 2005;271:6–10.

Kuczkowski KM. Marijuana in pregnancy. *Ann Acad Med Singap.* 2004;33:336–339.

Mallat AM, Roberson J, Broch-Utne JG. Preoperative marijuana inhalation and airway concern. *Can J Anaesth.* 1996;43:691–693.

Miscellaneous

Kuczkowski KM. Herbal ecstasy: cardiovascular complications of khat chewing in pregnancy. *Acta Anaesthesiol Belg.* 2005;56:19–21.

Kuczkowski KM. Liquid ecstasy during pregnancy. *Anaesthesia.* 2004;59:926.

Kuczkowski KM. Mothballs and obstetric anesthesia. *Ann Fr Anesth Reanim.* 2006;25:464–465.

Opioids

Bauer CR, Langer JC, Shankaran S, et al. Acute neonatal effects of cocaine exposure during pregnancy. *Arch Pediatr Adolesc Med.* 2005;159:824–834.

Birnbach DJ. Anesthesia and maternal substance abuse. In: Norris MC, ed. *Obstetric Anesthesia.* Lippincott; 1999491–499.

Burns L, Mattick RP, Lim K, Wallace C. Methadone in pregnancy: treatment retention and neonatal outcomes. *Addiction.* 2007;102:264–270.

Committee Opinion No. 711 opioid use and opioid use disorder in pregnancy. *Obstet Gynecol.* 2017;130:e81–e94.

Fajemirokun-Odudeyi O, Sinha C, Tutty S, et al. Pregnancy outcome in women who use opiates. *Eur J Obstet Gynecol Reprod Biol.* 2006;126:170–175.

Goff M, O'Connor M. Perinatal care of women maintained on methadone. *J Midwifery Womens Health.* 2007;52:23–26.

Kashiwagi M, Arlettaz R, Lauper U, et al. Methadone maintenance program in a Swiss perinatal center: (I): management and outcome of 89 pregnancies. *Acta Obstet Gynecol Scand.* 2005;84:140–144.

Mawhinney S, Ashe RG, Lowry J. Substance abuse in pregnancy: opioid substitution in a Northern Ireland maternity unit. *Ulst Med J.* 2006;75:187–191.

Sander SC, Hays LR. Prescription opioid dependence and treatment with methadone in pregnancy. *J Opioid Manag.* 2005;1:91–97.

Screening

Williamson S, Jackson L, Skeoch C, et al. Determination of the prevalence of drug misuse by meconium analysis. *Arch Dis Child Fetal Neonatal Ed.* 2006;91:291–292.

Tobacco

Anblagan D, Jones NW, Costigan C, et al. Maternal smoking during pregnancy and fetal organ growth: a magnetic resonance imaging study. *PLoS One.* 2013;8(7):e67223.

Coleman T, Cooper S, Thornton JG, et al. A randomized trial of nicotine-replacement therapy patches in pregnancy. *N Engl J Med.* 2012;366:808–812.

Cooper S, Taggar J, Lewis S, et al. Effect of nicotine patches in pregnancy on infant and maternal outcomes at 2 years: follow-up from the randomized double-blind, placebo-controlled SNAP trial. *Lancet Respir Med.* 2014;2(9):728–737.

Meyer MB, Tonascia JA. Maternal smoking, pregnancy complications, and perinatal mortality. *Am J Obstet Gynecol.* 1977;128(5):494–502.

Miles DR, Lanni S, Jansson L, Svikis D. Smoking and illicit drug use during pregnancy: impact on neonatal outcome. *J Reprod Med.* 2006;51:567–572.

35

The Placenta

Helen Jones, PhD

The placenta is the central player of the maternal–fetal interface, able to communicate with both the fetus and the mother and to regulate signals from one to the other. Consequently, disturbing its development, growth, or function can have major impacts on both the maternal response to pregnancy and the development of the fetus. Currently, very little is known about the effects of maternal cardiac conditions on the placenta, but what we do know highlights the need to investigate this topic further and to consider the contribution of the placenta during pregnancies with mothers who have cardiac disease. This chapter discusses placental–maternal communication, placenta and fetal outcomes, substance abuse and the placenta, and congenital vascular dysfunction.

PLACENTAL–MATERNAL COMMUNICATION

Although maternal adaptation to pregnancy is generally thought of as a response to pregnancy hormones that alter the maternal heart, blood volume, and kidneys, the bigger picture includes the critical communication between the placenta and the maternal environment.

In early pregnancy, the interplay between the maternal immune cells resident in the decidua (e.g., uterine natural killer cells) and the invading placental trophoblast is finely balanced, and if disrupted, it can result in early pregnancy loss or aberrant invasion of the trophoblast. The consequences of disrupted trophoblast invasion can manifest as preeclampsia or an overinvasive placenta (percreta, accreta, or increta). Recent research has identified multiple communication pathways between the placenta and the mother that occur throughout pregnancy. These include both secreted factors and placental "debris." Secreted factors consist of many placenta-specific molecules but also include factors typically expressed by adipose tissue or immune cells, such as leptin, adiponectin, and cytokines. "Placental debris" is used to describe the trophoblast-derived material that is composed of extracellular vesicles of various sizes, including exosomes and apoptotic bodies. These are intentionally shed by the placenta and are found circulating in maternal blood. In the future, they may be used as biomarkers for the diagnosis of pregnancy pathologies. Currently, cell-free nucleic acids are commonly assessed during the first trimester in high-risk patients undergoing noninvasive prenatal testing.

One proposed mechanism of placental–maternal communication goes so far as to propose "placentalization" of the maternal endothelium by targeted exosomes and extracellular vesicles, expanding the placental output of secreted factors to the entire maternal circulation. Recently, targeted communication in this manner has been proposed to occur between the placenta and the maternal kidneys, with a potential application for this system to impact the maternal heart, which, when successful, enables proper maternal adaptation to pregnancy.

PLACENTA AND FETAL OUTCOMES

The fetal outcomes from a pregnancy complicated by maternal cardiac conditions can vary significantly but include higher incidences of preterm birth, preeclampsia, and low birth weight. There is significant evidence that improper placentation plays a significant role in these sequelae. Although preeclampsia is a syndrome involving multiple factors, the underlying mechanism is attributed to poor trophoblast invasion and limited remodeling of the maternal spiral arteries in early pregnancy. This improper remodeling results in malperfusion of the placenta and may cause abnormal maternal responses to the placenta. Placental insufficiency, thought to underlie more than 75% of all cases of intrauterine growth restriction, is a defect in placental function (transfer of oxygen and nutrients) and is commonly associated with underperfusion and impaired placental blood flow. Both oxygen and nutrient transfer rely on a properly invaded placenta and remodeled maternal spiral arteries or villous vascular branching and remodeling.

SUBSTANCE ABUSE AND THE PLACENTA

Many drugs affect placental metabolism and induce fundamental changes affecting the fetus. Furthermore, drugs and their metabolites can cross the placenta to the developing fetus and can sometimes be detected at higher concentrations in fetal tissues than in the mother. Metabolites thus produced could be more active or more toxic than the parent compound. Drug-metabolizing enzymes with oxidative, deaminating, hydroxylating, and hydrolytic activity have been demonstrated in placentas.

CONGENITAL VASCULAR DYSFUNCTION

By analyzing placentas delivered by healthy women carrying a fetus with congenital heart disease, we have started to identify changes in the fetal vasculature. Despite surgery to restore cardiac function, the vasculature may remain abnormal throughout the child's life. If that child is a girl, if she becomes pregnant later in life, the abnormal vasculature may be a significant impairment to normal communication between the placenta and the maternal vasculature, resulting in maternal endothelial dysfunction, which is commonly associated with preeclampsia.

BIBLIOGRAPHY

Beaconsfield P. Drugs and the placenta—a personal view. *Placenta: A Neglected Experimental Animal.* 1979:105–108.

Cuffe JSM, Holland O, Salomon C, Rice GE, Perkins AV. Placental derived biomarkers of pregnancy disorders. *Placenta.* 2017;54:104–110.

Jones HN, Olbrych SK, Smith KL, et al. Hypoplastic left heart syndrome is associated with structural and vascular placental abnormalities and leptin dysregulation. *Placenta.* 2015;36(10):1078–1086.

Pieper PG, Balci A, Aarnoudse JG, et al. Uteroplacental blood flow, cardiac function, and pregnancy outcome in women with congenital heart disease. *Circulation.* 2013 3;128(23): 2478–2487.

Pijnenborg R, Robertson WB, Brosens I, Dixon G. Trophoblast invasion and the establishment of haemochorial placentation in man and laboratory animals. *Placenta.* 1981;2(1):71–91.

Tong M, Chamley LW. Placental extracellular vesicles and feto-maternal communication. *Cold Spring Harb Perspect Med.* 2015 29;5(3):a023028.

Appendix

Normal Lab Values In Pregnancy

	Test or Analysis	Reference Range in Non-Pregnant Women	Reference Range in Pregnancy
Cardiac function	B-type natriuretic peptide (BNP)[a]	<50 pg/mL	<126 pg/mL ↑
	Troponin I	0–0.08 ng/mL	0–0.06 ng/mL ↓
	Creatine kinase	40–240 units/L	12–102 units/L ↓
Coagulation	Bleeding time	1–5 min	1–5 min
	Fibrinogen	200–500 mg/dL	300–650 mg/dL ↑
	Platelet count	160–400 × 10⁹/l	140–400 × 10⁹/l
	Prothrombin time (PT)	12–16 sec	9–13 sec ↓
	Partial thromboplastin time (aPTT)	26–39 sec	22–39 sec
	D-dimer[b]	0.2–0.75 mcg/mL	0.1–1.7 mcg/mL ↑
	INR	0.9–1.1	0.8–1.1
	Factor VIII	50%–150%	90%–350% ↑
	von Willebrand factor antigen	75%–125%	60%–422% ↑
	Protein S (free)	70%–140%	20%–130% ↓
Hematology	Hemoglobin	12–15.8 g/dL	9.5–15 g/dL ↓
	Hematocrit	35%–45%	28%–40% ↓
	White blood cell (WBC) count	3.5–9.1 × 10³/mm³	5.6–16.9 × 10³/mm³ ↑
	Mean corpuscular volume (MCV)	80–93 fL	81–99 fL ↑
	Red cell distribution width (RDW)	<14.5%	12.5%–15%
	Neutrophils	1.4–4.6 × 10³/mm³	3.6–13.1 × 10³/mm³ ↑
Chemistry	Alanine transaminase (ALT)	7–41 units/L	3–30 units/L ↓
	Aspartate transaminase (AST)	12–38 units/L	3–32 units/L ↓
	Albumin	4.1–5.3 g/dL	2.3–5.1 g/dL ↓
	Amylase	20–96 units/L	15–90 units/L
	Bicarbonate	22–30 mmol/L	20–24 mmol/L ↓
	Blood urea nitrogen (BUN)	7–20 mg/dL	3–12 mg/dL ↓
	Calcium (total)	8.7–10.2 mg/dL	8.2–10.6 mg/dL
	Chloride	102–109 mEq/L	97–109 mEq/L
	Creatinine	0.5–0.9 mg/dL	0.4–0.9 mg/dL ↓
	Lactate dehydrogenase (LDH)	115–221 units/L	80–525 units/L ↑
	Lipase	3–45 units/L	21–112 units/L ↑
	Magnesium	1.5–2.3 mg/dL	1.1–2.2 mg/dL
	Phosphate	2.5–4.3 mg/dL	2.5–4.6 mg/dL
	Potassium	3.5–5.0 mEq/L	3.3–5.1 mEq/L ↓
	Prealbumin	17–34 mg/dL	14–27 mg/dL ↓
	Sodium	136–146 mEq/L	129–148 mEq/L ↓
	Uric acid	2.5–5.6 mg/dL	2.0–6.3 mg/dL

Continued

	Test or Analysis	Reference Range in Non-Pregnant Women	Reference Range in Pregnancy
Endocrine	Thyroid-stimulating hormone (TSH)	0.34–4.25 mIU/mL	0.1–3.0 mIU/mL ↓
	Free thyroxine (free T_4)	0.8–1.7 ng/dL	0.5–1.2 ng/dL ↓
	Free triiodothyronine (free T_3)	2.4–4.2 pg/mL	4.0–4.4 pg/mL ↑
	Renin (plasma activity)	0.3–9.0 ng/mL/hr	6–60 ng/mL/hr ↑
	Aldosterone	2–9 ng/dL	6–104 ng/dL ↑
	Cortisol	0–25 mcg/dL	7–50 mcg/dL ↑
Inflammatory	C-reactive protein (CRP)	0.2–3 mg/L	0.4–20 mg/L ↑
	Erythrocyte sedimentation rate (ESR)	0–20 mm/hr	4–70 mm/hr ↑
Blood gas	pH	7.38–7.42	7.36–7.52 ↑
	PO_2	90–100 mm Hg	90–110 mm Hg ↑
	PCO_2	38–42 mm Hg	25–33 mm Hg ↓
	Bicarbonate (HCO_3^-)	22–26 mEq/L	16–22 mEq/L ↓

[a]Fibrin split products, such as D-dimer, increase markedly in pregnancy with levels in late pregnancy up to 10-fold higher than in the nonpregnant state. Therefore, D-dimer levels are not reliable in predicting thromboembolism in pregnant patients. D-dimer levels increase during normal pregnancy and increase with complications such as preeclampsia and placental abruption. Furthermore, false-negative D-dimer results have also been reported during pregnancy.

[b]BNP levels normally increase in pregnancy. However, a level above 126 pg/mL has been shown to be predictive of cardiovascular complications. We believe this test is useful in pregnancy, but a different upper limit of normal must be taken into account.

INDEX

Page numbers followed by '*f*' indicate figures, '*t*' indicate tables, '*b*' indicate boxes.